Convergent Strabismus

Monographs in Ophthalmology 6

Dr W. JUNK PUBLISHERS THE HAGUE - BOSTON - LONDON

Convergent Strabismus

edited by

L. EVENS

Dr W. JUNK PUBLISHERS THE HAGUE - BOSTON - LONDON

REPRINTED FROM Bull. Soc. belge Ophtal. 196, 1982

Distributors:

for the United States and Canada

Kluwer Boston Inc.
190 Old Derby Street
Hingham, MA 02043
USA

for all other countries

Kluwer Academic Publishing Group
Distribution Center
P.O. Box 322
3300 AH Dordrecht
The Netherlands

ISBN-13: 978-94-009-8026-6 e-ISBN-13: 978-94-009-8024-2
DOI: 10.1007/978-94-009-8024-2

PREFACE

When the Board of Directors of the Belgian Ophthalmological Society, in its session of November 26th 1978, asked me to prepare a report on strabismus to be presented at the joint meeting of the Dutch and Belgian Ophthalmological Societies to be held on June 13th 1981, I felt greatly honored but still more overwhelmed by the immensity of the task.

I took advantage of the complete liberty given to me by the Board of Directors, first to limit the work to one particular form of strabismus, i.e. the convergent comitant form; second, to seek the help of what I thought to be the best strabologists in the Low Countries; third, to aim not at an encyclopedic treatise but at a practical volume destined to the general ophthalmologist.

This volume is thus limited to the various aspects of convergent strabismus, more accurately of comitant convergent strabismus. The omission of the word "comitant" is purposely made to avoid the difficulties accompanying the explanation of this term and all the acrobatics needed to explain that most comitant strabismus are not completely comitant. The choice of this particular form of strabismus seems logical. First of all, it is the most common form of strabismus. On the other hand, most principles concerning examination and treatment can with some modifications be applied to other forms of strabismus.

Prof. R.C. Crone and Prof. A. Th.M. van Balen of the Netherlands, Dr. H. De Corte, Dr. M. Gobin and Dr. E. Vereecken of Belgium did me the great honor of accepting to collaborate in this entreprise. This volume then is the product of the cooperative efforts of these six authors, each of whom is entirely responsible for the chapters he has written. As strabismus treatment is an empirical matter and at the same time in full evolution, it cannot be expected that six independent authors have exactly the same ideas on each aspect of this treatment. If not all, many roads lead to Rome. In strabismus, different ways of treatment can lead to acceptable results and therapeutic variations can even be useful for progress in this still controversial field.

It was neither the goal of the authors to present an encyclopedic work nor to produce a volume so complicated as to be readable only by the elite of the strabological world. To the contrary, the purpose of this undertaking was to present a work that would be useful to the general ophthalmologist. I express the hope that this work will effectively help him to diagnose more accurately the different forms of esotropia, to elucidate the causes and contributing factors of each form, to define the aims and treatment possibilities of each form and to approach complete healing.

This volume will not be the last book on convergent strabismus but the efforts of the authors would be rewarded if it could bring us one step nearer to the "land where all is clarity, all is simplicity, all is logic..."

Brussel, June 13th, 1981.

Dr. Leo Evens, Editor
Lakenselaan 36
1090 Brussels, Belgium

Mr. Vanhove of Janssen Pharmaceutica, 2340 Beerse, Belgium, corrected linguistic errors in chapters 1, 2, 6, 8, 9, for which we are most grateful.

TABLE OF CONTENTS

CHAPTER III

NORMAL BINOCULAR VISION

R.A. CRONE

CHAPTER IV

NEUROMECHANICS OF THE HUMAN PERIPHERAL OCULOMOTOR SYSTEM

H. DE CORTE

CHAPTER V

SYMPTOMATOLOGY

R.A. CRONE

CHAPTER VI

EXAMINATION METHODS

E. VEREECKEN

CHAPTER VII

AMBLYOPIA

A.Th.M. VAN BALEN

CHAPTER VIII

CONSERVATIVE TREATMENT

E. VEREECKEN

CHAPTER IX

SURGICAL MANAGEMENT OF ESOTROPIA

M.H. GOBIN

Bull. Soc. belge Ophtal., **195**, 1-17, 1981.

CHAPTER I

INTRODUCTION

L. EVENS (*)

I. *Definition. Classification*

The subject of this book being the manifest forms of convergent comitant strabismus (esotropia), with the exclusion of the latent forms (esophoria), we can define our topic as the study of the different aspects of the misalignment in a convergent sense of the visual axes, existing either permanently or intermittently during fixation at a distant and/or near object. This misalignment is accompanied by various sensorial phenomena: suppression (inhibition), anomalous correspondence, diplopia, amblyopia, eccentric fixation (6, 7, 22, 27, 80, 104).

As our subject is limited to the comitant esodeviations, we will not consider:

a. incomitant deviations due to a paralysis of one or more of the external ocular muscles or due to structural anomalies of these muscles as in fibrosis and in the Duane retraction syndrome;
b. secondary deviations as sensory esotropia accompanying cataract, optic atrophy, etc.;
c. consecutive esotropia (after surgical overcorrection of an exodeviation).

The esodeviations have varied characteristics that are used singly or in combination for classification purposes (68):

— age of onset: congenital, infantile, late;
— intermittency;
— relationship to accommodation: accommodative and non accommodative;

(*) Lakenselaan 36, 1090 Brussels (Belgium).

- relationship to the accommodative convergence/accommodation (AC/A) ratio: esodeviation greater at near or distance;
- comparison of up and down gaze: A and V patterns;
- size of deviation: microstrabismus, large angle squint.

Fletcher and Silverman (31) adopt the following classification for all cases of esodeviations: a) esophoria; b) esodeviations with associated diseases; c) consecutive esotropia; d) intermittent or constant esotropia. This last group, the only one which we are interested in, is subdivided into: 1) accommodative; 2) partially accommodative; 3) nonaccommodative esotropia.

Burian and von Noorden (107) classify the comitant esodeviations in four categories: a) accommodative (refractive with normal AC/A, non-refractive high AC/A, partially accommodative); b) non-accommodative (congenital or acquired); c) microtropia; d) nystagmus blockage syndrome. Lang (59) also adopts four categories: a) congenital strabismus; b) accommodative strabismus; c) normosensorial late strabismus; d) microstrabismus. Ward and Hughes (108) distinguish the following four categories: a) accommodative squint with convergence excess; b) intermittent convergent squint with divergence weakness; c) partially accommodative squint; d) nonaccommodative squint. Accentuating the arbitrary aspect of all forms of classification, Hugonnier and Hugonnier (51) adopt the following classification for convergent comitant strabismus: a) accommodative strabismus; b) essential strabismus (early or late); c) strabismus with amblyopia (organic or functional); d) rare forms (congenital myopia, psycho-somatical forms); e) strabismus of the adult.

Since the various characteristics may overlap, all types of classification will not be entirely accurate. For reasons more extensively outlined by Crone (chapter V), the authors of this book have adopted a classification which has the great advantage of being in direct relationship to the possibilities of treatment and of prognostic evaluation. They classify their cases of comitant esotropia in:

a) early strabismus convergens;
b) late strabismus convergens;
c) microstrabismus convergens;

While Malbran (67) already noted that the prognosis for successful treatment is worst for early forms, better for accommodative and best for late essential squints, Duke-Elder (27) also mentioned that the pathological anomalies in ocular motility may be of two fundamental types: they are either a failure in the development of the fixation reflexes or a disruption of reflexes already formed. Corcelles (16) makes a distinction between the innate and the acquired in strabismus and Goddé-Jolly (43) in accordance with others (35, 57, 64, 72) states that the prognosis of each case depends on the age of apparition of the strabismus, its duration, the visual acuity, the alternating or monocular aspect and the quality of the retinal correspondence.

II. *Goals of treatment*

To put it ideally, the goal of treatment must be a return to the normal alignment of the eyes and a replacement of the various sensorial adaptations by normal binocular vision. Ardouin and Coll. (3) observe that the final objective of treatment of strabismus is the realisation of: 1) bifoveolar fixation in all directions of gaze; 2) a good fusional amplitude; 3) a stereoscopic acuity of less than 20 seconds. The aim should thus be the obtainment of normal binocular vision and stereopsis in normal conditions; necessary for their obtainment is full visual acuity in both eyes and parallel position. It is certain that this perfect healing cannot be expected in most forms of strabismus. What certainly must be attained is a good cosmetic result without amblyopia and without diplopia.

In order to assess the functional results of operation, Ward and Hughes (108) divide their postoperative cases into three groups: 1) orthophoric or with fully controlled heterophoria; 2) heterophoria intermittently breaking down to manifest deviation; 3) manifest deviation. A first class result or cure was considered to be achieved postoperatively if binocular visual acuity was 6/6 with and without glasses in cases in which the hypermetropic correction was +3 d. or less. Where the correction was higher, these conditions had to be present with −3 d. clip-ons added to the spectacles. The percentage of the total number of their cases attaining binocular single vision was disappointingly small.

Other standards of cure mentioned in the literature are: "eyes straight with comfortable fusion", "binocular single vision with and without glasses". Fletcher and Silverman (31) see it as the alleviation of symptoms, an acceptable cosmetic appearance, good vision in both eyes and fusion if possible.

The evaluation of results of strabismus treatment is a difficult matter. As Fletcher, Silverman and Albott (30) state, in clinical research there exist many factors influencing the outcome of the experiment. These cannot always be accurately controlled and must be taken into account in interpreting results. Among them are: 1) variations in examiner's technique, 2) variations in patient's disease and 3) unreliability of history or specific tests. To give some examples: of the 119 parameters which the authors examined, different examiners reached 80% to 90% agreement in measuring horizontal and vertical deviations within 10 prism diopters in long-standing strabismus; agreement as to the fusion status was only 68%. According to the "Standards for discharge as orthoptically satisfactory in cases of binocular anomaly", published by the British Orthoptic Society, the requirements for binocular single vision are as follows. "When the refractive error is corrected, comfortable binocular single vision should be present for all distances and in all directions of gaze without the adaptation of an abnormal head posture. If hypermetropia is present, binocular single vision should be maintained when correction of the manifest hypermetropia is reduced by 3 dioptre sphere. "The results of tests for binocular single vision should be:

- cover test: binocular fixation should be resumed for all positions of gaze immediately after removal of the cover;
- Worth's lights test (near and distance): the patient should see four lights in correct formation;
- bar reading: bar reading should be attained for print of the size of N5 or of a size read by the weaker eye and maintained when the manifest hypermetropia, if present, is under-corrected by 3 dioptre sphere;
- convergence: near point of convergence should be 8 cm or better and should be well maintained;
- accommodation: amplitude should be equal in each eye when the refractive error is corrected and should be at least as great binocularly as uniocularly.

Nonetheless, to test the results, the unilateral cover-test (56) is still the first to be done: it allows detection of all deviations superior to 1 to 2 prism diopters. When no movement occurs and if good vision is present in both eyes, the quality of binocular vision will be examined by various procedures which will be outlined later. For Romano and von Noorden (93), two prism diopters should be considered the smallest deviation routinely detectable by the cover-test. Absence of a detectable shift on the cover-test means only that a deviation, if present, is probably less than two prism diopters. A negative result on the cover-test does not necessarily rule out strabismus nor does it imply that normal binocular single vision or bifoveal fixation is present. The cover-test will also be negative in cases of microstrabismus with parafoveal fixation and identity between the degree of eccentricity of fixation under monocular and the angle of anomaly under binocular conditions. Crone and Hardjowijoto (22) recently stressed the lessening distinction between normal binocular vision and squint. They appropriately stated that the upper limit of microstrabismus has been fixed at 6° (5° for others) but that the lower limit has never been determined.

In consequence, it would also be possible to classify the esotropias according to the angle of strabismus:

1. From 0 to 10 minutes of arc, for which the term "fixation disparity" has already been coined (71).
2. From 10 minutes of arc to 1°: these cases, clinically difficult to detect, could be called "microstrabismus".
3. From 1° to 5°, for which the term ministrabismus could be used.
4. More than 5°: manifest esotropia.

We are also in complete agreement with Arruga and Downey (5) who state that "during the last few years, it has been found that many patients presumed to have normal binocular single vision after optical, orthoptic and/or surgical treatment, have in fact a small angle of anomaly".

We have ourselves (28) analysed the long-term results in 55 non-amblyopic subjects operated on for different forms of strabismus. 12 had an angle of 0° but 5 of them presented a phoria, 4 had a normal Worth-test but only 2 of them had normal stereoscopic vision with the Titmus-test. We think however that it is better to bring the goals and the possibilities of treatment in relation to the three categories of convergent strabismus which we have mentioned earlier.

III. *Goals and possibilities of treatment in the different forms of convergent comitant esotropia*

A. *Early esotropia*

It is still an open question if comitant esotropia can really be congenital, that is existing at birth. To solve this problem, American authors tend to use the term "congenital esotropia" synonymously with "infantile esotropia" to designate all esotropias with an onset between birth and six months of age. French authors use the term "essential strabismus" of early onset (51).

This form of esotropia has to be differentiated from the early forms of accommodative esotropia, from the very rare cases of bilateral abducens paralysis and from Moebius-syndrome (65). It has also to be distinguished from esotropia associated with brain damage or dysfunction (cerebral palsy, mongolism, mental retardation) but most of all from pseudoesotropia where the appearance of esotropia is due to prominent epicanthal folds or a broad flat nasal bridge.

The deviation is usually large (35-50$^{\Delta}$ or more) and constant for distance and near. Abduction is often apparently defective with cross fixation; vertical deviations, especially overaction of the inferior oblique muscles, are often associated. Some authors have the impression that the vertical deviations are of late onset, whereas for Gobin (36) sagittalization of the oblique muscles is considered to be responsible for nearly all forms of comitant strabismus. Dissociated vertical deviations (19) and nystagmus (41) are also frequent findings.

Certain cases of congenital esotropia give the impression that they are caused by a bilateral abducens muscle paralysis where in fact they are due to a nystagmus that is blocked by adduction. Hence the name "Nystagmus blockage syndrome", introduced by Adelstein and Cüppers (1) and "Nystagmus compensation syndrome", proposed by von Noorden (106). Several symptoms can be recognised: diminution of abduction of the non-fixing eye (the stop-sign of Corcelle (15)), pseudoparalysis of the external recti and nystagmus in abduction. Burian and von Noorden (107) diagnosed this syndrome in 5% of their cases of infantile esotropia while Quéré et Coll. (87) find elements of blockage or spastic components in 60% of their cases. Weiss (110) however attributes most of the symptoms to the existence of a large angle and stresses the fact that the pseudoabducens paresis disappears spontaneously with age. The electro-oculographic study of this entity has extensively been done by French authors (10, 85, 86, 109).

Without going into the discussion on the question if normal retinal correspondence is innate or empirically acquired (70) and if the loss of binocular vision results from the lack of synergy of the imputs from the two eyes to the visual cortex (11, 49, 52), it is undeniable that the functional results of strabismus treatment are less favorable as the age of onset is earlier. The question even arises if congenital esotropia is fundamentally curable (102). Nonetheless, the goal of treatment must be to achieve the most perfect alignment with negative cover-test; for Parks (76) it means: after elimination of any existing amblyopia, the surgical correction within 10 diopters of straight, done at an early age. Bifoveal fixation with stereopsis seems to be unobtainable in these cases although it is difficult to determine stereoacuity in young children (97). The goal of extramacular, peripheral fusion with normal retinal correspondence seems more easily attained if the eyes are straight at an early age (92). Perfect alignment can be attained in 10% of all cases according to Burian and von Noorden (107); in the remaining cases, a small angle esotropia is the most common end result. In these small angles (up to 8 diopters), peripheral binocular vision is possible and the smallest deviation should be aimed at to obtain the most stable results. Results far better than any heretofore described were reported by Taylor (103): by early surgery, 60% of his cases received a functional cure, this means conversion from a tropia to a phoria with normal retinal correspondence and stereopsis.

Most authors agree that the treatment is essentially a surgical one, preceded by alternate occlusion according to some, by sectorized glasses (occlusive sectors on nasal side of corrective lenses) according to others (96). Whereas Fletcher and Silverman (32) found that asymmetrical surgery is just as effective as symmetrical surgery and whereas a recession-resection procedure still has its advocates (105), most authors seem to prefer a symmetrical approach. Resection of both external recti (89) seems to be increasingly abandoned in favor of a bimedial recession, possibly augmented by resection of one or two external recti (44). Surgery to remediate the erroneous diagnosis of lateral rectus palsy leads to unwanted results (33).

Bimedial recessions, done at an early age, are advocated by most American authors (53). Recession or tenotomy of the inferior oblique is done simultaneously if overaction of the inferior oblique can be demonstrated. Gobin (see chapter IX) on the other hand always does an intervention on two or four oblique muscles. When the horizontal deviation is large, this same author combines the bimedial recession of 5 mm with a loop of 2 to 3 mm (37). French authors recently recommended the use of bilateral loops of up to 8 mm instead of recessions (12); others, also mostly French, defend the superiority of the Faden-operation, alone or in combination with recession and resection in cases where blockage or spasmodic elements are present (88).

Contrary to the "uniform approach" (bimedial recession, standard four- or six-muscles surgery of Gobin (38, 39, 40)) done before 12 months of age, Fisher, Flom and Jampolsky (29) and also Taylor (101) prefer the "selective approach" (adapted to each particular case), done between 12 and 24 months of age. Taylor himself advises surgery from 6 to 18 months after birth for congenital strabismus and within 3 months after onset for acquired strabismus.

Concerning the earliness of the operation (105), some authors recommend operation before one year of age (76), others before two years (29). The study of Hiles, Watson and Bliglan (48) to the contrary seems to demonstrate that the absolute age of the ocular alignment and its influence on the development of fusion is probably not as crucial. These authors practised a bimedial recession before one year of age and combined this operation with various non-surgical modalities. Their goal was to align the eyes within 10 prism diopters, to correct significant refractive errors and to eliminate amblyopia. Their results fell into three groups: those who remained stable following their initial alignment (39 %), those who were well aligned and remained stable for prolonged periods of time and then decompensated and those who were unstable throughout the observation period. Including the initial operation, the study population required 1.8 operations per patient to align the eyes within 10 prism diopters of orthophoria. 69 % of the patients required a secondary operation and 11 % of these required a third operation between the second and ninth year of life.

While some authors use prisms postoperatively for correction of residual small angles (33), Pigassou (79) uses them systematically as the primary treatment. While she considers the "binocular union", the supreme goal of some (13) as a failure, her prismatic treatment, done between 1 and 3 years, can lead to binocular single vision in all cases of normal and abnormal retinal correspondence! If retinal correspondence is normal, the treatment consists of exact prismatic correction; if retinal correspondence is anomalous, the treatment must first destroy the abnormal correspondence by the prescription of overcorrecting prisms of about 15 diopters.

B. *Late esotropia*

If not related to aggravation of a pre-existing microtropia, binocular vision may have been normal until the onset of the squint and the possibilities of complete healing are markedly greater.

1. Accommodative esotropia

It was Donders (26) who first made the relation between convergent strabismus and the frequently accompanying hypermetropia. The hypermetrope who wants to see clearly, even for distance, must use his accommodation; the convergence which is coupled to this accommodation forces the eyes in a convergent position. The logical treatment of this strabismus lies in the correction of the hypermetropia which effectively often cures the deviation. This nice explanation does not fit for all forms of convergent squint but only for a small group, called the "purely accommodative strabismus". Much more frequent are the "partially accommodative strabismus" in which the spectacle correction only diminishes the angle. For some authors the accommodative factor counts for 15% of the cases of convergent strabismus, for Rethy (90, 91) on the contrary, it counts for 80%.

It has since long been recognized that most children are hypermetropic but do not have strabismus, whereas most of the individuals having an esotropia are hypermetropic. This led to the theory that hypermetropia was only a provoking factor in an individual already predisposed to strabismus; thus Worth (11) in 1906 believed that strabismic individuals had a defect in their fusion faculty that allowed the esotropia to develop.

On the other hand, is has also been recognized that the parallelism of the eyes obtained with glasses, does not mean cure of the sensory defects; only one third of the cases develop normal binocular vision together with parallelism (45).

While accommodative esodeviations may thus be the result of the need to clear the blurred vision caused by hypermetropia, they may also be caused by the exaggerated accommodative convergence associated with normal accommodation in a patient who has a high accommodative convergence ratio (14, 75, 98, 113). This AC/A ratio expresses the relationship between the amount of convergence produced by the stimulus to accommodate (accommodative convergence in prism diopters) and the amount of accommodation (in diopters) which produces that convergence (50). A high accommodative convergence ratio is generally identified by the near esotropia exceeding the distance esotropia by 10 prism diopters. The near fixation has to be stimulated by an accommodative fixation target which requires identification of small details and the refractive error must be fully corrected (107).

In opposition to infantile esotropia with its usually large and stable deviation, accommodative esotropia starts at a later age, mostly between 1.5 and 3 years, and the deviation is at first intermittent and variable. Exceptions exist and recently attention has been drawn to early-onset accommodative esotropia (8, 82).

Therapy is antiaccommodative in nature and may be of two types: 1) optical: single vision lenses or bifocals; 2) medical: miotics. In some children both of these may be used. Besides the treatment of an often existing amblyopia, supportive orthoptic treatment is directed at the elimination of suppression and the development of fusional divergence amplitudes. The recently rediscovered techniques of penalisation, although primarily designed to cure the amblyopia, can have a beneficial effect on the angle of strabismus, especially if this treatment is combined not only with the exact correction of the hypermetropia but more so with the penalizing overcorrection of one eye (40).

Concerning the optical corrections, most textbooks explain how to prescribe them (51, 84): all insist on the necessity of maximal correction after complete cycloplegia which has to be repeated from time to time. While one can agree with Kettesy (53) that the spectacles have to be worn as soon as possible, have to correct the hypermetropia completely and have to be worn continuously, it is not possible for everybody to follow Rethy (90, 91) and overcorrect progressively when no parallelism is obtained.

If the child has a high AC/A ratio, further antiaccommodative therapy will be required at near in the form of bifocals. In general, the addition rarely exceeds +2.5 d. and an executive-type of bifocal is preferred with the dividing line at level with the lower border of the pupil. Miotics, especially DFP and Phospholine iodide, are used by some authors, generally for short periods of time.

While for some authors (107), surgery is only indicated for the nonaccommodative component of the strabismus, others (38, 39, 40) advocate surgery instead of glasses or to reduce a strong correction. In cases where a firm degree of control exists preoperatively, a single muscle operation can be envisaged (108); Gobin (38) on the contrary, who never uses glasses except when needed for vision purposes, prefers his four-muscle surgery in all cases. The "Fadenoperation" has recently been introduced as an alternative for bifocals or miotics in the treatment of the hyperconvergence for near.

The term deteriorated accommodative strabismus (69) is used to indicate that the esotropia was initially accommodative and then became nonaccommodative. This can be caused by neglect, insufficient correction or even despite correct antiaccommodative therapy. Besides the treatment of the often present amblyopia, the treatment is surgical. Recession-resection on the deviating eye or bilateral recessions can be done. In later life, a phoria can always break down into a tropia with symptoms of diplopia (decompensated strabismus (47)).

2. Acquired non-accommodative esotropia

Besides some cases of non-accommodative convergence excess and of esotropia in myopia, most of these cases belong to a group called "Essential esotropia of late onset" by the Hugonniers, "Acquired tonic esotropia" by Costenbader (17) and "Normosensorial essential late strabismus" by Lang (62).

In this group, onset is after the age of 6 months but it usually starts suddenly in the 4th year of life. The refractive error is insignificant and the angle can be small at the onset but tends to increase; the near deviation equals the distance deviation. There is normal retinal correspondence and no amblyopia; diplopia and confusion are frequently occurring early symptoms. Under anesthesia, the eyes are straight or divergent.

The treatment consists of prisms and surgery. Overcorrection during the immediate postoperative period resulted in a higher incidence of fusion than in those who were initially orthophoric or undercorrected. Such deliberate overcorrection, experimented by de Decker (24) in cases of early convergent strabismus but mostly to change the sensorial status, is only advocated in late cases when a good fusional potential is present preoperatively (23).

C. *Microstrabismus (microtropia)*

Although between normal alignment with bifoveal fixation and large angle squint a whole spectrum of deviations exists and although the dividing line between normal and abnormal binocular vision is blurred (22), a group has been separated in which the angle does not exceed 5°. Lang (58, 60) coined the term microstrabismus for this cosmetically non disturbing deviation. It would perhaps have been better to speak of microstrabismus when the angle is inferior to 1 prism diopter and of ministrabismus when the angle lies between 1 and 5 prism diopters; nevertheless, it seems not appropriate to add more confusion to the terminology of this entity which is already called "fixation disparity", "fusion disparity", "monofixational esophoria", "retinal slip", "flicker cases", "small angle esotropia", "microtropia".

American authors (66) tend to use the term fixation disparity in the sense given by Ogle (73). In a person with heterophoria, inexactness of fixation of the fovea may be associated with fusion of disparate retinal images (not falling on corresponding retinal elements of the two eyes) on the condition that the disparity is not too great, which is 6 to 10 minutes of arc. This phenomenon is also called "retinal slip" (66), "fusional disparity" (99), "cortical slip" (73). It has extensively been studied by Crone (20, 21).

We will use the term convergent microstrabismus synonymously with monofixational esotropia.

Besides the fact that all these cases have an angle smaller than 5°, they have wide variations in many other respects. According to their origin, cases exist where the deviation is primary and often hereditary but more often they are the final result of surgical or nonsurgical treatment of large angle squints. This form of strabismus can often be found in amblyopia with anisometropia and can also be at the basis of amblyopia in cases where there seems to be no strabismus. With regard to the deviation, this can be so small as to be undetectable by ordinary methods or great enough to be visible by the unilateral cover test; von Noorden however does not include heterotropias with a positive cover test (107). On the other hand, the fixation can be excentric in the deviating eye which renders the cover test useless.

This strabismus is mostly monolateral and amblyopia is a frequent finding. Under binocular circumstances, one eye fixates while there is a small tropia of the other with suppression of its fovea (monofixation). The method of binocular fixation pattern has shown that patients with small angles of esotropia demonstrate strong grades of fixation preference, even in the absence of amblyopia (113). In a series of 62 patients with primary microsquint, Lang (63) found no scotoma in 21, a fixation or zero point scotoma of 0.5-1° in 15 and a large scotoma of 3.7° in 26. In binocular vision two regions of the strabismic eye are inhibited: the fovea and the region which receives the same image as the fovea of the fixing eye. The first is called the foveal or central scotoma, the other the diplopia point scotoma or zero point scotoma.

Concerning the binocular situation, it is generally accepted that nearly all patients with fixed small-angle convergent strabismus and bilateral central fixation show harmonious anomalous retinal correspondence when examined in normal surroundings under non-dissociating test conditions (54, 71, 77). De Decker and Haase (25) however found that 7% of their cases were corresponding normally whereas one third remained unstable in their sensory behavior. For them, four sensopathological principles allow a better description of the clinical findings in cases showing a more complicated state: 1) haziness of cortical connections; 2) rivalry of more than one correspondence; 3) horror fusionis; 4) inherited amblyopia.

As the anomalous retinal correspondence seems to be untreatable, all efforts in these cases are directed to the prevention or the healing of the amblyopia (61). Not all authors agree with this conception. Rubin (95) found that a reverse 5 prism-diopter prism base in lens with calibrated occlusion of the fixing eye is an effective tool for the correction of small-angle esotropia, especially if this small-angle esotropia is the result of undercorrection of a pre-existing larger esotropia. Nearly 60% of his cases became parallel with no residual angle of deviation.

Jampolsky (54) writes that surgical treatment of small esotropias of 15 diopters or less is usually not indicated and results at best in a newer, smaller angle of strabismus and more often in the same preoperative angle. Pollard and Manley (81) practised unilateral medial rectus muscle recession of 5 mm for small angle esotropia; it has to be said that all their cases measured from 14 to 18 prism diopters preoperatively and fell in fact outside the limits of this entity. Bedrossian (9), in discussing small angle strabismus thought that if surgery was performed on one muscle, incomitant strabismus would probably occur. He also believed that operating on two muscles posed the danger of overcorrection. He recommended a marginal myotomy combined with a resection of the direct antagonist.

BIBLIOGRAPHY

(1) ADELSTEIN, F., CÜPPERS, C. — Zum Problem der echten und scheinbaren Abducenslähmung (das sogenannte "Blockierungssyndrom"). In: Augenmuskellähmungen, Bücherei des Augenarztes. Stuttgart. *F. Enke Verlag*, 1966, *46*, 271-278.

(2) AMES, A., GLIDDON, G.H. — Ocular measurements. *Trans. Sec. Ophthal. Amer. Med. Ass.*, 1928, 102-175.

(3) ARDOUIN, M., URVOY, M., SALMON, D., ELIET, F. — Traitement non chirurgical du strabisme convergent. L'Année thérapeutique et clinique en Ophtalmologie. Tome XXXI, Marseille, Diffusion Générale de Librairie, 1980, 139-162.

(4) ARNOULT, J.B., YESHURUN, O., MAZOW, M.L. — Comparative study of the surgical management of congenital eostropia of 50^{Δ} or less. *J. Pediat. Ophthal.*, 1976, *13*, 129-131.

(5) ARRUGA, A., DOWNEY, R. — Anomalous sensory relationship in apparently cured squints. *Brit. J. Ophthalmol.*, 1960, *44*, 492-502.

(6) BAGOLINI, B. — Anomalous correspondence: definition and diagnostic methods. *Doc. Ophthalmol.*, 1967, *23*, 346-386.

(7) BAGOLINI, B. — Sensorische und sensomotorische Abweichungen bei Schielen. In: Aktuelle Ophthalmologische Probleme. *Bücherei des Augenartzes*, *86*, 155-169. Stuttgart, F. Enke Verlag, 1981.

(8) BAKER, J.D., PARKS, M.M.M. — Early-onset accommodative esotropia. *Amer. J. Ophthalmol.*, 1980, *90*, 11-18.

(9) BEDROSSIAN, H. — Management of small-angle strabismus. *Amer. Orthop. J.*, 1968, *18*, 35-38.

(10) BÉRARD, P.V., TASSY, A., DERANSART-FERRERO, J.C., MOUILLAC-GAMBARELLI, N. — Valeur séméiologique de l'électro-oculographie motrice de poursuite dans les ésotropies de l'amblyopie strabique. *J. Fr. Ophtalmol.*, 1980, *3*, 719-730.

(11) BLAKEMORE, C. — The conditions required for the maintenance of binocularity in the kitten's visual cortex. *Journ. of Physiol.*, 1976, *261*, 423-444.
(12) BOULAD, L., CREHANGE, J., DELLER, M., HOROVITZ, G., LASSER-VIDAL, C., LAULAN, J., MAWAS, J., RICHON, J., SCHILOVITZ, G., WEISS, J.B. — Opération du strabisme avec anses. *J. Fr. Orthopt.*, 1980, *12*, 101-107.
(13) BRAUN-VALLON, S., LUCA, F. — Les petits angles d'anomalie. Étude clinique. *Ann. Oculist.*, 1967, *200*, 1129-1141.
(14) BREININ, G.M. — Accommodative strabismus and the AC/A ratio. *Amer. J. Ophthalmol.*, 1971, *71*, 303-311.
(15) CORCELLE, L. — Les formes pseudo-paralytiques du blocage. *J. Fr. Orthopt.*, 1978, *10*, 27-33.
(16) CORCELLE, L. — Strabisme de l'inné et de l'acquis. *J. Fr. Ophtalmol.*, 1980, *3*, 281-289.
(17) COSTENBADER, F.D. — Clinical course and management of esotropia. In: Allen, J.H. Strabismus Ophthalmic Symposium, II. St. Louis, The C.V. Mosby Company, 1958, 325-353.
(18) COSTENBADER, F.D. — Infantile esotropia. *Trans. Amer. Ophthalmol. Soc.*, 1961, *59*, 397-429.
(19) CRONE, R.A. — Alternating hyperphoria. *Brit. J. Ophthalmol.*, 1954, *38*, 591-604.
(20) CRONE, R.A. — The kinetic and static function of binocular disparity. *Investigative Ophthalmology*, 1969, *8*, 557-560.
(21) CRONE, R.A. — Diplopia. Amsterdam, Excerpta Medica & New York, American Elsevier Publishing Cy., Inc., 1973.
(22) CRONE, R.A., HARDJOWIJOTO, S. — What is normal binocular vision? *Doc. Ophthalmol.*, 1979, *47-1*, 163-199.
(23) DANKNER, S.R., MASH, A.J., JAMPOLSKY, A. — Intentional surgical overcorrection of acquired ésotropia. *Arch. Ophthalmol.*, 1978, *96*, 1848-1852.
(24) DE DECKER, W. — Kurze Bilanz der Behandlung mit artifizieller Divergenz. *Klin. Mbl. Augenheilk.*, 1975, *166*, 619-623.
(25) DE DECKER, W., HAASE, W. — Subnormales Binokularsehen. Versuch einer Einteilung des Mikrostrabismus. *Klin. Mbl. Augenheilk.*, 1976, *169*, 182-195.
(26) DONDERS, F.C. — On the anomalies of accommodation and refraction of the eye. London, The New Sydenham Society, 1864.
(27) DUKE-ELDER, S. — Ocular motility and strabismus. System of Ophthalmology, vol. VI. London, Henry Kimpton, 1973.
(28) EVENS, L. — Résultats à long terme du traitement des strabismes. *Bull. Soc. Belge Ophtalm.*, 1971, *159*, 686-690.
(29) FISCHER, N.F., FLOM, M.C., JAMPOLSKY, A. — Early surgery for congenital esotropia. *Amer. J. Ophthalmol.*, 1968, *65*, 439-443.
(30) FLETCHER, M.C., SILVERMAN, S.J., ABBOTT, W.P. — Strabismus. Reliability of recorded data used in clinical research. *Amer. J. Ophthalmol.*, 1965, *60*, 1047-1055.
(31) FLETCHER, M.C., SILVERMAN, S.J. — Strabismus: I. A summary of 1110 consecutive cases. *Amer. J. Ophthalmol*, 1966, *61*, 86-94.
(32) FLETCHER, M.C., SILVERMAN, S.J. — Strabismus: II. Findings in 472 cases of partially accommodative and nonaccommodative esotropia. *Amer. J. Ophthalmol.*, 1966, *61*, 255-265.
(33) FORTIER, E.G. — Infantile comitant esotropia. A new diagnostic test and results of early surgery. *Amer. J. Ophthalmol., 1962, 54*, 804-806.
(34) FOSTER, R.S., PAUL, T.O., JAMPOLSKY, A. — Management of infantile esotropia. *Amer. J. Ophthalmol., 1976, 82*, 290-299.
(35) FRANÇOIS, J., JAMES, M. — Traitement du strabisme concomitant. Étude comparative des résultats dans différents groupes d'âge. *Ann. Ocul., 1956, 189*, 771-777.
(36) GOBIN, M.H. — Sagittalization of the oblique muscles as a possible cause for the "A", "V" and "X" phenomena. *Brit. J. Ophthalmol.*, 1968, *52*, 13-18.
(37) GOBIN, M.H. — Récession avec anse du droit interne. *Bull. Soc. Belge Ophtalm.*, 1975, *171*, 789-795.
(38) GOBIN, M.H. — Nouvelles conceptions sur la pathogénie et le traitement du strabisme. I. Pathogénie du strabisme. *J. Fr. Ophtalmol.*, 1980, *3*, 541-556.

(39) GOBIN, M.H. — Id. II. Traitement du strabisme. Introduction. Chirurgie primaire. Chirurgie secondaire. *J. Fr. Ophtalmol.*, 1981, *4*, 7-18.

(40) GOBIN, M.H. — Id. III. Traitement du strabisme. Introduction. Complications. Conclusions. *J. Fr. Ophtalmol.*, 1981, *4*, 297-305.

(41) GODDÉ-JOLLY, D., LARMANDE, A. — Les nystagmus, 2 Vol. Paris, Ed. Masson et Cie, 1973.

(42) GODDÉ-JOLLY, D. — Les pénalisations dans le traitement du strabisme convergent. *J. Fr. Ophtalmol.*, 1978, *1*, 607-614.

(43) GODDÉ-JOLLY, D. — Le strabisme. Encycl. Méd. Chir. Paris, *Ophtalmol.*, 21550 A 10 et A 15, *2*, 1981.

(44) GOLDSTEIN, J.H. — Large-angle esotropia. *Ann. Ophthal.*, 1974, *6*, 1025-1027.

(45) HAMBURGER, F.A. — Das akkommodative Moment beim Begleitschielen. *Klin. Mbl. Augenheilk.*, 1972, *160*, 113-118.

(46) HELVESTON, E.M., VON NOORDEN, G.K. — Microtropia: a newly defined entity. *Arch. Ophthalmol.*, 1967, *78*, 272-281.

(47) HIATT, R.L., BOYER, S.L., COPE-TROUPE, C. — Decompensated strabismus. *Ann. Ophthalmol.*, 1979, *11*, 1581-1588.

(48) HILES, D.A., WATSON, B.A., BIGLAN, A.W. — Characteristics of infantile esotropia following early bimedial rectus recession. *Arch. Ophthalmol.*, 1980, *98*, 697-703.

(49) HUBEL, D.H., WIESEL, T.N. — Binocular interaction in striate cortex of kittens reared with artificial squint. *J. Neurophysiol.*, 1965, *28*, 1041-1059.

(50) HUGHES, A. — AC/A ratio. *Brit. J. Ophthalmol.*, 1967, *51*, 786-787.

(51) HUGONNIER, R., HUGONNIER, S. — Strabismes. Hétérophories. Paralysies oculo-motrices. Paris, Éd. Masson et Cie, 1965.

(52) IKEDA, H., TREMAIN, K.E. — Amblyopia resulting from penalisation: neurophysiological studies of kittens reared with atropinisation of one or both eyes. *Brit. J. Ophthalmol.*, 1978, *62*, 21-28.

(53) ING, M., COSTENBADER, F.D., PARKS, M.M., ALBERT, D.G. — Early surgery for congenital esotropia. *Amer. J. Ophthalmol.*, 1966, *61*, 1419-1427.

(54) JAMPOLSKY, A. — Retinal correspondence in patients with small degree strabismus. *Arch. Ophthalmol.*, 1951, *45*, 18-26.

(55) KETTESY, A. — Die Brille als Heilmittel des Schielens. *Klin. Mbl. Augenheilk.*, 1972, *161*, 160-164.

(56) KRIMSKY, E. — The corneal-light reflex: a guide to binocular disorders. Springfield, Charles C. Thomas Co, 1972.

(57) LANG, J. — Welche Schielfälle können geheilt werden? *Ophthalmol.*, 1968, *156*, 190-195.

(58) LANG, J. — Evaluation in small angle strabismus or microtropia. In: Strabismus, Symposium Giessen, August 1966. p. 219-222. Basel, New York, Karger, 1968.

(59) LANG, J. — Einfache Differentialdiagnostik und gezielte Behandlung des Strabismus convergens. *Klin. Mbl. Augenheilk.*, 1969, *155*, 457-475.

(60) LANG, J. — Mikrostrabismus; Bücherei des Augenartztes 62. Stuttgart, Ferd. Enke Verlag, 1973.

(61) LANG, J. — Management of microtropia. *Brit. J. Ophthalmol.*, 1974, *58*, 281-292.

(62) LANG, J. — Das normosensorische essentielle konvergente Spätschielen, eine Schielform "sui generis". *Klin. Mbl. Augenheilk.*, 1978, *172*, 807-824.

(63) LANG, J. — Die Skotome im binokularen Gesichtsfeld bei hochgradiger Amblyopie und bei Mikrostrabismus. *Klin. Mbl. Augenheilk.*, 1978, *173*, 470-474.

(64) LAVAT, J. — Peut-on guérir tous les strabiques? *Bull. Soc. Ophtalm. Fr.*, 1968, *68*, 183-208.

(65) LEGRAND, J., GILLOT, F. — Syndrome de Moebius. A propos d'un cas. *J. Fr. Ophtalmol.*, 1980, *3*, 579-582.

(66) LINKSZ, A. — Physiology of the eye. New York, Grune & Stratton Inc., 1952.

(67) MALBRAN, J. — Strabismes et paralysies (Ed. 1949); traduction Sevrin, G. Charleroi, Ed. Héraly, 1953.

(68) MANLEY, D.R. — Classification of esodeviations. In: Manley, D.M.: Symposium on horizontal ocular deviations (p. 3-48). Saint Louis, The C.V. Mosby Cy, 1971.

(69) MANLEY, D.R. — Accommodative esodeviations. In: Manley, D.R.: Symposium on horizontal ocular deviations (p. 49-71). Saint Louis, The C.V. Mosby Cy, 1971.

(70) MARAINI, G., PASINO, L. — Development of normal binocular vision in early convergent strabismus after orthophoria. *Brit. J. Ophthalmol.*, 1965, *49*, 154-158.
(71) MARAINI, G., PASINO, L. — Variations in the angle of anomaly and fusional movements in cases of small-angle convergent strabismus with harmonious anomalous retinal correspondence. *Brit. J. Ophthalmol.*, 1964, *48*, 439-443.
(72) MOLNAR, L. — Über die Behandlung und das Resultat der verschiedenen Schielformen. *Klin. Mbl. Augenheilk.*, 1974, *165*, 898-902.
(73) OGLE, K., MUSSEY, F., PRANGEN, A. de H. — Fixation disparity and the fusional processes in binocular single vision. *Amer. J. Ophthalmol.*, 1949, *32*, 1069-1087.
(74) OGLE, K.N., MARTENS, T.G., DYER, J.A. — Oculomotor imbalance in binocular vision and fixation disparity. Philadelphia, Lea and Febiger, 1967.
(75) PARKS, M.M. — Abnormal accommodative convergence in squint. *Arch. Ophthalmol.*, 1958, *59*, 364-380.
(76) PARKS, M.M. — Early strabismus care. *Amer. J. Ophthalmol.*, 1964, *57*, 854-855.
(77) PARKS, M.M. — The monofixation syndrome. *Trans. Amer. Ophthal. Soc.*, 1969, *67*, 607-657.
(78) PARKS, M.M. — Management of acquired esotropia. *Brit. J. Ophthalmol.*, 1974, *58*, 240-247.
(79) PIGASSOU, R. — "Entente cordiale" in the early treatment of squint. *Brit. J. Ophthalmol.*, 1977, *61*, 16-22.
(80) PIGASSOU-ALBOUY, R. — Les processus d'inhibition dans le strabisme convergent. *J. Fr. Ophtalmol.*, 1980, *3*, 45-56.
(81) POLLARD, Z.F., MANLEY, D. — Unilateral medial rectus recession for small-angle esotropia. *Arch. Ophthalmol.*, 1976, *94*, 780-781.
(82) POLLARD, Z.F. — Accommodative esotropia during the first year of life. *Arch. Ophthalmol.*, 1976, *94*, 1912-1913.
(83) POULIQUEN, P. — Surcorrection optique et angle strabique. *Bull. Soc. Opht. Fr.*, 1964, *64*, 742-745.
(84) QUÉRÉ, M.A. — Le traitement précoce des strabismes infantiles. Paris, Ed. Doin, 1973.
(85) QUÉRÉ, M.A., DELPLACE, M.P. — Les troubles optomoteurs dans les strabismes et les paralysies oculomotrices. *Ann. Ocul.*, 1973, *206*, 449-475.
(86) QUÉRÉ, M.A., CLERGEAU, G., FONTENAILLE, N. — Die Lähmungsdyssynergien. Die Schieldyssynergien und das Cüppersche Syndrom. *Klin. Mbl. Augenheilk.*, 1975, *167*, 162-178.
(87) QUÉRÉ, M.A., CLERGEAU, G., FONTENAILLE, N., GOURAY, A., SPIELMANN, A., LLEDO, M. — Les syndromes de blocage dans les strabismes infantiles. *Ann. Ocul.*, 1976, *209*, 339-349, 417-433, 483-500.
(88) QUÉRÉ, M.A., PECHEREAU, A., CLERGEAU, G. — La nouvelle chirurgie des ésotropies fonctionnelles (opération du fil et techniques classiques). *J. Fr. Ophtalmol.*, 1978, *1*, 56-60, 151-161, 221-228.
(89) RASKIND, R.H., BURIAN, H.M. — Bilateral resections. *Amer. J. Ophthalmol.*, 1967, *64*, 78-89.
(90) RETHY, S., GÁL, S. — Ergebnissen der konservativen Schielbehandlung durch Überkorrektur der manifesten Hypermetropie. *Klin. Mbl. Augenheilk.*, 1967, *150*, 170-175.
(91) RÉTHY, S., GÁL, S. — Results and principles of a new method of optical correction of hypermetropia in cases of esotropia. *Acta ophthalmol.*, 1968, *46*, 757-766.
(92) RIISE, P. — The importance of early treatment of esotropia. *Amer. J. Ophthalmol.*, 1961, *51*, 634-643.
(93) ROMANO, P.E., VON NOORDEN, G.K. — Limitations of cover test in detecting strabismus. *Amer. J. Ophthalmol.*, 1971, *72*, 10-12.
(94) ROSENBAUM, A.L., JAMPOLSKY, A., SCOTT, A.B. — Bimedial recession in high AC/A esotropia. *Arch. Ophthalmol.*, 1974, *91*, 251-253.
(95) RUBIN, W. — Reverse prism and calibrated occlusion in the treatment of small angle esotropia. *Amer. J. Ophthalmol.*, 1965, *59*, 271-277.
(96) SARNIGUET-BADOCHE — Traitement du blocage par les secteurs. *J. Fr. Orthopt.*, 1979, *11*, 117-121.
(97) SIMONS, K. — Stereoacuity. Norms in young children. *Arch. Ophthalmol.*, 1981, *99*, 439-445.

(98) SLOAN, L.L., SEARS, M.L., JABLONSKI, M.D. — Convergence-accommodation relationships. *Arch. Ophthalmol., 1960, 63*, 283-306.
(99) SWAN, K. — Nature of normal binocular visional-fusional process. In: Allen, J.H. Strabismus, Ophthalmic Symposium, vol. 2. St. Louis, The C.V. Mosby Cy, 1958.
(100) TAYLOR, D.M. — How early is early surgery in the management of strabismus. *Arch. Ophthalmol.*, 1963, *70*, 752-756.
(101) TAYLOR, D.M. — Congenital strabismus. The common sense approach. *Arch. Ophthalmol.*, 1967, *77*, 478-484.
(102) TAYLOR, D.M. — Is congenital esotropia fundamentally curable? *Trans. Amer. Ophthalmol. Soc.*, 1972, *70*, 529-576.
(103) TAYLOR, D.M. — Congenital esotropia: management and prognosis. New York, Intercontinental Medical Book Corp., 1973.
(104) VERFECKEN, E., FLYNN, J. — Amblyopia: part I. Diagnosis. *J. Ped. Ophthal.*, 1967, *4*, 33-44. Part II: Therapy. *J. Ped. Ophthal.*, 1967, *4*, 45-56.
(105) VON NOORDEN, G.K. — Strabismus surgery: early and very early. *Arch. Ophthalmol.*, 1964, *71*, 759.
(106) VON NOORDEN, G.K. — The nystagmus compensation (blockage) syndrome. *Amer. J. Ophthalmol.*, 1976, *82*, 283-290.
(107) VON NOORDEN, G.K. — Burian-von Noorden's Binocular vision and ocular motility. Theory and management of strabismus. St. Louis, Toronto, London, The C.V. Mosby Cy, 1980.
(108) WARD, B.A., HUGHES, A. — The functional results in cases of convergent squint. *Amer. J. Ophthalmol.*, 1964, *58*, 258-261.
(109) WEISS, J.B. — Étude électro-oculographique des déséquilibres oculo-moteurs. *Bull. Mém. Soc. Fr. Ophtal.*, 1977, *88*, 122-128.
(110) WEISS, J.B. — Le «blocage» existe-t-il? *J. Fr. Ophtalmol.*, 1979, *2*, 715-722.
(111) WORTH, C. — Squint. 6th Ed. London, Bailliere, Tindall & Cox, 1929.
(112) WYBAR, K. — Relevance of the AC/A ratio. *Brit. J. Ophthalmol.*, 1974, *58*, 248-254.
(113) ZIPF, R.F. — Binocular fixation pattern,- *Arch. Ophthalmol.*, 1976, *94*, 401-405.

Bull. Soc. belge Ophtal., **195**, 19-52, 1981.

CHAPTER II

HISTORY OF STRABISMUS TREATMENT

L. EVENS (*)

„Keine Realität ist wesentlicher für unsere Selbstvergewisserung als die Geschichte. Mitten in der Geschichte stehen wir und unsere Gegenwart. Der Blick auf die Menschheitsgeschichte führt uns an das Geheimnis unseres Menschseins."

K. Jaspers

I. *Introduction*

Although it would have been interesting to present a history of the ideas on strabismus, of the evolution of the opinions concerning the causes and contributing factors, of the philosophical and empirical foundations of treatment (43, 46, 58, 96, 105, 129, 145, 179), we will limit this chapter to the history of the therapeutical approaches to convergent squint. Not without mentioning that the theoretical insight into strabismus has in recent years substantially been deepened by work carried out in the fundamental sciences. The awareness of neurons ready for binocular input in the early weeks of life has completely changed our ideas concerning the treatment possibilities in the early forms of strabismus.

Most historical surveys on strabismus treatment start with the chevalier Taylor and the strabismus operations he performed around 1750; generally the authors hesitate about the qualification which he deserves. Was he a crook or was he the father of strabismus surgery? Recently, Berg (22), on the basis of newly discovered papers, tries to put Taylor in a more correct perspective. It seems that he cut off a strip

(*) Lakenselaan 36, 1090 Brussels (Belgium).

of conjunctiva over the medial rectus muscle thinking (erroneously) that he was cutting through the nerves supplying this muscle, which he held responsible for the deviation. It is possible that in doing this he sometimes accidentally sectioned the rectus internus, resulting of course in a dramatic change in the ocular position.

From this period of interventions on the conjunctival tissues (excision of a piece of this tissue or cauterisation with lapis infernalis) arises the great figure of Dieffenbach who really deserves the honour of having performed the first strabismus operation (96, 145, 179) on October 26, 1839. The patient was a seven-year-old boy with a convergent

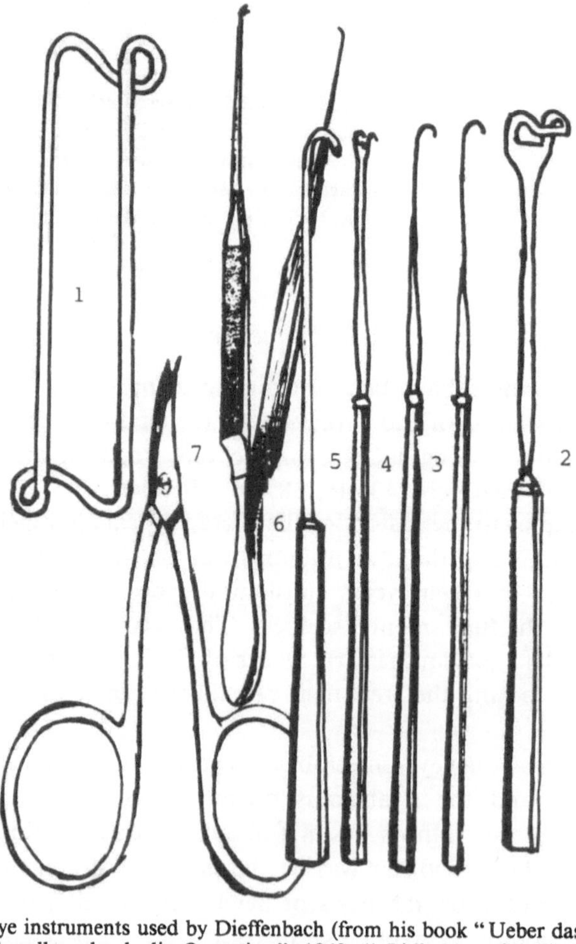

Fig. 1. — Eye instruments used by Dieffenbach (from his book "Ueber das Schielen und die Heilung desselben durch die Operation", 1842. 1) Lidholder of Pellier for the upper eyelid. 2) Lidholder for the lower eyelid. 3) Two conjunctival pointed hooks. 4) Double hook. 5) Blunt muscle hook. 6) Forceps. 7) Scissors.

squint on whom Dieffenbach performed a section of the musculus rectus internus. With the instruments shown in figure 1 he used the following technique: 1. incision of the conjunctival tissue; 2. placement of a muscle hook and liberation of the muscle from the underlying sclera; 3. section of the muscle 3 to 4 lines after its insertion (i.e. 6 to 8 mm after its anterior insertion, as the old measure of length called line (ligne, Linie) has a length of approximatively 2 mm) (fig. 2).

The idea of myotomy came from an orthopedic surgeon, Stromeyer (194), who used this operation for the correction of torticollis and clubfoot; he had also demonstrated on the cadaver that tenotomy of the ocular muscles was possible (while myotomy is the section of the muscle itself and tenotomy the section of the tendon, both terms are often interchanged).

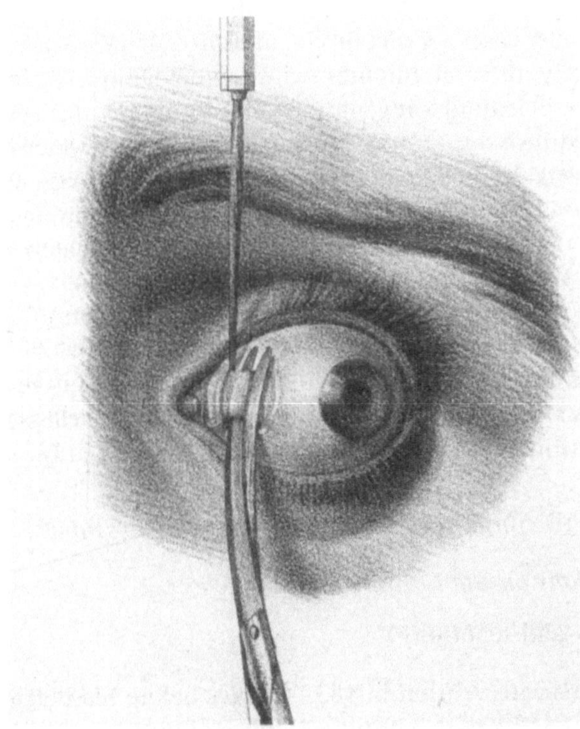

Fig. 2. — Myotomy of Dieffenbach, modified by Sichel (from the Atlas of Bourgery (30)).

It has to be mentioned that Dieffenbach used his myotomy on all six ocular muscles. But whereas he never saw overcorrections after section of the rectus externus, he noted himself that the major complication of his technique for convergent squint was a secondary divergent squint. These secondary exodeviations were given the meaningful name of "old Dieffenbachs". In the following years, Dieffenbach and his contemporaries tried numerous technical variations to improve the myotomy and to avoid or to correct the secondary exotropias.

While A. von Graefe saw the cause of strabismus in a muscular disease (116), the role of hypertropia was recognised by F.C. Donders who wrote in 1864 (57): "Strabismus convergens almost always depends upon hypermetropia... In general, it is not the highest degrees of hypermetropia with which strabismus is combined... So long as strabismus occurs only intermittently with fixing an object, its development may be prevented by wearing convex glasses, which neutralise the existing hypermetropia". The same Donders had already very surprising recommendations for the treatment of amblyopia; in the same work he writes: "In such cases I generally confine myself to advising them to look twice daily for some minutes, with the deviating eye alone, which practice is sufficient to prevent the diminution of the acuteness of vision... Mydriasis by atropia (atropine) of the eye which is usually properly directed immediately causes the other to be used and is therefore sometimes recommended in the case of young squinting children". In this way, the basis of refraction, occlusion and penalisation in the treatment of squint were laid more than 100 years ago.

Although Dieffenbach already mentions the treatment of strabismus by ocular gymnastics without operation, it is the merit of E. Javal to have explored the possibilities of all kinds of exercises in the treatment of strabismus and to have divulged his experiences in a classic textbook "Manuel théorique et pratique du strabisme" (1896, 113).

II. *Surgical procedures for convergent squint*

A. *Interventions on the medial rectus muscle*

1. Myotomy and tenotomy

After his first intervention in 1839 (3 days before his Belgian colleague Cunier), Dieffenbach continued his strabismus operations with such an enthusiasm that in 1842 he could already publish his book in which he gives his experience on 1200 cases (56). But whereas this myotomy can give excellent results for the lateral and especially the inferior oblique muscle, the section of the medial rectus leads too often to divergent squint with complete absence of adduction. Von Graefe (1857, 80) tried to improve the method by displacing the section nearer to the anterior insertion and leaving intact all the adherences of the muscle with the conjunctiva and the sclera. He hoped that the muscle would more posteriorly fix itself to the sclera. He writes: "The strabotomy exists in a posterior displacement of the tendon whereby the muscle keeps its full length".

2. Partial tenotomy

In the same study of 1857, von Graefe advises partial tenotomy in cases where only a small effect is desired. He states that the incision has to divide three fourths of the muscle to be effective but the buttonhole he made had little effect. Afterwards this technique fell into oblivion before being reintroduced by Abadie in 1880. All kinds of variations have been described by Stevens, Ziegler, Verhoeff, Todd, O'Connor, Blaskovics, Astruc, Bishop-Harman, Terrien, etc. (see Van der Hoeve, 205).

Although this partial or marginal myotomy is a seldom-used extraocular muscle weakening procedure, it should not be completely abandoned. It is useful when an already recessed muscle requires additional weakening; in rare cases it may be the primary procedure of choice. Rintelen (178) advises a unilateral or bilateral partial tenotomy in comitant convergent strabismus of less than 12°. He advises two cuts of two thirds of the muscle width with an interspace of 6 mm. This procedure gives him a change in angle of 6°. Helveston and coworkers (89) and also Kennedy (115) think that those myotomies which failed to section all fibres, allowing some of them to run continuously between the origin and the insertion of the muscle, produced no significant lengthening. They advise an incision on each side of the muscle; each incision should cross the midline and section 60 to 85% of the width of the muscle or tendon. This double incomplete marginal myotomy was originally described by Blaskovics (26) (fig. 3) but seems only to have lasting results when combined with resection of the antagonist. Gobin (73) still uses central tenotomy in which 8/10 of the tendinous insertion is severed from the globe, leaving only the two lateral extremities in place.

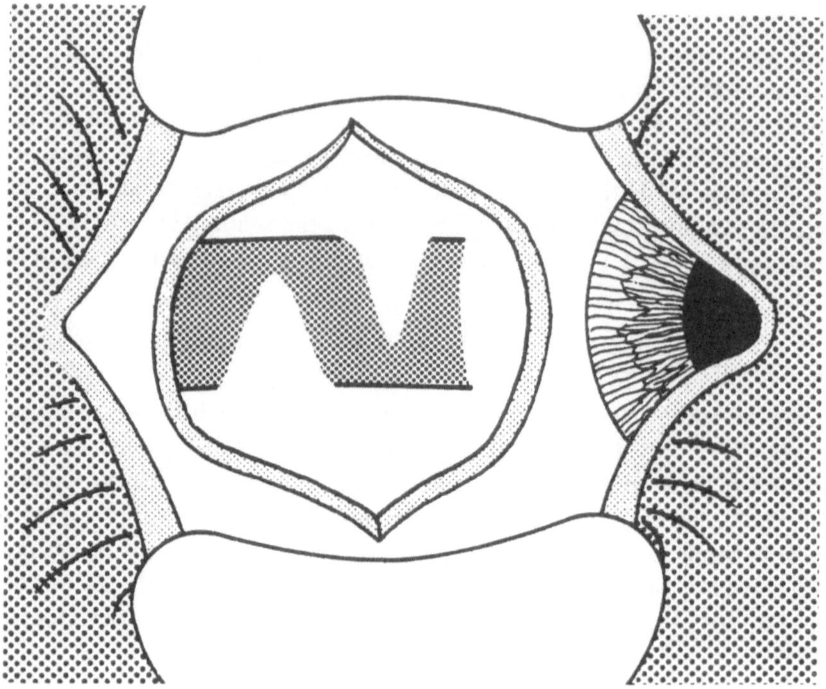

Fig. 3. — Partial or marginal myotomy.

3. Controlled (bridled) tenotomy

In 1895, Beard, after performing a tenotomy, put a suture through the muscle, brought it through Tenon and conjunctiva and knotted it externally, thus preventing the muscle to slip too far away. Bielschowsky (24) brought the suture through the scleral insertion stump before tying it in the same manner. By tightening or loosening this external knot, it was even possible to change the operative result in the first days after the operation.

This technique merits our attention as its two variations are widely used today.

In the first variation, which really deserves the name of controlled, or bridled tenotomy (or tenotomy with retention sutures (Arruga, 7)), the muscle after tenotomy remains attached to its previous scleral insertion by one or more suture loops of various lengths. These loops are covered by Tenon and conjunctiva and cannot be modified. Stallard (188) considers it an alternative operation to recession of the medial rectus, appropriate for either the infrequent operator or the beginner... "until precision is acquired in passing a suture through the superficial layers of the sclera". On the other hand, Hass in 1965 (85) considers his technique of recession with fixation sutures to be the best and safest way to achieve a recession. In his method, two 3.0 catgut loops knotted over a special spatula fix the muscle to the original insertion and allow it to realize an new scleral insertion 3 to 5 mm from the original one. While some authors criticize this method as being unreliable concerning the new insertion and think that the muscle can reattach at any point between the original insertion and the maximum width of the loop, others on the contrary consider it the method of choice. They contend that the muscle does not reattach to the sclera but that the space separating it from the original insertion is filled by fibrous tissue, thus lenthening the muscle.

Recently, Gobin (68, 73) renewed the interest for loops. After doing a classical recession of the internal rectus of 5 mm with scleral insertion, he tied the knot over a probe with a diameter of 2 mm for great loops, of 1.5 mm for small loops (fig. 4). Silk sutures (Ethicon 5/0) were used at the beginning, actually Vicryl 6/0 has taken its place. Primary loops are used as the first procedure in large angle esodeviations and they are mostly combined with displacement of both inferior obliques (four

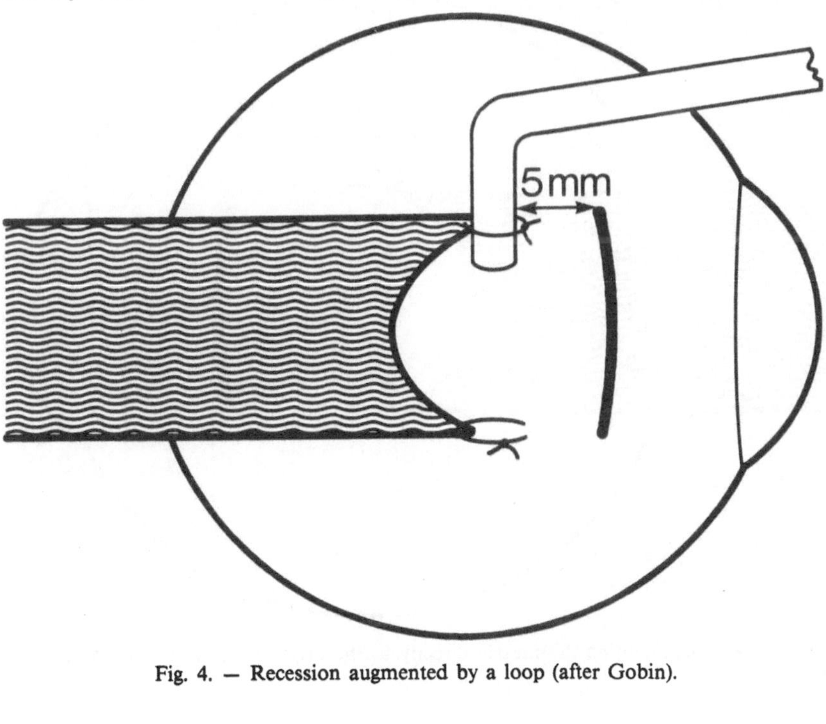

Fig. 4. — Recession augmented by a loop (after Gobin).

muscle surgery, see chapter IX). Secondary loops are used for reinterventions; the already recessed muscle is disinserted and fixed at the same place but with a loop. Even a new loop can be placed on a muscle which had before been recessed with a first loop. Gobin states that the space existing between the muscle and the sclera is filled with fibrous tissue; an elongation of the recessed muscle is thus realised. A bilateral 5 mm recession of both medial recti is always done but a unilateral or bilateral, small or large loop is used according to the angle of the deviation.

Weiss, Horovitz and Vergne (208) extended this technique by using large loops which unite the muscle directly to its original insertion (fig. 5). Two Vicryl 5/0 or 6/0 sutures are tied over one of their probes creating a loop of 2 to 8.5 mm. Taking into account that it is always difficult to give strict indications, it takes roughly 1 mm of loop for 3 diopters of deviation (for a deviation of 30 diopters, one can make a bilateral loop of 5 mm; for a deviation of 45 diopters one of 7 and one of 8 mm). The collective experience of ten strabismus surgeons has recently favored this technique (29).

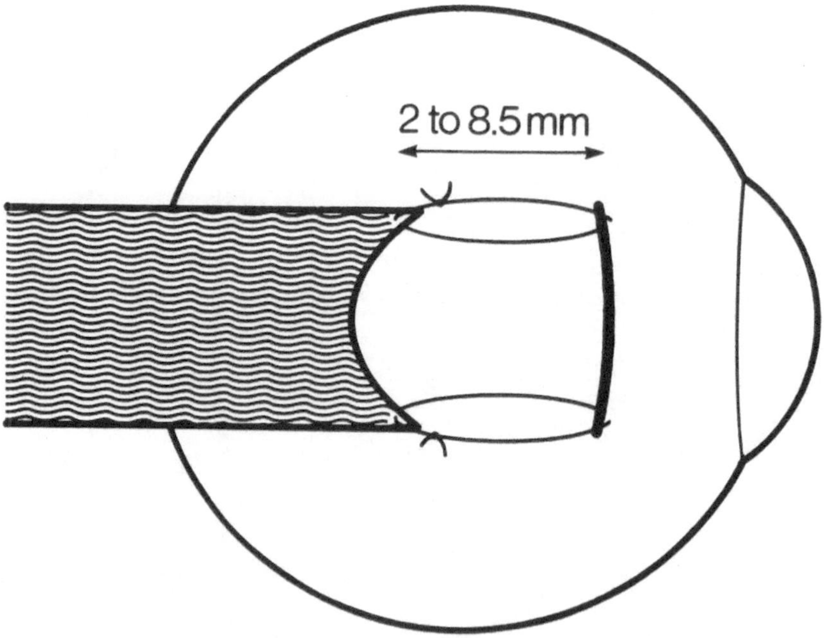

Fig. 5. — Loops uniting the muscle directly to the original insertion (after Weiss and coll.).

In the second variation of tenotomy with retention sutures, the end of the sutures uniting the cut muscle with the initial insertional stump cross the conjunctiva and are knotted externally. This makes it possible to remove them afterwards. It also allows some adjustments in the first days after the operation, either by pulling the muscle up to minimize the recession, or by loosening the loop to allow the muscle to recess further. Recently, Jampolsky revived the interest in adjustable strabismus surgery (111, 112, 141, 180). Although this technique can be used in concomitant convergent squint, especially if a larger than usual recession is necessary, it is more often used in complicated strabismus cases, as in thyroid myopathy, difficult reinterventions, etc. In Jampolsky's technique, the rather complicated sutures are placed during general anesthesia whereas the adjustements are made in the conscious state.

This procedure thus permits the surgeon to enhance or diminish the amount of muscle recession on the evening after the surgery or the first postoperative day if the covertesting indicates an inappropriate amount of undercorrection or overcorrection. It has to be stated that most cases treated in this way are complicated reoperation problems and that additional muscle surgery is usually performed on each patient in conjunction with the adjustable procedure (resection of the antagonist). Also, while adjustment is effective in altering the deviation between 1 and 23 prism diopters, it requires a cooperative patient and is not feasible in young children. Most children under 14 are unable to cooperate in this adjustment.

4. Recession of the medial rectus muscle

The actual technique of recession is derived from Jameson's procedure (106, 107, 108). The detached muscle is refixed to the sclera by two or three sutures, some millimeters (generally 3 to 6) behind the original insertion.

For a purely horizontal action, both extremities of the detached muscle have to be fixed to the globe at the same distance from the original insertion. Some authors put a third suture in the middle of the muscular section to counteract the tendency of the center of the tendon to bow backwards.

If an effect on an accompanying vertical deviation is desired, both muscular extremities can be refixed at a different distance from the initial insertion or the whole recessed muscle can be moved upwards or downwards. For a more important horizontal action, it is possible to combine a recession with the placement of a loop.

Non-absorbable and absorbable sutures are used and the design of needles has constantly been improved to prevent scleral perforation. Jameson already stressed the importance of superficial sutures and the necessity to always have the needle visible during its way through the scleral layers; perforation however and its sometimes disastrous consequences is the major complication of this technique. McLean, Galin and Baras (138), examining the retinal periphery in patients who had undergone strabismus surgery, found 16 cases which had unequivocal, surgically caused retinal tears at the site of the extraocular muscle manipulation. Havener and Kimball (87) reported four cases of scleral perforation, one resulting in panophthalmitis, phtisis and enucleation, one leading to cataract, one with massive hyphema and secondary glaucoma and one without complications after diathermy of the perforation site had been performed. Endophthalmitis was also described by Knobloch and Lorenz (120) and lens dislocation by Hittner (97). Gottlieb and Castro (79) consider perforation of the choroid and retina during strabismus surgery to be the etiology in two cases of retinal detachment, a case of vitreal hemorrhage and a case of endophthalmitis. Among 65 other children who had undergone corrective surgery for strabismus, six (9.2%) had funduscopic lesions indicating perforation of the globe with a needle. Perforation was not limited to recessions but also occurred in cases of resection.

The sclera is generally very thin at the site where the sutures have to be placed in a recession procedure. The sclera is of normal thickness, however, immediately adjacent to the thin area, above and below the medial rectus position. In cases where the sclera is excessively thin, the sutures are to be placed in the adjacent sclera of normal thickness (88).

Besides corneal dellen (15, 146, 203) which are frequently observed after muscle surgery, a case of hypopion keratitis was described (16) and two cases of orbital cellulitis (149).

5. Muscle lengthening

The idea of weakening the action of an ocular muscle by lengthening it comes from Stephenson (1902, 193). He realised this lengthening by two different techniques. In the first, the myotomy was done in an oblique way and the points of the two ends were united; in the second,

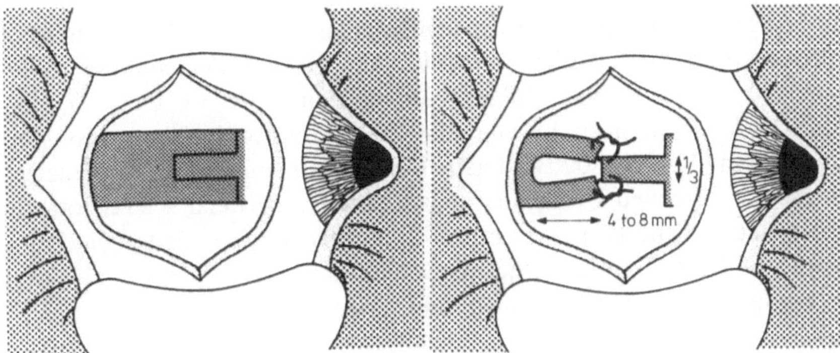

A B

Fig. 6A and B. — Muscle lengthening technique of Gonin.

the myotomy was done by a bayonet-like section and the two extremities were joined.

Gonin (1911, 77) describes a lengthening technique in which the normal insertion and the normal direction of the muscle are maintained (fig. 6). Klein, Muchnich and Raskind (117) recommend it as an alternative to recession in cases of abnormally thin sclera; they suggest the application of cyanoacrylate adhesive to the sclera under the muscle as a barrier to the formation of adhesions.

A different approach was made by Kuhnt (1908, 124, 125) (fig. 7). He dissected in the muscular tendon a tongue-like flap which after complete tenotomy was inverted and fixed to the insertion line; Bangerter and Bamert (13) actualised this procedure and Hollwich uses both the techniques of Gonin and Kuhnt (98, 99, 100).

Lengthening by a graft of fascia lata was proposed by Focosi and Ruzzi (1978, 64) and endorsed recently by Salvi, Frosini and Bos-

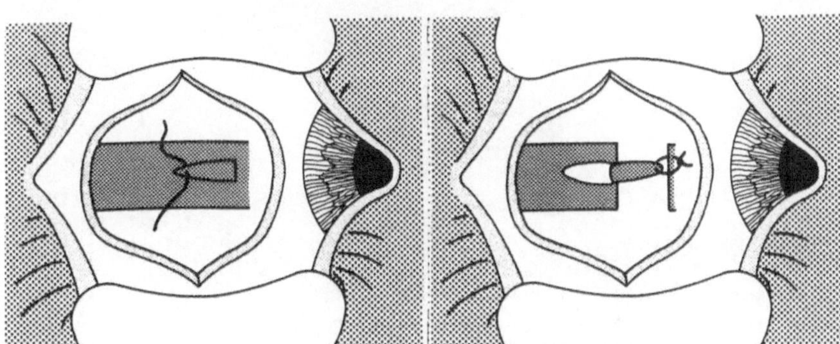

A B

Fig. 7A and B. — Lengthening technique of Kuhnt.

chi (181). We mention the experimental use of a small thin sheet of silicone rubber to lengthen an extraocular muscle which could be useful in large angle tropias, in strabismus fixus and in Duane's syndrome (76). Tenoplasty by marginal scleral division had been proposed by Vancea (204) and by Bordeianu (28). Lengthening of the hyperactive muscle is obtained by means of two small superficial scleral tongues positioned at the two extremities of the insertion; each tongue has a width of 1.5 to 2 mm, a thickness of 0.2 mm and a length that varies according to the degree of deviation to be corrected.

6. Faden-Operation

Synonyms are: " Opération du fil ", " retroequatorial myopexy " and " posterior fixation suture ".

Without entering into the discussion on " blockage-phenomena " (49, 172, 206), " nystagmus compensation " (150), " static and dynamic angle " (173, 175), it must be stated that this operation devised by Cüp-

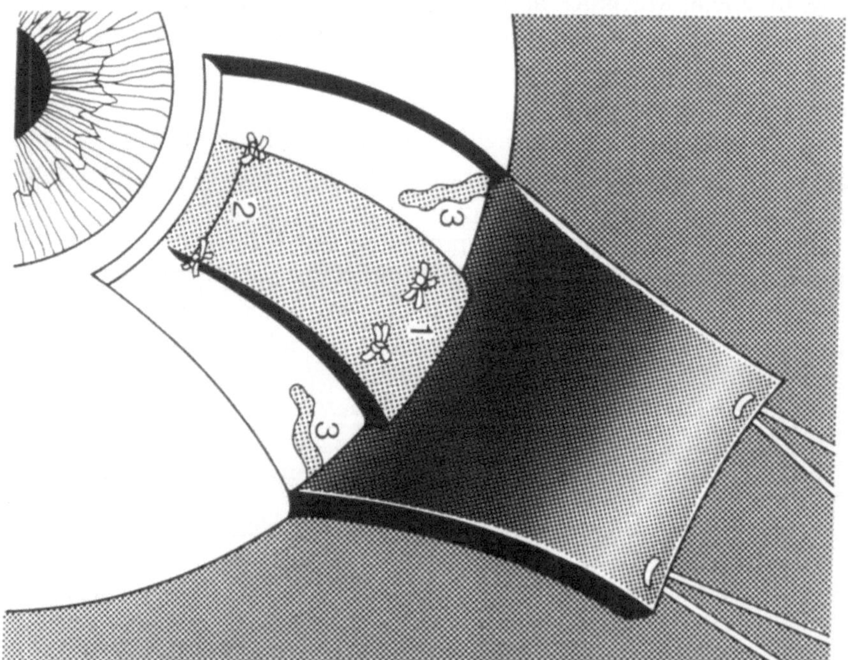

Fig. 8. — Faden-Operation (after Cüppers).
1) sutures fixing the muscle to the sclera;
2) replacement of the muscle at its original insertion;
3) vorticose veins.

pers (47) constitutes an entirely new approach in strabismus surgery (fig. 8). For horizontal muscles, this author prefers a limbal conjunctival incision, a temporary section of the muscle at its insertion, the placement of sutures far behind to fix the muscle to the sclera after which the muscle is sutured again to its original insertion (48). Cüppers draws attention to the dangers of injury to the vorticose veins which are in the neighborhood of these sclero-muscular sutures and the long ciliary artery which is underneath the muscle (102).

Thomas, Spielmann and Bernardini (1976, 197) state that for the medial rectus muscle, the posterior fixation suture should never be less than 13 mm from the original insertion; it can go to 14 mm in infants and 15 mm in adults. These authors saw four scleral perforations. Whereas Cüppers uses two U-shaped sutures sparing the center and the lateral parts of the muscle, de Decker and Conrad (52) and Deller (54) on the contrary include on both sides the lateral third of the muscle. They do not detach the muscle unless a recession or resection is realised at the same time. A variation of the original technique has been presented by Queré, "le sanglage musculaire rétro-équatorial", which the author recommends for cases with nystagmus blockage, with variable angles and with convergence excess (174).

Acting only against the active part of the angle, this technique has to be completed by classical procedures of recession and resection for correction of the passive part of the angle (175). Quéré finds spastic phenomena in the medial rectus of most strabismus cases; he favors the "Faden-Operation" in pseudo-paralysis of the abduction, in pronounced incomitancies and in nystagmus. This author also advises placing the sutures at least 12 mm behind the original insertion, going sometimes to 15-16 mm. While the procedure has in 80% of his cases an effect on the strabismus angle in the primary position, recession and resection often have to be combined to cure the basic deviation. Its usefulness in cases with a non-accommodative variable angle is stressed by Spielmann (187) and Mühlendyck (144).

7. Other weakening procedures

a. *Supramaximal recessions.* It is generally accepted that the recession of the medial rectus muscle should not be larger than 5 mm. In recent years however, some authors have increased the amount of recession. Helveston et al. (91), Hess and Calhoun (95) did recessions of 6 to 8 mm in large angle esotropia and found weakness of the medial rectus only in a small percentage of cases. In early esotropia with bilateral limitation of abduction, Prieto-Diaz (169) reports excellent results with large bilateral medial rectus recessions of up to 8 mm; adduction and convergence were not significantly affected.

b. *Stretching of eye muscles.* In the technique presented by Huysmans (104), a very strong silk thread is led under the tendon of the rectus internus. After hyaluronidase is injected around the muscle, the latter is stretched for some minutes in a temporal direction by a force of about 300 g. The silk thread is then fixed on a rod of stainless steel which is fixed to the temporal side of the palpebral opening by a plaster-of-Paris bandage. A resection of the lateral rectus is practised at the same time. The thread is removed after five days and the operated eye is in an extremely divergent position. The temporary paresis decreases slowly, orthoptic training is started in the second week and after a few weeks, the eye is in the right position. In convergent squint, nearly 50% of cases are straight with normal correspondence, adequate range of fusion and more or less stereoscopic vision. It seems that this method has not received great popularity. Nevertheless, stay sutures (with bare sclera conjunctival closure) are still of value in difficult cases of strabismus surgery as in generalised fibrosis of the extra-ocular muscles (5).

c. *Botilinum toxin* injection into extra-ocular muscles. Scott (1980, 185) relates excellent results with injection of Botilinum A toxin into an individual extra-ocular muscle. This results in a temporary paralysis. No systemic complications of any kind were encountered.

B. *Interventions on the lateral rectus muscle*

The secondary exodeviations after myotomy of the rectus internus already obliged Dieffenbach (56) to find ways for reinforcement of this severely weakened muscle. The sectioned muscle then had to be localised, freed from all adhesions and, after the eye was rotated maximally inwards by a thread fixed in the temporal region, it was hoped that the muscle would contract a new insertion nearer to the cornea. Besides this "Vorlagerung", suturing of the cut ends of the myotomized muscle was practised as was a displacement of the muscle towards the cornea where it was fixed to the conjunctiva ("Vornähung"); Critchett (1855, 42) got the paternity of this procedure. Afterwards, the terms "Vorlagerung" and "Vornähung" were used indiscriminately to designate all methods by which a muscle was given a new insertion nearer the cornea. Progressively, this technique of advancement was used on the lateral rectus muscle as a primary procedure in convergent squint.

1. Simple advancement

In this procedure, the lateral rectus muscle is freed from its insertion, advanced towards the cornea and fixed with a suture to the conjunctiva, the episclera, the tendon of other eye muscles or finally to the sclera. A multitude of techniques were developed differing in the number of sutures, the way in which they hold the muscle and their anchorage. A much employed procedure was the one described by Meller (140): the disinserted muscle is fixed to the sclera in a similar manner as in the recession of Jameson, but on a place very near to the cornea. Other procedures were the "avancement musculaire" de Lagrange (127) or "l'avancement en Y" de Gonin (1911, 77).

These techniques were designed to obtain an advancement of the muscular insertion; this goal not always seems to have been obtained and some authors think that the portion of the muscle which is in contact with the old insertion contracts an adherence at this site. In this way, only a muscle shortening is obtained whereby the anterior part of the muscle is functionally excluded. At any rate, the correction obtained in this way is not very significant. As moreover this technique leaves a raised, unsightly mass between the original insertion and the limbus, it is likely to become an obsolete operation.

2. Resection

The just described advancement was often combined with the resection of a part of the muscle. In our days, most resections of the rectus externus are done without changing the insertion site.

Resection (myectomy, tenectomy) was first described by Vieusse in 1875; he resected a piece of tendon at 1 mm from the sclera and sutured both ends together. Most techniques used today are derived from those of Reese (1911) and of Blaskovics (26).

3. Tucking of the lateral rectus muscle

This procedure in which a fold is made in the not disinserted muscle goes back to Savage (1893). A very simple technique for shortening a muscle without cutting it was devised by Peter; another, in which the knots are tied externally, was proposed by Lagrange. Recently, an other folding technique was proposed by Küper (1964, 126).

It has to be mentioned that various instruments have been proposed to perform musculotendinous tucking more easily; we mention the tucking apparatus of Wesley Bishop and of Speas. Briggs used a silver ring instead of threads to hold the muscle fold.

A very unique procedure is that of O'Connor (154). In his cinch-procedure, the muscle is divided into four or six strands over an extent of 10 to 12 mm. A special suture is woven around these strands and by stretching it, a fold is realised. Notwithstanding reviews by McCool (1930, 137) and Durr (1937, 60), the cinch operation was nearly forgotten but it has recently been revived by Jampolsky (211) in a modified form as a method of adjustable resection.

A variation of these folding techniques is proposed by Hollwich (99): he proceeds as in resection but instead of cutting the proximal part of the muscle, he simply folds it backwards and sutures it to the muscular body.

The disadvantage of all these techniques is that they do not have a great effect and that they leave a disgracious nodule.

4. Malbran's screwlike twisting

In 1965 Malbran (136) described a technique in which a muscular reinforcement is obtained by twisting the muscle on its axis in a screw-like fashion. The operation consists of cutting and reattaching the muscle to its original insertion after twisting it along its longitudinal axis for one or two turns; one turn gives a shortening of 6 mm, two turns a shortening of 12 mm. A recession is always carried out on the antagonist.

Good results with this technique were reported by Damato (50) who thinks that it should replace muscular resection; negative results however were reported by Staples and Jackson (191). The correction was found to be variable, minimal and not stable; these authors also found fibrosis of the twisted muscle.

C. *Interventions for A and V Phenomena*

Comitant strabismus is by no means always strictly comitant since there is frequently an elevation during adduction. Also, during upward gaze the eyes may be more divergent (or less convergent) than during downward gaze; this is called a V syndrome (V pattern, V phenomenon). If this is combined with esotropia, one speaks of V esotropia. In the opposite picture, the A syndrome (A phenomenon, A pattern or A esotropia if combined with esotropia), the eyes are more convergent in upward gaze than in downward gaze; depression in adduction is often combined (59, 199, 207).

When the difference in divergence, recorded when the eyes look down 25° and then look up 25°, is less than 15^{Δ}, then this difference is considered to be within physiologic limits. Although these vertical incomitancies exist in 25 to 50% of all cases of horizontal strabismus, it was not until the 1950's that they were extensively studied. Different names were used: "horizontal squint with secondary vertical deviations" (Urist, 1951, 198), "vertically incomitant horizontal strabismus" (Knapp, 1959, 119) and finally "A and V syndromes" after a discussion between Jampolsky, Albert and Costenbader (109).

V pattern esotropia, in which the eyes are more convergent in downward than in upward gaze, can be associated with an elevation in adduction (called upshoot or hyperaction of the inferior oblique muscle); but this association does not always exist. In a similar way, A pattern esotropia, in which the eyes are more convergent in upward than in downward gaze, can be associated with a depression in adduction (called hyperaction of the superior oblique muscle).

Numerous explanations have been given for these A and V phenomena: anatomical anomalies, ocular muscle palsies and supranuclear disturbances have been invoked to explain this entity. But in fact, no definitive interpretation of the incomitance has been given (45).

Although the exact cause of A and V patterns is not known, empirical surgical treatments of the ocular muscles have been devised. However, if in primary position, the eyes are straight and more so if fusion exists in downward gaze, great care must be taken not to make the patient worse (148). Concerning the surgical treatment, it must be stated that some surgeons only intervene if there are gross vertical disturbances, whereas others intervene systematically on the oblique muscles even if there is little or no vertical incomitancy (72, 73, 74). But interventions on the horizontal muscles and to a lesser extent on the vertical recti, are also in common use.

1. *Interventions on the horizontal recti*

Costenbader and Albert (1962) expressed the opinion that while the A phenomenon responds well to oblique muscle surgery, the V phenomenon requires only horizontal surgery (40). Urist (1963, 200) also initially preferred a simple bilateral 5 mm medial rectus recession in V pattern esotropia (esotropia of less than 30° in primary position and of at least 16° looking up) and a bilateral 8-10 mm lateral rectus resection in A pattern esotropia (of 10-15° in primary position, eyes straight looking down); he later changed for recession and upward displacement of the medial rectus muscles in A pattern esotropia (1968, 201). If there exists however an elevation in adduction (or overaction of the inferior obliques), then this author recommends recession of the inferior obliques of 8 mm whenever the amount of elevation exceeds 20°. In fact, many authors combine their horizontal muscle surgery with vertical displacement of these horizontal recti or with oblique suturing.

a. Vertical displacement of the horizontal recti

Hugonnier (101, 103) prefers the vertical displacement of the horizontal recti which he associates with the classical surgery for esotropia; he thus often combines recession and vertical displacement of both internal recti for A and V esotropia. He also thinks that overcorrection of the esotropia is more frequent if an A or V pattern is associated. Reinecke (176) also thinks that if an A or V pattern of less than 25^{Δ} is present, pure correction of the horizontal squint will usually correct the A or V pattern; as already mentioned, Urist (1968, 201) advises in A pattern the recession of one or both medial recti with upward displacement of their insertion for 5 mm. In V esotropia, together with the recession of the recti interni, the new insertion is displaced downward, 5 to 6 mm (21, 101). Goldstein (75) even tries to correct the A and V patterns by doing monocular surgery: in recession the insertion is moved in the direction in which the maximum weakening effect is desired, in resection it is moved in the opposite direction.

b. Oblique displacement of the horizontal recti

Although this technique was already proposed by Bietti (25), it is more generally known as Lavat's procedure (131). For V esotropia during recession, the inferior point is recessed more than the superior point. Initially, the difference between the two points was 2-3 mm, later it became 5 mm. This technique however can only be used in cases of A and V without clear indication of a perturbance of the oblique muscles (55).

2. *Interventions on the vertical recti*

Miller (1960, 142) displaced the insertion of the vertical recti. In V esotropia with only slight overaction of the inferior oblique he demonstrated that lateral transplantation of the inferior rectus augments abduction in downward gaze. Von Noorden (1963, 147) also saw good results with this technique.

3. *Interventions on the oblique muscles*

If there are signs of malfunctioning obliques in A and V syndromes, then the treatment has to be directed against these oblique muscles (94). For the inferior oblique this means generally a weakening procedure to counteract the overelevation of the adducting eye although no one has ever demonstrated any change in the inferior oblique (which never appears as a tight or contracted muscle). Dieffenbach (56) already described the myotomy of the inferior oblique near its scleral insertion. Procedures near the scleral insertion are much more in general use than procedures near the orbital origin although Landolt (128) already advised the section near the orbital insertion in 1885 and although good results were reported by Stuart (195) after excision of 3-5 mm of muscle and sheath near its origin. But ocular surgeons are still devided on what to do after the muscle is cut near its scleral attachment (which is close to the macula, to the optic nerve and in the vicinity of a vortex vein).

Finck (63) pioneered the recession technique. After section of the muscle close to its insertion, the anterior point of the new insertion line (in a 8 mm recession) is found by using Finck's localiser; this point is situated beneath and behind the inferior point of the insertion of the lateral rectus muscle; a posterior suture is placed at a point 6 mm posterior to the anterior point. Apt and Call (4) prefer to use the inferior rectus muscle as a landmark for the recession of the inferior oblique; they prefer to start the reinsertion at a point 4 mm posterior and 4 mm superior to the lateral insertion of the inferior rectus muscle.

For Parks (156), the three most frequent complications in inferior oblique muscle weakening procedures are: 1. inadvertently dividing only a portion of the entire muscle; 2. inadvertently cutting the lateral or inferior rectus muscle; 3. producing an adherence syndrome manifest by hypotropia and restricted elevation in the operated eye. His personal preference goes to the recession procedure, the action of which he has compared to the one obtained by free disinsertion, by myectomy at the origin and by myectomy of the terminal 8 mm (1972, 155).

Gobin (66, 71, 73) uses either a posterior tenotomy, an anteroposition or a disinsertion according to the importance of the deviation. In anteroposition, the new insertion site is not measured; it is situated at the equator midway between the insertion of the lateral and the inferior rectus muscles. Only the anterior part of the muscle is sutured. A similar recession technique is proposed by Gillies (65).

In 1962, Dyer (61) redirected attention to a simple procedure for the correction of overaction of the inferior oblique muscle: the tenotomy at its scleral insertion. After a horizontal incision is made through the conjunctiva and Tenon's capsule in the lower temporal region of the globe, the muscle is severed flush with the sclera along its entire attachment using Stevens scissors. This procedure gives excellent results and does not lead to complete paralysis as Lockwood's ligament, the muscle sheath and other membranous attachments remain intact; this allows the muscle to reattach to the sclera. Cooper (38) also prefers free myotomy to recession. Costenbader and Kertesz (41) are also in favor of tenotomy or disinsertion (section flush with the sclera, freeing any adherences to the lateral rectus and the optic nerve sheath); they find it as effective as myectomy (in which the belly of the muscle and its sheath are completely transected near the insertion) and as recession. Von Noorden (153) prefers a myectomy of approximately 8 mm in its temporal course; so do McNear, Scott and Jampolsky (139): they advise cauterisation of the clamped ends of the muscle.

Partial or marginal myotomy is also used: several cuts are made through the sheath and halfway through the muscle on both sides and at different levels (Brown, 33); the cuts can also be made by cautery (De Decker, 51).

A lengthening procedure was proposed by Corcelle: the muscle is divided in its longitudinal direction, the two halves are sectioned at different places and sutured together (36, 157).

It is obvious that actually most ocular surgeons are in favor of a weakening procedure on the inferior oblique muscle for the V phenomenon with elevation in adduction. In 1962 however, Sevrin (186) preferred a tucking procedure on the superior oblique. Strengthening operations on the superior oblique muscle were also favored by Haase (84) and by Krzystkowa (123). Deller (1968, 53) to the contrary did not have good results with strengthening of the superior oblique in V-esotropia.

The same Sevrin favored a resection and advancement of the inferior obliques in the A phenomenon. However in cases of A phenomenon with "down-shoot" in adduction, most authors prefer a weakening procedure on the superior oblique muscles (37).

Berke introduced the intrasheath tenotomy (23). In this procedure, the superior oblique is exposed on the medial side of the superior rectus. The tendon is peeled out of its sheath and simply sectioned (90) or a tenectomy of up to 9 mm is done (17). Urist (202) saw the development of a V pattern deviation after a bilateral 5 mm intrasheath tenectomy. For Fink (63), the most efficient procedure aimed at weakening an overactive superior oblique muscle is tenotomy of its reflected tendon. His technique is similar to that advocated by Berke.

Gobin (69, 70) first did disinsertions of the superior oblique in A pattern esotropia, combined with a 5 mm recession of both medial recti (eventually augmented by a loop). He abandoned this complete section of the tendon at its insertion because he saw too great a percentage of A becoming V and of pareses of the superior obliques. He later changed for a posterior tenotomy of the superior oblique muscle where only the posterior part of the tendon is cut at its scleral insertion and where the anterior point of the insertion is left in place. Prieto-Dias (168) also favors this posterior tenectomy. In some cases, Gobin (73) will do a complete disinsertion of the superior oblique but will keep it attached to the anterior point of the previous insertion with a 3 mm loop.

D. *Combined surgical procedures*

Success in strabismus depends more on accurate diagnosis and choice of the proper operation than on surgical techniques. Nevertheless, superior surgical technique helps in obtaining good results.

While it is seldom indicated in convergent comitant strabismus to operate on only one muscle, it is not easy to give strict indications on what to do in each particular case. We illustrate this with a statement of Urist (200): "The problem on which muscles to operate and how much to do in cases of strabismus has been a difficult one, even for the experienced surgeon with a large motility practice. For the beginner in ophthalmology, for the occasional muscle surgeon and for the expert surgeon who wants to learn from the experiences of others, the literature has been of little help. This is because, while general principles of muscle surgery are widely disseminated, detailed information concerning on which muscles to operate and the amounts in mm of muscle to move or remove is usually not given".

It would be out of the scope of this chapter to go into a detailed description of what to do in each particular situation. We personally favor bimedial recessions of 5 mm or bilateral loops of 5 to 8 mm. We also favor unilateral recession of 5 mm combined with a resection of

8 mm of the rectus externus. We do not systematically combine this operation with an intervention on the oblique muscles as does Gobin; Gobin's system of surgical treatment is found in chapter IX. For other surgical systems we refer to the literature on this subject (3, 7, 83, 90, 92, 101, 114, 118, 133, 151, 153, 162, 188, 212).

III. *Non-surgical procedures*

This aspect of strabismus treatment will only summarily be treated here, as it is extensively developed in chapter VIII and as there has not been much evolution since the beginning of these forms of treatment and the actual situation.

A. *Optical corrections*

1. Positive glasses

In 1845 Böhm (27) wrote a book on strabismus in which it is stated that "to ameliorate the vision of distant objects, convex glasses have to be given to the squinting eye". Although at the time of that publication, it was known that the majority of patients with convergent squint have hyperopia, it is Donders who merits the honor of having popularized the relationship between esotropia and hyperopia. He wrote (57): "Strabismus convergens almost always depends upon hypermetropia... It occurs in about 77% of the cases (?)... Since in strabismus convergens hypermetropia in general exists, no other connection is conceivable than that hypermetropia is the cause of the deviation. Hypermetropia is, indeed, the primary anomaly... Strabismus is the secondary condition which does not arise until some years after birth". Donders stated that in intermittent cases the development of strabismus may be prevented by wearing convex glasses and that in confirmed cases the operation of tenotomy may be performed. But "where the patient preferred obviating the strabismus by wearing spectacles, I willingly consented to it and almost invariably the object was thus attained".

Since this time, it has become a classical procedure to prescribe convex glasses in convergent squint. "It is evident", writes Duke-Elder (58) "that as soon as the squint appears in a young child, spectacles become a therapeutic necessity no matter what the age. The child should be atropinized... and initially the fullest possible correction should be worn constantly... But in all cases when the spectacles do not completely abolish the deviation and allow binocular vision, they will never be curative; other more effective methods of treatment must be adopted and the sooner these are embarked upon the better". For more detailed information on optical treatment, we refer to chapter VIII. But it must be said that, while most authors find convex glasses an absolute necessity in convergent strabismus, others, as Gobin (see chapter IX) have a different opinion and do not use them at all. For others, as Urist (200), "the wearing of glasses should be temporarily to encourage binocular vision and should be discarded as soon as possible, just as with a splint in a fracture". This discarding can be done after progressively reducing their strength.

2. Bifocals

The first model of bifocals was suggested by Benjamin Franklin about 1775 and consisted merely of two separate segments, held together is a frame (the split or two piece bifocal). But it is the modern one-piece version of Franklin's bifocals, called the executive bifocal that is still preferred in strabismus treatment.

Bifocals emerge as a powerful and effective tool in the management of esotropia with a high AC/A ratio (convergence excess). But they are useless if they only diminish the angle for near; they have to suppress it completely (34, 184). Bifocals also have to be used as a temporary treatment; it is often mentioned that an attempt should be made to wean the patient from the bifocal segment at the age of 10 years. But it is only in 1/3 of the cases that healing can be obtained and the bifocal segment eliminated (152).

3. Prisms

On January 31, 1853, A. von Graefe held a lecture in Berlin on the use of prisms in cases of diplopia and of strabismus; he considered them of great value in the ocular "orthopedics". He mentioned that it was a Dutch scientist, F. W. C. Krecke, who was the first to have published a case healed by this method (121). The thickness and the weight of the prisms used at that time made that Javal (113) saw only a limited use for them: he used them for correction of deviations not greater than 12° and on the condition that fusion exists. He also used them occasionally for the correction of an imperfect surgical result.

While prisms are thus used to maintain single binocular vision in the presence of a deviation, following Sattler (182, 183) they are also used to modify an abnormal sensory state such as anomalous retinal correspondence or eccentric fixation. Since the application of the principles formulated by Fresnel more than 150 years ago has permitted the realisation of prisms much thinner and lighter than the ones formerly used, a renewed interest in prismotherapy has taken place (12, 18, 82, 93). Pigassou (161, 163, 164) is a great proponent of their use as a permanent treatment in free space; she applies either the exact prismatic correction or, more often, a temporary overcorrection.

Prisms are also used: 1. as a preoperative measure (158) which often leads to an increase of the deviation (9) but can enforce bifoveal stimulation before operation (18); 2. for correction or overcorrection of a residual angle of esotropia after surgery (11) or treatment of a subsisting convergence excess (14); 3. in decompensated heterophorias (19).

B. *Other procedures*

1. Orthoptics

Although in the broader sense, all non-surgical treatment is considered orthoptic treatment, in the narrower sense it is the treatment employed to combat suppression, amblyopia and anomalous retinal correspondence and to enhance the development of fusional amplitudes and improvement of stereopsis (153). Orthoptics are thus aimed at achieving normal fusion, or as Pigassou states (163): "In orthoptics binocular single vision is solicited and bifoveal stimulation is even provoked (flash or massage) by means of a device such as the "amblyoscope". The sessions last from 20 to 30 minutes and take place two or three times a week over a period of 2 to 6 months... This method leads to binocular single vision only in cases with underlying normal retinal correspondence, that is to say, in about 30% of cases".

The possibilities of orthoptic treatment are clearly outlined by Duke-Elder (58): "The development of the binocular reflexes concerned with the establishment of fusion is a process which takes place naturally in the early formative period of life and there is no evidence that it can be acquired in later years when neural habits have become fixed. If however fusion is present or potentially present, even if it is of an anomalous type, it is possible to strengthen and consolidate it by various forms of orthoptic measures... Now that the popular impression that orthoptics is a procedure designed to exercise the extrinsic muscles of the eye and so to correct an ocular deviation has been completely abandoned and now that it is used for its proper purposes, i.e. to awaken a dormant or stimulate a weakened capacity of fusion and stereopis, the technique has assumed its proper place as a valuable adjuvant to other methods of treatment". From the foregoing it is clear that in convergent comitant strabismus, orthoptics are essentially useful in the late normosensorial forms.

First suggested by du Bois-Reymond (1852) and Mackenzie (1854), this form of treatment has been elaborated into an established technique by Javal who used a mirror-stereoscope derived from the stereoscope of Wheatstone (1833). Successive modifications have led to the actually used amblyoscope (86, 190).

For details of orthoptic treatment we refer to the literature on this subject (8, 31, 35, 78, 134, 177) not without mentioning that orthoptic treatment has known periods of high popularity and of neglect. The uncertainty regarding orthoptic treatment has remained until now and there still exist, as Crone remarked (44) "on the one hand the youthful enthusiasts and perfectionists and on the other the distrustful pragmatists". We fully agree with von Noorden that "a comprehensive, well-designed collaborative study of the various forms and methods is urgently needed to definitively determine the value of such training and to define specifically the type of patients who may benefit from it" (153).

2. Penalisation

While penalisation is essentially a method against amblyopia (170)—and for some only a modified form of occlusion—it also has an effect on the angle of squint and on the retinal correspondence (10); hence its use in alternating strabismus, especially in its early stages as it prevents the constitution of abnormal correspondence. The principle consists of utilising the dominant eye for distance vision (giving it the exact correction and atropine), the amblyopic eye for near vision (giving it a hypercorrection of + 1 d.).

Besides the penalisation for near of Pouliquen (167), other modalities are in use (171): penalisation for distance (atropine and overcorrection for the dominant eye, exact correction for the amblyopic one); complete penalisation (dominant eye made useless for distance and near), alternating, selective and mild penalisation.

The French naturalist Buffon is considered to be the inventor of the method; in the 18th century he already advised to diminish the function of the best eye by giving it a positive glass. Donders, for the same reason, recommended the use of atropine. Pfandl in 1958 (159) revived this procedure after observing cases of convergent strabismus in which one eye was myopic, the other emmetropic (thus creating an alternation which prevented amblyopia and conserved normal retinal correspondence); Pouliquen (166) popularised it recently.

3. Miotics

After the calabar-bean became known in Europe in 1840 and after the plant which produced the bean had been identified and christened Physostigma venenosum in 1846, it was not until 1863 that the miotic effect of its extract was described by Fraser (132). The active alkaloid was isolated in 1864 and called physostigmine; it was called eserine by others. These extracts were introduced in the treatment of glaucoma in 1876. Pilocarpine, extracted from an other plant (Pilocarpus jaborandi) became known in 1875 and was introduced for glaucoma treatment in 1876 (213); another miotic, arecoline, was isolated in 1888. Synthetic miotics followed: neostigmin in 1929, metacholine in 1931, carbachol in 1932, isofluorphate (DFP) in 1946, demecarium bromide (Humorsol) in 1959 and echothiophate (Phospholine Iodide) in 1959.

The use of eserine and pilocarpine in strabismus treatment was well known to Javal who wrote in 1896: "... in observation no. 302, I had obtained a temporary alignment by use of eserine... Pilocarpine also was several times of great use to me. Contrary to atropine, the action of eserine and of pilocarpine (which is preferable) can be explained by the unvoluntary augmentation of accommodation; thanks to this, the subject no longer needs to converge to see clearly..." (pag. 81).

This treatment was reintroduced in 1949 by Abraham (1), especially for convergent strabismus of the intermittent type and for high AC/A ratio (convergence excess (2, 32, 143)). Miotics are also used for diagnostic purposes, to distinguish accommodative from non-accommodative esotropia (6). Actually, the parasympathomimetics (pilocarpine, carbachol (210)) are not in great favor; the anti-cholinesterases drugs Echothiophate (Phospholine) Iodide (165) and Isofluorophate (DFP) (135, 209) seem to be preferred.

BIBLIOGRAPHY

(1) ABRAHAM, S.V. — The use of miotics in the treatment of convergent strabismus and anisometropia. *Amer. J. Ophthalmol.*, 1949, *32*, 233-240.

(2) ABRAHAM, S.V. — Present status of miotic therapy in nonparalytic convergent strabismus. *Amer. J. Ophthalmol.*, 1961, *51*, 1249-1255.

(3) ADELSTEIN, F.E., CÜPPERS, C. — Probleme der operativen Schielbehandlung. Ber. dtsch. ophthal. Ges. 1968. München, Verlag J.F. Bergmann, 1969 (580-593).

(4) APT, L., CALL, N.B. — Inferior oblique muscle recession. *Amer. J. Ophthalmol.*, 1978, *85*, 95-100.
(5) APT, L., AXELROD, R.N. — Generalised fibrosis of the extraocular muscles. *Amer. J. Ophthalmol.*, 1978, *85*, 822-829.
(6) ARDOUIN, M., CATROS, A., FEUVRIER, Y.-M., URVOY, M., DAULEUX, M.L. — L'iodure de phospholine dans le traitement des ésotropies. *Bull. Soc. Opht. Fr.*, 1966, *66*, 74-89.
(7) ARRUGA, H. — Ocular Surgery. 1953, New York, Toronto, London, McGraw-Hill Book Co, Inc.
(8) AUST, W. — Pleoptik und Orthoptik. Basel, New York, Verlag S. Karger, 1966.
(9) AUST, W., WELGE-LÜSSEN, L. — Prä- und postoperative Schielwinkeländerungen nach längerem präoperativem prismatischen Schielwinkelausgleich. *Klin. Mbl. Augenheilk.*, 1969, *155*, 494-503.
(10) AUST, W., ROESEN, K. — Der Einflusz der Totalokklusion auf Schielwinkel und anomale Netzhautkorrespondenz bei Alternansschielern. *Klin. Mbl. Augenheilk.*, 1974, *165*, 180-184.
(11) BAGOLINI, B. — Postsurgical treatment of convergent strabismus, with a critical evaluation of various tests. *Int. Ophthalmol. Clin.*, 1966, *6*, 633-642.
(12) BAGOLINI, B. — Sensory anomalies in strabismus. *Brit. J. Ophthalmol.*, 1974, *58*, 313-318.
(13) BAMERT, W. — Erfahrungen mit den Sehnenverlängerung nach Kuhnt-Bangerter. *Ophthalmologica*, 1956, *131*, 257-261.
(14) BARANOWSKA-GEORGE, T. — Hypercorrection prismatique dans le traitement du symptôme de surconvergence paraissant dans les strabismes convergents. *Arch. Opht. (Paris)*, 1968, *28*, 745-750.
(15) BAUM, J.L., MISHIMA, S., BORUCHOFF, S.A. — On the nature of dellen. *Arch. Ophthalmol.*, 1968, *79*, 657-662.
(16) BEDROSSIAN, E.H. — Hypopion keratitis following muscle surgery. *Amer. J. Ophthalmol.*, 1966, *61*, 1530-1532.
(17) BEDROSSIAN, E.H. — Bilateral superior oblique tenectomy for the A-pattern in strabismus. *Arch. Ophthalmol.*, 1967, *78*, 334-336.
(18) BÉRARD, P.V., PADOVANI, J. — Les prismes. Leur utilisation thérapeutique dans les strabismes concomitants. *Ann. Oculist.*, 1967, *200*, 1142-1155.
(19) BÉRARD, P.V., NOAT-BERGAZZY, J. — Les prismes: leur utilisation thérapeutique dans les hétérophories. *Arch. Opht. (Paris)*, 1968, *28*, 641-656.
(20) BÉRARD, P.V. — V-ésotropie et chirurgie des muscles horizontaux. *Bull. Soc. Ophtal. Fr.*, 1968, *68*, 368-373.
(21) BÉRARD, P.V., JEAN, M., DELANGLADE, O. — La valeur relative du recul oblique et de l'abaissement de l'insertion des muscles droits internes dans la chirurgie des V-ésotropies. *Bull. Soc. Opht. Fr.*, 1976, *76*, 581-586.
(22) BERG, F. — The Chevalier Taylor and his strabismus operation. *Brit. J. Ophthalmol.*, 1967, *51*, 667-673.
(23) BERKE, R.N. — Tenotomy of the superior oblique muscle for hypertropia. *Trans. Amer. Ophthal. Soc.*, 1946, *44*, 304-342.
(24) BIELSCHOWSKY, A. — Die neueren Anschauungen über Wesen und Behandlung des Schielens. Beihefte zur Med. Klinik, 1907, 12.
(25) BIETTI, B.B. — Su un accorgimento tecnico (recessione e reinserzione obliqua a ventaglio dei muscoli retti orizzontali) per la correzione di atteggiamenti a V o A di grado modesto negli strabismi concomitanti. *Boll. Ocul.*, 1970, *49*, 581-588.
(26) BLASKOVICS, L. von, KREIKER, A. — Eingriffe am Auge. Stuttgart, F. Enke, 1943.
(27) BÖHM, L. — Das Schielen. Berlin, Duncker und Humbolt, 1845.
(28) BORDEIANU, C.D. — La ténoplastie par clivage scléral marginal. *J. Fr. Ophtalmol.*, 1980, *3*, 671-674.
(29) BOULAD, L., CREHANGE, J., DELLER, M., HOROVITZ, G., LASSER-VIDAL, C., LAULAN, J., MAWAS, J. RICHON, J., SCHILOVITZ, G., WEISS, J.B. — Opération du strabisme avec anses. *J. Français d'Orthoptique*, 1980, *12*, 101-107.
(30) BOURGERY, J.M. — Iconographie d'Anatomie chirurgicale et de médecine opératoire. Paris, Ed. C.A. Delaunay, 1837 et suiv.

(31) BREDEMEYER, H.G., BULLOCK, K. — Orthoptics (Theory and Practice). St. Louis, The C.V. Mosby Company, 1968.
(32) BREININ, G.M., CHIN, N.B., RIPPS, H. — A rationale for therapy of accommodative strabismus. *Amer. J. Ophthalmol.*, 1966, *61*, 1030-1037.
(33) BROWN, H.W. — Surgery on the oblique muscles. In: Allen, J.H. Ed.: Strabismus. Ophthalmic Symposium II (p. 428-452). St. Louis, The C.V. Mosby Company, 1958.
(34) BURIAN, H.M. — Use of bifocal spectacles in the treatment of accommodative esotropia. *Brit. Orthopt. J.*, 1956, *13*, 3-6.
(35) CASHELL, G.T.W., DURRAN, I.M. — Handbook of orthoptic principles. Edinburgh and London, E. & S. Livingstone Ltd., 1967.
(36) CAZENAVE, P. — Contribution à l'étude du traitement chirurgical de l'hyperaction de l'oblique inférieur. Allongement du petit oblique. Bordeaux, Impr. Gaudy et Fils, 1964.
(37) CLERGEAU, G. — La chirurgie du grand oblique. Indications et techniques. *Ann. Oculist.*, 1977, *210* (supplément au n° 4), 3-60.
(38) COOPER, E.L. — Recession versus free myotomy at the insertion of the inferior oblique muscle. *J. Ped. Ophthalmol.*, 1969, *6*, 6-10.
(39) COSTENBADER, F.D. — Clinical course and management of esotropia. In: Allen, J.H.: Strabismus Ophthalmic Symposium II (p. 325-353). St. Louis, The C.V. Mosby Company, 1958.
(40) COSTENBADER, F.D., ALBERT, D.G. — Surgery of Strabismus. *International Ophthalmology Clinics*, 1962, *2*, 815-1042. Boston, Little, Brown and Co, 1962.
(41) COSTENBADER, F.D., KERTESZ, E. — Relaxing procedures of the inferior oblique. A comparative study. *Amer. J. Ophthalmol.*, 1964, *57*, 276-280.
(42) CRITCHETT, A, — Practical remarks on strabismus with some novel suggestion respecting the operation. *Lancet*, 1855, *1*, 479-507.
(43) CRONE, R.A. — Scheelzien. Openbare les. Amsterdam, N.V. Swets en Zeitlinger, 1964.
(44) CRONE, R.A., VAN DEN BOSCH, J.G. — The sweet and bitter fruits of orthoptic exercise. In: Perspectives in Ophthalmology II (p. 172-178). Amsterdam, Excerpta Medica, 1970.
(45) CRONE, R.A. — Diplopia. Excerpta Medica, Amsterdam & American Elsevier Publ. Cy., Inc., New York, 1973.
(46) CRONE, R.A. — Anomale Korrespondenz und anomales Binokularsehen. In: Remky, H.: Aktuelle Ophthalmologische Probleme; Bücherei des Augenarztes, 72 (p. 49-62). Stuttgart, Ferd. Enke Verlag, 1978.
(47) CÜPPERS, C. — The so called Fadenoperation (surgical corrections by well-defined changes of the arc of contact). The second Congress of the International Strabismological Association (p. 395-400). Paris, Marseille, Diffusion Générale de Librairie, 1976.
(48) CÜPPERS, C., THOMAS, C. — «L'opération du fil» sur un œil pour le traitement du ptosis de l'autre œil par la provocation d'une impulsion d'élévation sur cet autre œil. *Bull. Mém. Soc. Fr. Ophthal.*, 1975, *87*, 318-328.
(49) CÜPPERS, C. — Historique et Physiopathologie des blocages. *J. Français d'Orthoptique*, 1978, *10*, 15-26.
(50) DAMATO, F.J. — Muscular reinforcement in strabismus (screwlike twisting of a rectus muscle). *The Eye, Ear, Nose and Throat Monthly*, 1968, *47*, 92-93.
(51) DE DECKER, W., KÜPER, J. — Obliquus-inferior-Schwächung durch marginale Myotomie (Thermoschwächung). *Klin. Mbl. Augenheilk.*, 1971, *159*, 183-
(52) DE DECKER, W., CONRAD, H.G. — Fadenoperation nach Cüppers bei komplizierten Augenmuskelstörungen und nichtakkommodativem Konvergenzexcesz. *Klin. Mbl. Augenheilk.*, 1975, *167*, 217-226.
(53) DELLER, M., SEDDIK, N., BRACK, B. — Le renforcement des obliques supérieurs dans les ésotropies obliques en V. *Bull. Mém. Soc. Fr. Ophtalm.*, 1968, *81*, 464-471.
(54) DELLER, M. — L'opération du fil. *Bull. Mém. Soc. Fr. Ophtal.*, 1976, *88*, 167-172.
(55) DELLER, M. — La place des reculs obliques des droits horizontaux dans la chirurgie des syndromes A et V. *J. Fr. Ophtalmol.*, 1981, *4*, 75-80.

(56) DIEFFENBACH, J.F. — Ueber das Schielen und die Heilung desselben durch die Operation. Berlin, Albert Förstner, 1842.
(57) DONDERS, F.C. — On the anomalies of accommodation and refraction of the eye. London, The New Sydenham Society, 1864.
(58) DUKE-ELDER, S., WYBAR, K. — Ocular motility and strabismus. In: System of Ophthalmology. Vol. VI. London, Henry Kimpton, 1973.
(59) DUNLAP, E.A.: Present status of the A and V syndromes. *Amer. J. Ophthalmol.*, 1961, *52*, 396-401.
(60) DURR, S.A. — The O'Connor cinch-operation technique. *Amer. J. Ophthalmol.*, 1937, *20*, 178-180.
(61) DYER, J.A. — Tenotomy of the inferior oblique at its scleral insertion. *Arch. Ophthalmol.*, 1962, *68*, 176-181.
(62) DYER, J.A. — Atlas of extraocular muscle surgery. Philadelphia, London, Toronto, W.B. Saunders Company, 1970.
(63) FINK, W.H. — Surgery of the vertical muscles of the eye. Springfield, Charles C. Thomas Publisher, 2° Ed., 1961.
(64) FOCOSI, M., RUZZI, P. — Su di una nuova tenica d'indebolimento muscolare mediante l'innesto tendino. *Boll. Oculist.*, 1978, *57*, 3-12.
(65) GILLIES, W.E. — Simple technique for recession of the inferior oblique muscle. *Brit. J. Ophthalmol.*, 1970, *54*, 736-739.
(66) GOBIN, M.H. — Anteroposition of the inferior oblique muscle in V-esotropia. *Ophthalmologica*, 1964, *148*, 325-341.
(67) GOBIN, M.H. — Cyclotropia and squint. Antwerpen, Krol & Courtin, 1969.
(68) GOBIN, M.H. — Récession avec anse du droit interne. *Bull. Soc. belge d'Ophtalmol.*, 1975, *171*, 789-795.
(69) GOBIN, M.H. — Desinsertion of the superior oblique in A-patterns. *Doc. Ophthal.*, 1977, *44*, 1, 193-202.
(70) GOBIN, M.H. — Ténotomie postérieure du grand oblique dans les syndromes en A. *Bull. Soc. belge Ophtal.*, 1978, *182*, 104-113.
(71) GOBIN, M.H. — Indications for surgery of the A and V Phenomena. *Brit. J. Ophthalmol.*, 1979, *36*, 45-56.
(72) GOBIN, M.H. — Nouvelles conceptions sur la pathogénie et le traitement du strabisme. I. Pathogénie du strabisme. *J. Fr. Ophtalmol.*, 1980, *3*, 541-556.
(73) GOBIN, M.H. — Nouvelles conceptions sur la pathogénie et le traitement du strabisme. II. Traitement du strabisme. Introduction. Chirurgie primaire. Chirurgie secondaire. *J. Fr. Ophtalmol.*, 1981, *4*, 7-18.
(74) GOBIN, M.H. — Nouvelles conceptions sur la pathogénie et le traitement du strabisme. III. Traitement du strabisme. Introduction. Complications. Conclusion. *J. Fr. Ophtalmol.*, 1981, *4*, 297-305.
(75) GOLDSTEIN, J.H. — Monocular vertical displacement of the horizontal rectus muscles in the A and V patterns. *Amer. J. Ophthalmol.*, 1967, *64*, 265-267.
(76) GOMEZ MORALES, A., POLACK, F.M., FERRER ARATA, A. — Silicone implant to extra-ocular muscles. *Brit. J. Ophthalmol.*, 1966, *50*, 235-244.
(77) GONIN, J. — Des procédés aptes à remplacer la ténotomie dans l'opération du strabisme. *Ann. Oculist.*, 1911, *146*, 340-350.
(78) GÖRTZ, H. — Binokularschulung — Orthoptik. In: Hollwich, F.: Schielen (Pleoptik, Orthoptik, Operation). Bücherei des Augenarztes, 38 (p. 116-134). Stuttgart, Ferd. Enke Verlag, 1961.
(79) GOTTLIEB, F., CASTRO, J.L. — Perforation of the globe during strabismus surgery. *Arch. Ophthalmol.*, 1970, *84*, 151-157.
(80) GRAEFE, A. von — Beiträge zur Lehre vom Schielen und von der Schieloperation. *Archiv für Ophthalmologie*, 1857, *3/1*, 177-386.
(81) GRAEFE, A. von — Symptomenlehre der Augenmuskellähmungen. Peters, Berlin, 1867.
(82) GUIBOR, G.P. — Some uses of ophthalmic prisms. In: Allen, J.H.: Strabismus Ophthalmic Symposium II. St. Louis, The C.V. Mosby Company, 1958 (p. 244-260).
(83) GUILLAUMAT, L., PAUFIQUE, L. DE SAINT-MARTIN, R., SCHIFF-WERTHEIMER, S., SOURDILLE, G. — Traitement chirurgical des affections oculaires.

Tome III: Traitement chirurgical des strabismes et des paralysies oculaires (p. 7-93). Paris, Ed. G. Doin & Cie, 1961.
(84) HAASE, W. — Zur operativen Behandlung horizontaler Inkomitanz im Rahmen des frühkindlichen Strabismus. (A-Syndrom). *Klin. Mbl. Augenheilk.*, 1972, *160*, 648-662.
(85) HASS, H.D. — Rücklagerung mit Fixationsnähten beim Strabismus concomitans convergens. *Klin. Mbl. Augenheilk.*, 1965, *146*, 44-50.
(86) HAUGWITZ, T. — Ophthalmologische optische Untersuchungsgeräte. Bücherei des Augenarztes, 85, Stuttgart, Ferd. Enke Verlag, 1981.
(87) HAVENER, W.H., KIMBALL, O.P. — Scleral perforation during strabismus surgery. *Amer. J. Ophthalmol.*, 1960, *50*, 807-808.
(88) HAVENER, W.H., ZEPP, C.E. — Prevention of scleral perforation during muscle recession. *Amer. J. Ophthalmol.*, 1965, *60*, 535-536.
(89) HELVESTON, E.M., COFIELD, D.M. — Indications for marginal myotomy and technique. *Amer. J. Ophthalmol.*, 1970, *70*, 574-578.
(90) HELVESTON, E.M. — Atlas of strabismus surgery. Saint Louis, The C.V. Mosby Company, 1973.
(91) HELVESTON, E.M., ELLIS, F.D., PATTERSON, J.H. — Augmented recession of the medial recti. *Trans. Amer. Acad. Ophthalmol.*, 1978, *85*, 507-511.
(92) HERVOUËT, F. — Atlas pratique de la chirurgie du strabisme. Paris, Ed. Masson et Cie, 1970.
(93) HERZAU, V. — Beobachtungen bei der Prismenbehandlung des frühkindlichen Strabismus convergens. *Klin. Mbl. Augenheilk.*, 1974, *165*, 724-732.
(94) HERZAU, V., KNEBL, U. — Über Schieloperationen beim A- und V-Phänomen. *Klin. Mbl. Augenheilk.*, 1978, *173*, 675-680.
(95) HESS, J.B., CALHOUN, J.H. — A new rationale for the management of large angle esotropia. *J. Pediatr. Ophthalmol. Strabismus*, 1979, *16*, 345-348.
(96) HIRSCHBERG, J. — Geschichte der Augenheilkunde. In: Graefe-Saemisch Handbuch der gesamten Augenheilkunde, 2° Aufl. Bd XII-XV. Engelmann und Springer, Leipzig-Berlin, 1899-1918.
(97) HITTNER, H.M. — Lens dislocation after strabismus surgery. *Ann. Ophthalmol.*, 1979, *11*, 1115-1119.
(98) HOLLWICH, F. — Die Sehnenverlängerung nach Gonin. *Ophthalmologica*, 1961, *142*, 412-417.
(99) HOLLWICH, F. — Die chirurgische Behandlung des Horizontalschielens. In: Hollwich, F.: Schielen (Pleoptik, Orthoptik, Operation). Bücherei des Augenarztes, 38 (p. 135-167). Stuttgart, Ferd. Enke Verlag, 1961.
(100) HOLLWICH, F., KREBS, W. — Erfahrungen mit der Sehnenverlängerung nach Gonin. *Klin. Mbl. Augenheilk*, 1965, *147*, 480-487.
(101) HUGONNIER, R., HUGONNIER, S. — Strabismes. Hétérophories. Paralysies oculo-motrices. Paris, Ed. Masson et Cie, 1965.
(102) HUGONNIER, R. — L'opération du fil: opération facile ou difficile? *J. Fr. Ophtalmol.*, 1978, *1*, 671-673.
(103) HUGONNIER, R. — Les syndromes alphabétiques (leur influence sur la surcorrection opératoire des ésotropies). In: Année Thérapeutique et Clinique en Ophtalmologie, Vol XXXI, p. 183-188. Marseille, Diffusion Générale de Librairie, 1981.
(104) HUYSMANS, J. — Stretching of eye muscles. Technique and results. In: Perspectives in Ophthalmology, Vol. II (p. 179-183). Amsterdam, Excerpta Medica, 1970.
(105) JAENSCH, P.A.: — Die Entwicklung der Diagnose und der Therapie beim Strabismus. In: Hollwich, F.: Schielen (Pleoptik, Orthoptik, Operation). Bücherei des Augenartztes, 38, p. 168-176. Stuttgart, Ferd. Enke Verlag, 1961.
(106) JAMESON, P.C. — Correction of squint by muscle recession with scleral suturing. *Arch. Ophthalmol.*, 1922, *51*, 421-430.
(107) JAMESON, P.C. — The surgical entity of muscle recession. *Arch. Ophthalmol.*, 1931, *6*, 329-361.
(108) JAMESON, P.C. — Some essentials and securities which stabilize operations on ocular muscles. *Arch. Ophthalmol.*, 1932, *8*, 654-669.
(109) JAMPOLSKY, A. — Bilateral anomalies of the oblique muscles. *Trans. Amer. Acad. Ophthal. Otolaryng.*, 1957, *61*, 689-700.

(110) JAMPOLSKY, A. — The A and V syndromes. In: Strabismus; Symposium of the New Orleans Academy of Ophthalmology, St. Louis, The C.V. Mosby Co, 1962.
(111) JAMPOLSKY, A. — Strabismus reoperation techniques. *Trans. Amer. Acad. Ophthalmol. Otolaryngol.*, 1975, *79*, 704-717.
(112) JAMPOLSKY, A. — Current techniques of adjustable strabismus surgery. *Amer. J. Ophthalmol.*, 1979, *88*, 406-418.
(113) JAVAL, E. — Manuel théorique et pratique du strabisme. Paris, G. Masson Ed., 1896.
(114) KAUFMANN, H., SOHLENKAMP, R., HARTWIG, H. — Ergebnisse der operativen Behandlung bei Strabismus convergens. *Klin. Mbl. Augenheilk.*, 1975, *167*, 237-244.
(115) KENNEDY, J.A. — Marginal myotomy of the medial rectus. *Arch. Ophthalmol.*, 1970, *84*, 625-626.
(116) KETTESY, A. — Die Polemik zwischen Albrecht von Graefe und F.C. Donders über die Schielgenese. *Klin. Mbl. Augenheilk.*, 1975, *167*, 785-791.
(117) KLEIN, R.M., MUCHNICK, R.S., RASKIND, R.H. — Measured tendon lengthening. *Arch. Ophthalmol.*, 1974, *92*, 309-311.
(118) KNAPP, P. — The surgical treatment of strabismus. In: Allen, J.H.: Strabismus Ophthalmic Symposium II. St. Louis, The C.V. Mosby Company, 1958 (p. 377-390).
(119) KNAPP, P. — Vertically incomitant horizontal strabismus: the so called "A" and "V" syndromes. *Trans. Amer. Ophthalmol. Soc.*, 1959, *57*, 666-669.
(120) KNOBLOCH, R., LORENZ, A. — Über ernste Komplikationen nach Schieloperationen. *Klin. Mbl. Augenheilk.*, 1962, *141*, 348-
(121) KRECKE, F.W.C. — Over eene nieuwe soort van brillen voor scheelzienden. *Neederlandsch Lancet*, 1847, 227-233.
(122) KROCZEK, S.E., HEYDE, E.L., HELVESTON, E.M. — Quantifying the marginal myotomy. *Amer. J. Ophthalmol.*, 1970, *70*, 204-209.
(123) KRZYSTKOWA, K. — Beiträge zur Chirurgie der Musculi obliqui. *Klin. Mbl. Augenheilk.*, 1972, *160*, 662-669.
(124) KUHNT, H. — Über die operative Behandlung des konkomittierenden Schielens. *Zeitschr. Augenheilk.*, 1908, *20*, 231-247.
(125) KUHNT, H. — Über ein einfaches Verfahren die Wirkung der Tenotomie zu dosieren. *Zeitschr. Augenheilk.*, 1912, *27*, 49-58.
(126) KÜPER, J. — Die Verstärkung gerader Augenmuskeln durch Faltung. *Klin. Mbl. Augenheilk.*, 1964, *145*, 716-720.
(127) LAGRANGE, H. — Principes de technique dans l'avancement musculaire. (Opération du strabisme). *Ann. Oculist.*, 1934, *171*, 587-596.
(128) LANDOLT, E. — La ténotomie de l'oblique inférieur. *Arch. Ophtalmol. (Paris)*, 1885, *5*, 402-405.
(129) LANG, J. — Schielbehandlung: gestern, heute, morgen. *Der Augenarzt*, 1974, *8*, 92-100.
(130) LANG, J. — Strabisme. Diagnostic. Formes cliniques. Traitement. Berne, Stuttgart, Vienne, Editions Hans Huber, 1981.
(131) LAVAT, J., BONS, G. — Reculs obliques dans la chirurgie des syndromes A et V. *Bull. Soc. Ophtal. Fr.*, 1972, *72*, 317-320.
(132) LEBENSOHN, J.E. — The first miotic. *Amer. J. Ophthalmol.*, 1963, *55*, 657-659.
(133) LYLE, K.T. — The principles and techniques of strabismus surgery. *Ann. Ophthalmol.*, 1970, *1*, 415-427.
(134) LYLE, K.T., WYBAR, K. — Practical Orthoptics in the treatment of Squint. 5° Ed. London, 1967.
(135) MALBRAN, E.S., NORBIS, A. — Le D.F.P. dans le traitement du strabisme convergent. *Ann. Oculist.*, 1955, *188*, 720-733.
(136) MALBRAN, J. — Une nouvelle méthode de renforcement musculaire. Le raccourcissement «en vis». *Ann. Oculist.*, 1965, *198*, 563-568.
(137) McCOOL, J.L. — Some original experiments with the O'Connor muscle shortening operation. *Amer. J. Ophthalmol.*, 1931, *13*, 491-495.
(138) McLEAN, J.M., GALIN, M.A., BARAS, I. — Retinal perforation during strabismus surgery. *Amer. J. Ophthalmol.*, 1960, *50*, 1167-1169.

(139) McNEAR, K.W., SCOTT, A.B., JAMPOLSKY, A. — A technique for surgically weakening the inferior oblique muscle. *Arch. Ophthalmol., 1965, 73*, 87-88.
(140) MELLER, J. — Augenärztliche Eingriffe. Berlin, Springer Verlag, 1938.
(141) METZ, H.S. — Adjustable suture strabismus surgery. *Ann. Ophthalmol.*, 1979, *11*, 1593-1597.
(142) MILLER, J.E. — Vertical recti transplantation in the A and V syndromes. *Arch. Ophthalmol.*, 1960, *64*, 175-179.
(143) MILLER, J.E. — A comparison of miotics in accommodative esotropia. *Amer. J. Ophthalmol.*, 1960, *41*, 1350-1355.
(144) MÜHLENDYCK, H., LINNEN, H.J. — Die operative Behandlung nystagmusbedingter schwankender Schielwinkel mit der Fadenoperation. *Klin. Mbl. Augenheilk.*, 1975, *167*, 273-290.
(145) MÜNCHOW, W. — Zur Vorgeschichte der Schielbehandlung. *Klin. Mbl. Augenheilk.*, 1973, *162*, 415-424.
(146) NAUHEIM, J.S. — Marginal keratitis and corneal ulceration after surgery on the extraocular muscles. *Arch. Ophthalmol.*, 1962, *67*, 708-711.
(147) NOORDEN, G.K. von — Temporal transplantation of the inferior rectus muscle in V-esotropia. *Amer. J. Ophthalmol.*, 1963, *56*, 919-922.
(148) NOORDEN, G.K. von, OLSON, C.L. — Diagnosis and surgical management of vertically incomitant horizontal strabismus. *Amer. J. Ophthalmol.*, 1965, *60*, 434-442.
(149) NOORDEN, G.K. von — Orbital cellulitis following extra-ocular muscle surgery. *Amer. J. Ophthalmol.*, 1972, *74*, 627-629.
(150) NOORDEN, G.K. von — The nystagmus compensation (blockage) syndrome. *Amer. J. Ophthalmol.*, 1976, *82*, 283-290.
(151) NOORDEN, G.K. von — A selection of surgical techniques in strabismus. *Highlights Ophthalmol.*, 1976, *14*, 64-104.
(152) NOORDEN, G.K. von, MORRIS, J., EDELMAN, P. — Efficacy of bifocals in the treatment of accommodative esotropia. *Amer. J. Ophthalmol.*, 1978, *85*, 830-834.
(153) NOORDEN, G.K. von — Burian-Von Noorden's Binocular Vision and ocular Motility. St. Louis, Toronto, London, The C.V. Mosby Company, 1980.
(154) O'CONNOR, R. — A new shortening technique with report of forty-two operations. *J. of the Amer. Med. Associat.*, 1916, *67*, 268-276.
(155) PARKS, M.M. — The weakening surgical procedures for eliminating overaction of the inferior oblique muscle. *Amer. J. Ophthalmol.*, 1972, *73*, 107-122.
(156) PARKS, M.M. — The overacting inferior oblique muscle. *Amer. J. Ophthalmol.*, 1974, *77*, 787-797.
(157) PERDRIEL, G., BIARD, L., DECROIX, G., TERZIAN, M. — Valeur relative des procédés d'affaiblissement du corps musculaire du petit oblique. *Bull. Mém. Soc. Fr. Ophtalmol.*, 1977, *88*, 209-214.
(158) PESTALOZZI, D. — Über neue präoperative Masznahmen zur Überwindung des Zentralskotoms und Normalisierung der Korrespondenz bei Schielern. *Klin. Mbl. Augenheilk.*, 1974, *164*, 192-197.
(159) PFANDL, E. — Ein neuer Weg zur Verhinderung der Ausbildung einer anomalen retinalen Korrespondenz bei Strabismus convergens concomitans. Acta XVIII Concilium Ophthalmologicum. Bruxelles, Imprimerie Médicale et Scientifique, 1959 (p. 202-203).
(160) PIETRUSCHKA, G. — Über Ergebnisse der exact dosierten Rücklagerung und Myektomie beim Horizontalschielen. *Klin. Mbl. Augenheilk.*, 1965, *146*, 628.
(161) PIGASSOU, R., GARIPUY, J. — Traitement du strabisme dans l'espace libre. *Arch. Ophtalmol. (Paris)*, 1966, *26*, 445-458.
(162) PIGASSOU-ALBOUY, R. — Die motorischen Störungen beim Strabismus. Pathogenese und Therapie. *Klin. Mbl. Augenheilk.*, 1976, *169*, 468-481.
(163) PIGASSOU, R. — "Entente cordiale" in the early treatment of squint. *Brit. J. Ophthalmol.*, 1977, *61*, 16-22.
(164) PIGASSOU ALBOUY, R. — Prisms in strabismus management. Past, present and future. *J. Pediatr. Ophthalmol. Strabismus*, 1980, *17*, 325-330.
(165) PINÇON, F., VERIN, Ph. — L'iodure de phospholine dans le strabisme accommodatif. *Bull. Soc. Opht. Fr.*, 1965, *65*, 790-796.

(166) POULIQUEN, P. — Surcorrection optique et angle strabique. *Bull. Soc. Ophtal. Fr.*, 1964, *64*, 742-745.
(167) POULIQUEN, P. — Zum Problem der Penalisation. *Klin. Mbl. Augenheilk.*, 1972, *161*, 130-139.
(168) PRIETO-DIAZ, J. — Posterior tenectomy of the superior oblique. *J. Ped. Ophthalmol. Strabismus*, 1979, *16*, 321-323.
(169) PRIETO-DIAZ, J. — Large bilateral medial rectus recession in early esotropia with bilateral limitation of abduction. *J. Ped. Ophthalmol. Strabismus*, 1980, *17*, 101-105.
(170) QUÉRÉ, M.A. — Les pénalisations optiques dans le traitement des amblyopies strabiques. *Arch. Ophtal. (Paris)*, 1971, *31*, 877-886.
(171) QUÉRÉ, M.A. — Die Methoden der Penalisation in der Behandlung des Strabismus convergens. *Klin. Mbl. Augenheilk.*, 1972, *161*, 140-155.
(172) QUÉRÉ, M.A., CLERGEAU, G., FONTENAILLE, N. — Die Lähmungsdyssynergien. Die Schieldyssynergien und das Cüppersche Syndrom. *Klin. Mbl. Augenheilk.*, 1975, *167*, 162-178.
(173) QUÉRÉ, M.A., CLERGEAU, G., FONTENAILLE, N., GOURAY, A., SPIELMANN, A., LLEDO, M. — Les syndromes de blocage dans les strabismus infantiles. *Ann. Oculist.*, 1976, *209*, 339-349, 417-433, 483-500.
(174) QUÉRÉ, M.A., CLERGEAU, G., PECHERAU, A. — Le sanglage musculaire rétroéquatorial, variante technique de l'opération du Fil de Cüppers (note préliminaire). *Arch. Ophtal. (Paris)*, 1977, *37*, 531-538.
(175) QUÉRÉ, M.A., PECHEREAU, A., CLERGEAU, G. — La nouvelle chirurgie des ésotropies fonctionnelles (Opération du Fil et techniques classiques). *J. Fr. Ophtalmol.*, 1978, *1*, 56-60, 151-161, 221-228.
(176) REINECKE, R.D., MILLER, D. — Strabismus. A programmed text. New York, Appleton-Century-Crofts, 1966.
(177) REVELL, M.J. — Strabismus. A history of orthoptic techniques. London, Barrie and Jenkins, 1971.
(178) RINTELEN, F. — Zur partiellen Tenotomie. *Ophthalmol.*, 1956, *131*, 254-256.
(179) RINTELEN, F. — Zur Geschichte der Lehre vom Strabismus. *Klin. Mbl. Augenheilk.*, 1978, *173*, 449-457.
(180) ROSENBAUM, A.L., METZ, H.S., CARLSON, M., JAMPOLSKY, A.J. — Adjustable rectus muscle recession surgery. A follow-up study. *Arch. Ophthalmol.*, 1977, *95*, 817-820.
(181) SALVI, G., FROSINI, R., BOSCHI, M.C. — L'allongement du tendon selon Focosi dans les syndromes de blocage. *J. Fr. Ophtalmol.*, 1981, *4*, 127-132.
(182) SATTLER, C.H. — Erfahrungen über die Beseitigung der Amblyopie und die Wiederherstellung des binokularen Sehakts bei Schielenden. *Zeitschr. Augenheilk.*, 1927, *63*, 19 .
(183) SATTLER, C.H. — Prismenbrillen zur Frühbehandlung des konkomittierenden Schielens. *Klin. Mbl. Augenheilk.*, 1930, *84*, 813-
(184) SCHÄFER, W.D. — Die Bifokalbrille in der Schielbehandlung. *Klin. Mbl. Augenheilk.*, 1974, *165*, 915-920.
(185) SCOTT, A.B. — Botulinum Toxin injection into extraocular muscles as an alternative to strabismus surgery. *J. Pediatr. Ophthalmol. Strabismus.*, 1980, *17*, 21-25.
(186) SEVRIN, G. — Sobre la cirugia de los sindromes en "A" y "V". *Arch. Soc. Oftal. Hisp.-Amer.*, 1962, *22*, 336-338.
(187) SPIELMANN, A. — Les strabismes variables non accommodatifs. In: Année Thérapeutique et Clinique en Ophtalmologie, Vol. XXXI; Marseille, Diffusion Générale de Libraire, 1981 (p. 207-237).
(188) STALLARD, H.B. — Eye Surgery. Bristol. John Wright & Sons, Ltd., 1965.
(189) STANGLER-ZUSCHROTT, E. — Prismen als Operationsvorbereitung beim Strabismus convergens alternans. *Klin. Mbl. Augenheilk.*, 1974, *165*, 909-914.
(190) STANWORTH, A. — Modified major amblyoscope. *Brit. J. Ophthalmol.*, 1958, *42*, 270-287.
(191) STAPLES, W.E., JACKSON, H. — A clinical assessment of Malbran's "en vis" operation for squint correction. *Amer. J. Ophthalmol.*, 1969, *67*, 380-382.
(192) STARK, N., POPP, E. — Resultate der Penalisation. *Klin. Mbl. Augenheilk.*, 1975, *167*, 227-232.

(193) STEPHENSON, S. — A short note on some cases of convergent strabismus healed by lengthening the tendon of the internal rectus muscle. *Trans. Ophthalm. Soc. U.K.*, 1902, *22*, 276.
(194) STROMEYER, L. — Beiträge zur operativen Orthopädik oder Erfahrungen über die subcutane Durchschneidung verkürzter Muskeln und deren Sehne. Hannover, 1838.
(195) STUART, J.A. — Myectomy of the inferior oblique muscle. *Amer. J. Ophthalmol.*, 1964, *57*, 118-121.
(196) TESSLER, H.W., URIST, M.J. — Corneal dellen in the limbal approach to rectus muscle surgery. *Brit. J. Ophthalmol.*, 1975, *59*, 377-379.
(197) THOMAS, C., SPIELMANN, A., BERNARDINI, D. — L'expérience de trois années de l'«Opération du fil» de Cüppers dans les interventions contre l'ésotropie avec phénomène innervationel de blocage. *Bull. Mém. Soc. Franç. Ophtal.*, 1976, *88*, 173-180.
(198) URIST, M.J. — Horizontal squint with secondary vertical deviations. *Arch. Ophthalmol.*, 1951, *46*, 245-267.
(199) URIST, M.J. — The etiology of the so-called A and V syndromes. *Amer. J. Ophthalmol.*, 1958, *46*, 835-844.
(200) URIST, M.J. — Surgery in horizontal strabismus. *Amer. J. Ophthalmol.*, 1963, *55*, 62-80.
(201) URIST, M.J. — Recession and upward displacement of the medial rectus muscles in A-pattern esotropia. *Amer. J. Ophthalmol.*, 1968, *65*, 769-773.
(202) URIST, M.J. — Complications following bilateral superior oblique weakening surgical procedures for A-pattern horizontal deviations. *Amer. J. Ophthalmol.*, 1970, *70*, 583-587.
(203) VANCEA, P., VAIGHEL, V., VANCEA, P.P. — L'ulcère trophique de la cornée consécutif aux opérations sur les muscles oculaires. *Ann. Oculist.*, 1960, *193*, 28-34.
(204) VANCEA, P.P., TUDOR, E., GALIN, A. — La ténotomie intra-sclérale controlée dans la chirurgie du strabisme concomitant. *Ann. Oculist.*, 1974, *207*, 769.
(205) VAN DER HOEVE, J. — Operationen an den Augenmuskeln. In: Von Elschnig, A.: Augenärztliche Operationslehre, Bd. 2. In: Graefe, A. und Saemisch, Th.: Handbuch der ges. Augenheilk, 2 u 3 Auflage, Berlin, Springer, 1922.
(206) VEREECKEN, E., ADELSTEIN, F. — Diagnostic et traitement de la «paralysie» du droit externe. *Ophthalmol*, 1966, *151*, 465-476.
(207) VILLASECA, A. — The A and V syndromes. *Amer. J. Ophthalmol.*, 1961, *52*, 172-194.
(208) WEISS, J.B., HOROVITZ, G., VERGNE, J.L. — Ténotomie quantifiée. *Bull. Soc. Opht. Fr.*, 1978, *78*, 677-678.
(209) WHEELER, M.C. — Isofluorophate (DFP) in the handling of esotropia. *Arch. Ophthalmol.*, 1964, *71*, 298-302.
(210) WILLIAMS, H.P. — Comparison of the accommodative effects of Carbachol and Pilocarpine with reference to accommodative esotropia. *Brit. J. Ophthalmol.*, 1974, *58*, 668-673.
(211) WILLIAMS, A.T., METZ, H.S., JAMPOLSKY, A. — The O'Connor cinch revisited. *Brit. J. Ophthalmol.*, 1978, *62*, 765-769.
(212) WOILLEZ, M. — Traitement chirurgical du strabisme convergent. Dans: Année thérapeutique et clinique en Ophtalmologie, Vol. XXXI (p. 163-182). Marseille, Diffusion Générale de Librairie, 1981.
(213) WOLLENSAK, J., KEWITZ, H. — 100 Jahre Pilocarpin in der Augenheilkunde. *Klin. Mbl. Augenheilk.*, 1976, *169*, 660-663.

Bull. Soc. belge Ophtal., **195**, 53-73, 1981.

CHAPTER III

NORMAL BINOCULAR VISION

R.A. CRONE (*)

I. *Introduction* (**)

All vertebrates have two eyes. They are thus able to observe a wider panorama than would be the case if they had only one. Binocular vision also offers a second advantage, namely depth perception. This " stereoscopic vision " arises from the fact that the two eyes observe the world from slightly different positions. Panoramic vision and stereoscopic vision involve conflicting requirements. For the widest panorama, the visual fields of the two eyes must meet, but without overlapping. Depth perception in as large as possible an area of the visual field, by contrast, requires that the visual fields overlap as far as possible. Some animals have opted for panoramic binocular vision and thus for laterally positioned eyes. These are mainly the herbivores, which need to escape as soon as they scent danger in their surroundings. Other species have abandoned panoramic vision in favor of depth perception in as large a binocular field of vision as possible; their eyes have adopted a frontal position. This group consists mainly of predatory animals, which must be able to accurately estimate the distance to their prey, and tree-dwelling species, which need to know how far it is to the next branch if they are to jump successfully. Among the animal species, the apes have the most highly developed visual co-ordination of front leg movements.

In the human species, too, the eyes are frontally positioned and panoramic vision has largely been sacrified for depth perception. In

---

(*) Director of the Department of Ophthalmology, Academic Medical Center, Amsterdam, The Netherlands.

(**) In this chapter many formulations and figures have been borrowed from the thesis of Dr. Maillette de Buy Wenniger (8). For an excellent review see Bishop (1).

primitive man, the upright posture freed the hands for all manner of operations which demanded accurate estimation of depth, such as picking fruit, making and using tools, and many other things. Depth perception has inestimable advantages for modern man also; indeed, it is indispensable for certain manual operations, e.g. a cataract operation. The accuracy of the human ability to perceive depth is revealed in the following Table.

At 20 cm	1/25 mm
At 1 m	1 mm
At 10 m	10 cm
At 100 m	10 m

This small Table teaches us an important fact, namely that the power of depth perception decreases as the distance increases.

Where modern men and women are concerned, depth perception has lost much of its survival value. Their greatest danger lies in traffic, and here the distances are so great that binocular depth perception can be of little assistance. The principal activity of people today is writing on paper, and for this, too, depth perception is superfluous. Their greatest source of pleasure lies in watching television—a pleasure which can only exist by reason of the fact that the absence of stereoscopic parallax does not ruin the suggestion of depth in the picture. These facts have a strange consequence for the pathology of binocular vision and thus for strabismus. One might perhaps expect loss of depth perception to be the most serious consequence of strabismus. In practice, however, this is not so, and it is secondary phenomena such as a disfiguring eye position, amblyopia and diplopia which drive patients to the ophthalmologist. One seldom hears a victim of strabismus complaining that he cannot perceive depth; in fact, of all the techniques to do so, he lacks only one—binocular stereopsis. Using motion parallax, apparent size and various other factors, the strabismus victim can perceive depth as well as a normal person. Those who lack binocular depth perception—and this applies to one in twenty people—find it hard to imagine that stereoscopic vision is a sensory quality sui generis, unique and irreducible. The specifically binocular character of stereoscopic vision is clearly revealed in the random dot stereograms of Julesz (7) (fig. 1). The two squares appear to contain nothing but randomly scattered dots; but if they are fused binocularly, a small square becomes visible within the figure and "nearer" than the remainder of it. Random dot stereograms also teach us something else, namely that our visual system commences to process the perspective data, which lead to stereoscopic vision, at an

A

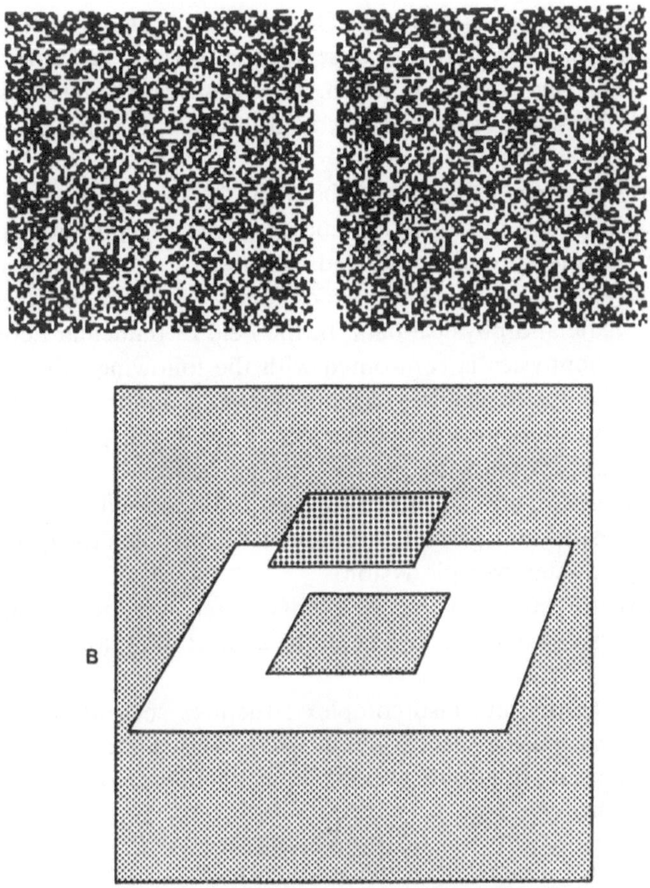

B

Fig. 1. — Random dot stereogram. When A is stereoscopically fused, a square appears in vivid depth above randomly textured surround, as indicated by perspective diagram B. (From Julesz, 1971).

early stage—at any rate before actual recognition of what we see, as a thing or a pattern, occurs. This hypothesis will be proved several times in the ensuing paragraphs, not only in connection with the psychophysics and neurophysiology of stereoscopic vision, but also in the discussion of the abnormal binocular vision which accompanies strabismus.

II. *Psychophysics of spatial vision*

Visual perception takes place in the psyche. For this reason, the space perceived is referred to as the "subjective space". It is the space within which the ego observes things in various directions and assigns a place to each ("relative localization"). The ego also assigns itself a place amid the things, from whence it observes the world ("egocentric localization"). For one visual direction, that observation has a special, intentional character; this is the direction in which the gaze is fixed on an object.

There is, of course, a connection between the subjective space which is the subject of the introspection and the objective physical space in which we can measure distances and directions.

Psychophysics is the science which deals with the interrelations between psychic and physical data. In the field of binocular depth perception, psychophysics is confronted with the following problems:

1. What is the position in the objective space of points which are seen in the same direction by both eyes? This is the problem of the horopter and of binocular vision without depth.
2. Which points in space can be observed to be more distant, or nearer, with respect to a given fixation point? This poses the question of the range of stereoscopic vision.
3. In which direction do we see points which are more distant, or nearer? This question brings us to the subject of cyclopean localization.
4. Not only points, but also complex structures such as random dot stereograms, can be seen in depth. How does this come about? In analysing such situations, we encounter phenomena such as rivalry and globality.

A. *The horopter. Binocular vision without depth*

Because we look with two eyes yet do not see two separate images, both eyes must be able to localize a certain point in space in the same direction, so that a single point is seen. This applies first and foremost to the point, at a given distance, at which one looks, the fixation point. But everywhere else in space there must be points, each of which, at the same fixation distance, are seen in the same direction by each eye. This certainly does not apply to all points in space, however. If one holds a finger close to the eyes and gazes into the distance, the finger is seen double, thus in a different direction by each eye.

The points which are seen in the same direction by both eyes can easily be investigated. A fixation point at a distance of, say, 1 metre is presented to the two eyes together, and in the peripheral field of vision a vertical strip of light, of which the upper half is visible only to one eye and the lower half to the other. With polaroid filters, a test of this

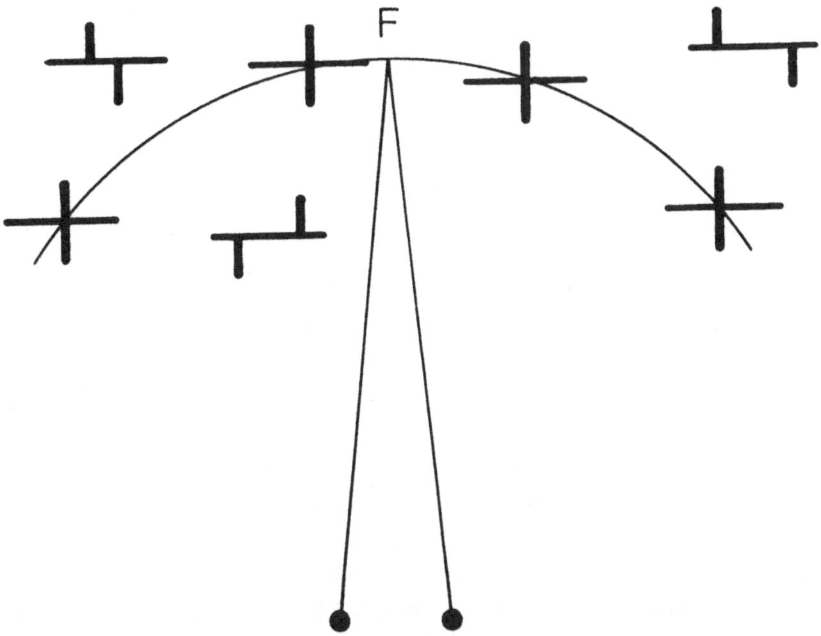

Fig. 2. — The longitudinal horopter. Both eyes are focussed on F. The points at which the nonius lines are seen as a continuous line are all at approximately the same distance from the observer.

nature can easily be carried out. In fact, the subject sees two vertical nonius lines, and only when the strip of light is neither too far away nor too close, but at exactly the correct distance, are these seen as one continuous line. This is the distance at which are situated the points which are seen in the same direction by both eyes.

The sum of the points referred to is known as the horopter (10). It is a plane which is concave in the direction of the observer and in which the fixation point is also located. The horizontal cross-section of the horopter plane, intersecting the fixation point, is known as the "longitudinal horopter" (fig. 2). The simple psychophysical test described above, in which the nonius horopter is determined, has produced an important result: all points which, at a given fixation distance, are seen in the same direction by both eyes are equally distant. Binocular vision without depth occurs in the horopter plane.

B. *Depth perception. Range of stereoscopic vision*

Points in front of and behind the horopter are seen in depth. The horizontal disparity, that is to say the difference in horizontal angle

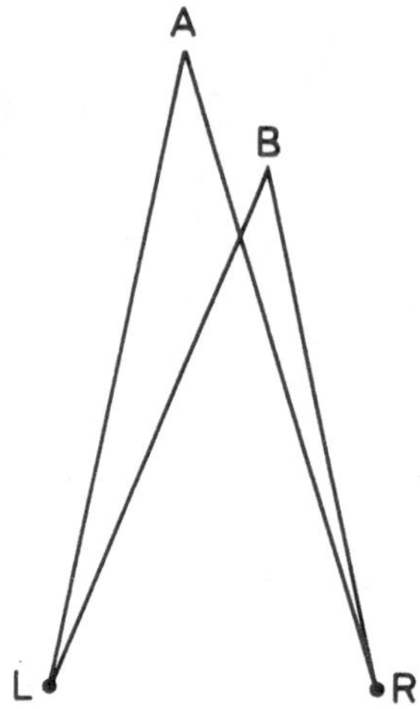

Fig. 3. — Horizontal disparity. The angular distance AB is not equal for both eyes.

between the visual directions in which two points are seen by both eyes, is decisive for the depth. If angle ALB is greater than angle ARB (fig. 3), B is nearer than A, and A farther away than B.

Our visual system is amazingly sensitive to horizontal disparity. Using carefully selected linear objects, and under optimum conditions, depth can still be perceived at a disparity of only a few seconds of arc. In simple clinical investigations to determine stereoscopic acuity, 15 seconds of arc constitute a low threshold, and a value of 40 seconds of arc is still regarded as normal. The acuity of stereoscopic vision cannot, of course, be greater than the monocular power of resolution. The monocular visual acuity decreases sharply towards the periphery, and the same happens to the stereoscopic acuity.

If the disparity increases, the visible difference in distance between A and B becomes correspondingly greater, but this is not in the first instance accompanied by diplopia. Here we encounter a fundamental characteristic of binocular vision, namely that not only all points on the horopter, but also others in front of and behind it, are observed in single vision. Single vision is sustained until the horizonal disparity reaches a certain maximum value, which may be termed the diplopia threshold. According to classical researches (9), the diplopia threshold in the centre of the visual field lies below 10 minutes of arc. The threshold is greater at the periphery of the visual field, where it is about 10% of the perimetric angle (4) (fig. 4). The magnitude of diplopia thresholds is governed not only by the position in the visual field, but

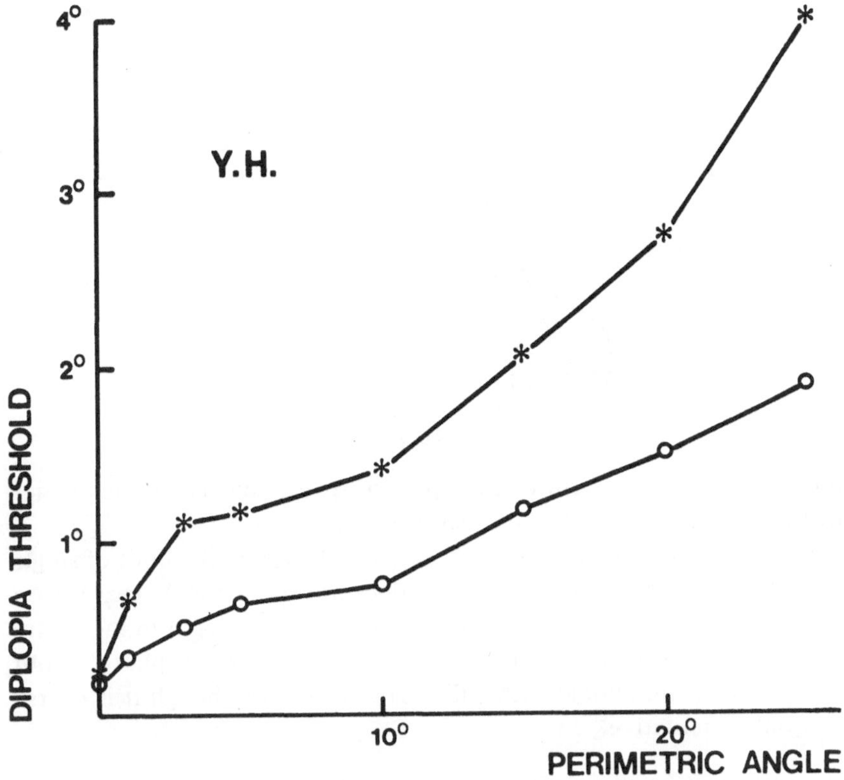

Fig. 4. — The relation between diplopia threshold and perimetric angle.
* Horizontal diplopia thresholds.
○ Vertical diplopia thresholds.
Subject: Y.H. (from Crone & Leuridan).

also by the nature of the objects used in tests. The data in figure 4 were obtained with two vertical strips of light in a darkened room. If random dot stereograms are used, the diplopia threshold, even in the centre of the visual field, is seen to be higher, perhaps by as much as a factor of ten. Similarly, with vertical disparity (of two horizontal strips of light presented monocularly), diplopia occurs only when a certain value is exceeded. As a rule, the vertical diplopia thresholds are lower than the horizontal. Vertical disparity is not of significance in relation to depth perception.

The sum of the diplopia thresholds in front of and behind the horopter, expressed as an angle of horizonal disparity, is described as the amplitude of horizontal sensory fusion. This is governed by the peri-

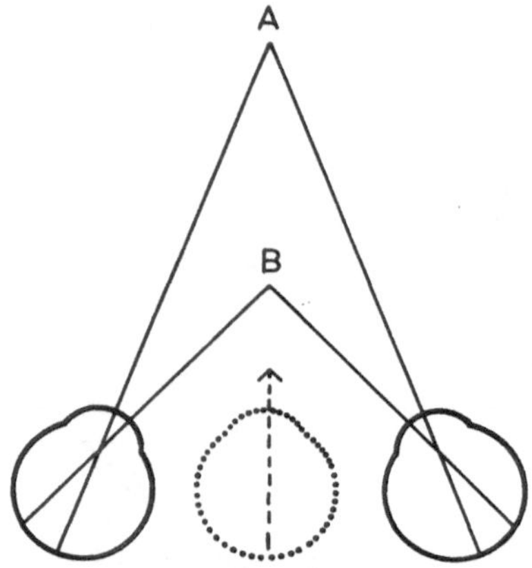

Fig. 5. — Cyclopean localization.

metric angle and the nature of the patterns presented. The same applies to the amplitude of vertical sensory fusion.

If, as a result of increasing the horizontal disparity, the limit of single vision is exceeded, depth perception does not immediately cease. At a disparity of 5°, or even 10°, an object can be seen in depth in the centre of the visual field, albeit it is seen double. At the periphery, depth perception is compatible with still greater disparity, though it is coarse and only qualitative.

C. *Cyclopean localization*

There is no problem concerning the direction in which we see things that are situated in the horopter plane, since every point of the horopter by definition represents a binocular direction of sight. But with points which lie in front of, or behind, the horopter, it is a different matter. In which direction are these seen? Figure 5 can help to explain the problem. The eyes fixate point A. To the left eye, point B lies to the right of point A, but to the right eye it is to the left of A. In reality, B is seen to be directly in front of A. The localization of point B is evidently midway between the two monocular localizations. It is as if A and B are viewed from a "cyclopean" eye equidistant from the two eyes. This cyclopean eye is the eye with which the ego—the visual egocentre—gazes into the subjective space.

D. *Local and global stereoscopic vision*

In the simplest depth perception situation, one eye sees a single dot, the other eye two dots. When the stereogram reproduced in figure 6 is

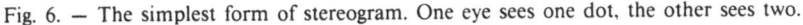

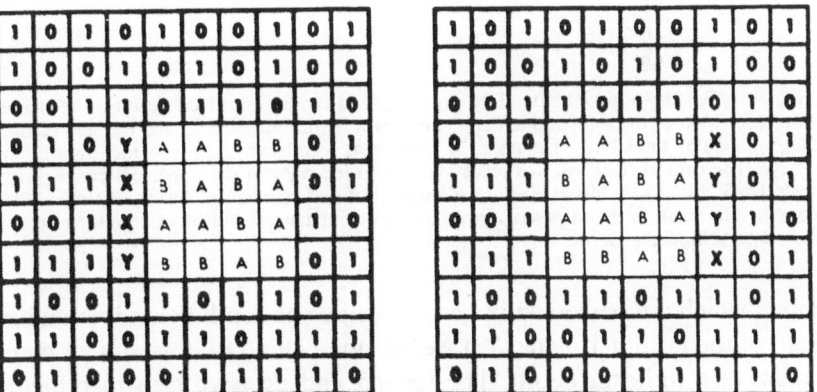

Fig. 6. — The simplest form of stereogram. One eye sees one dot, the other sees two.

fused by convergence, the right-hand dot of the near pair appears to be slightly closer than the left-hand one. With random dot stereograms, the situation is much more complicated, because these involve a very large number of dots. When the outer contours of these stereograms are fused by convergence, the dots in the innermost square do not correspond. The explanation for this lies in a lateral shift in the inner field of the random dot pattern which is seen by one eye, with respect to the pattern which is seen by the other (7) (fig. 7). As a result of this shift, dots appear in the centre, in the horopter plane (the plane in which the outer contour lies), which appear white to one eye and black to the other. Such dissimilar image elements do not lead to binocular vision. The elements repress each other, a phenomenon known as *rivalry*. Anticipating the language of strabismus, one could also describe it as alternating suppression. The phenomenon is illustrated in figure 8. Rivalry is the first step towards the achievement of the depth effect in the random dot stereogram, inasmuch as erroneous fusion of white and black dots is rejected.

Rivalry does not, however, fully explain the depth effect, for in principle innumerable combinations of black (or white) dots are possible in each of the figures (see fig. 9). The single squares in the stereogram seen by the left eye can be combined in many ways with the squares in the stereogram viewed by the right eye. This multiplicity of possible combinations ought a priori to lead to a chaotic mixture of all sorts of

1	0	1	0	1	0	0	1	0	1
1	0	0	1	0	1	0	1	0	0
0	0	1	1	0	1	1	0	1	0
0	1	0	Y	A	A	B	B	0	1
1	1	1	X	B	A	B	A	0	1
0	0	1	X	A	A	B	A	1	0
1	1	1	Y	B	B	A	B	0	1
1	0	0	1	1	0	1	1	0	1
1	1	0	0	1	1	0	1	1	1
0	1	0	0	0	1	1	1	1	0

1	0	1	0	1	0	0	1	0	1
1	0	0	1	0	1	0	1	0	0
0	0	1	1	0	1	1	0	1	0
0	1	0	A	A	B	B	X	0	1
1	1	1	B	A	B	A	Y	0	1
0	0	1	A	A	B	A	Y	1	0
1	1	1	B	B	A	B	X	0	1
1	0	0	1	1	0	1	1	0	1
1	1	0	0	1	1	0	1	1	1
0	1	0	0	0	1	1	1	1	0

Fig. 7. — Principle of the random dot stereogram (from Julesz).

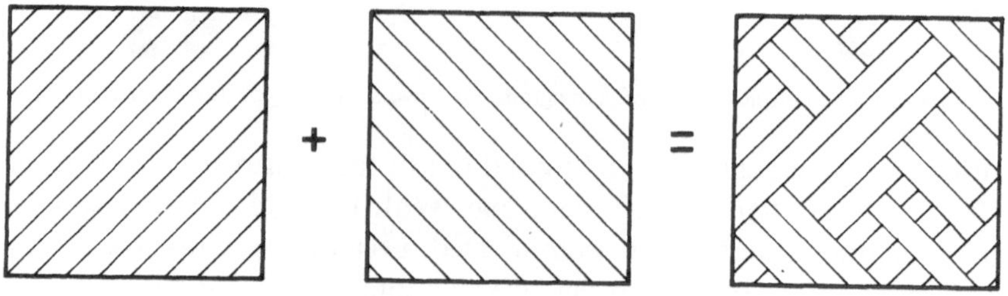

Fig. 8. — Rivalry.

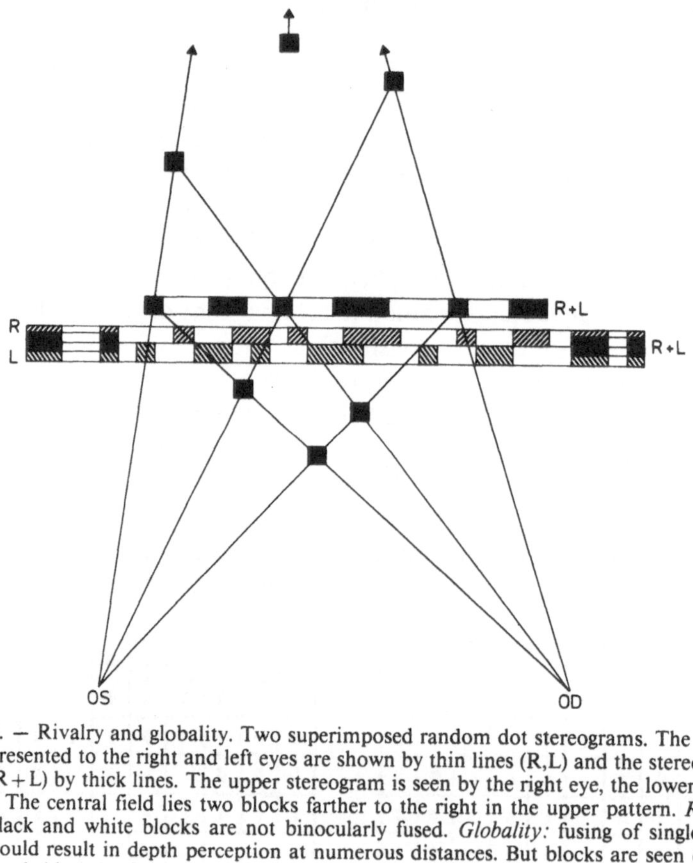

Fig. 9. — Rivalry and globality. Two superimposed random dot stereograms. The stereograms presented to the right and left eyes are shown by thin lines (R,L) and the stereoscopic image (R + L) by thick lines. The upper stereogram is seen by the right eye, the lower by the left eye. The central field lies two blocks farther to the right in the upper pattern. *Rivalry:* single black and white blocks are not binocularly fused. *Globality:* fusing of single black blocks could result in depth perception at numerous distances. But blocks are seen only in one plane behind the frame.

points which are perceived in various degree of depth behind, in and in front of the horopter plane. Yet we see not a cloud of dots, but an inner square at a uniform depth. The second and decisive step in bringing about this depth effect is *globality*, a term introduced by Julesz. By means of this mechanism, erroneous fusion of black (or white) dots, leading to ambiguity, is rejected and priority given to an interpretation with, as far as possible, identical disparity from place to place. With the aid of rivalry and globality, we achieve global stereoscopic vision in which, taking the example of the random dot stereograms, the inner square is seen in depth as a single plane.

III. *Neuroanatomy of binocular vision*

The neuroanatomy of binocular vision commences in the one hundred million or so receptors in the retinae. For the purposes of this study, we need not go into the microscopic anatomy of the retina; it suffices to use the general term "retinal elements" to describe the components of the retina which in binocular vision operate independently. Binocular vision requires close co-operation between the retinal elements of one eye and those of the other. This applies especially to the two retinal elements on which is imaged a spatial point that is seen in the same direction by both eyes and thus lies on the horopter. *Retinal elements on which a point of the horopter is imaged are described as corresponding elements.* In a somewhat wider sense, co-operation is demanded between non-corresponding retinal elements on which disparate but singly observed points are imaged. The "*Panum area*" is the retinal area of one eye, in which each element can co-operate with a certain retinal element of the other eye to produce single vision.

The nerve fibres from two corresponding elements lead, via the optic nerves, to the chiasma opticum. The structure in the optic paths which is essential for binocular vision is the semi-decussation in the optic chiasma. There, the fibres leading from the nasal halves of the retinae cross, while the fibres from the temporal halves of the retinae continue their path without crossing. The result is that fibres from corresponding elements of both retinae come together. The fibres of each optic nerve terminate behind the chiasma in the left and right lateral geniculate bodies. According to current opinion, this nucleus plays no part in depth perception. The corpus geniculatum contains six layers of cells which alternately represent the right and left retinae. Each layer of cells contains its own retinotopic chart of the contralateral field of vision, the representations of corresponding retinal elements being arranged in six-high stacks. After synapse, the optic fibres pass via the radiatio optica to the area striata. The retinal elements of the right halves of the retinae are represented in the right hemisphere, and those of the left halves in the left hemisphere.

In a narrow vertical strip which passes through the central foveae, the angular width of which is estimated to be 1° and which widens in the foveal area to about 3°, corresponding elements have a representation in both hemispheres. The bilateral representation is due partly to the fact that the fibres of the optic nerve which emerge from the medial raphe of the temporal half of the retina are not all uncrossed (nor those from the nasal half of the retina all crossed), and partly because fibres in the radiatio optica do not all terminate in the area striata on the same side but, via the corpus callosum, in the crossed area striata. The bilateral representation of the foveal area is functionally important because without this double representation, co-operation between a foveal element in the one eye and a slightly disparate element in the other eye would be difficult.

In the area striata, the representations of the corresponding elements are close together. This fact is known to clinicians. Scotomas in perimetry never "correspond" more exactly than when the lesion is situated in the occipital lobe. The spatial relations in the lobe differ from those in the retina. In proportional terms, the central part of the retina occupies the most space in the cortex. A foveal area 0.005 mm in diameter has a cortical projection with a diameter of 0.5 mm and thus an area 10,000 times as large.

In order to analyse the anatomical basis for binocular vision in the area striata, or perhaps even in the higher visual centres, it is necessary to examine the microscopic anatomy of the visual cortex. Our present knowledge is decidedly inadequate for such an analysis. The reader will have to be satisfied with a few facts which serve to indicate the unimaginable complexity of the neural network. Its complexity is not entirely unexpected: binocular vision results from co-operation between corresponding elements, disparate elements and even significant disparities. The links which serve binocular vision must be innumerable. And binocular vision is but one aspect of vision; to it may be added colour vision, the ability to distinguish movement, etc., etc. The complexity of the cortex is, for example, revealed in the number of cells and their connections. Whereas each of the optic nerves contains at most one million fibres, the primary visual cortex has approximately 400 million neurons, each of which has numerous synapses with other neurons. The cortex, which has a thickness of about 3 mm, consists of six layers, each with characteristic cell types and connections. The structural and functional entity is the module, a column 3 mm in length and a fraction of a millimeter in diameter, which is situated at right

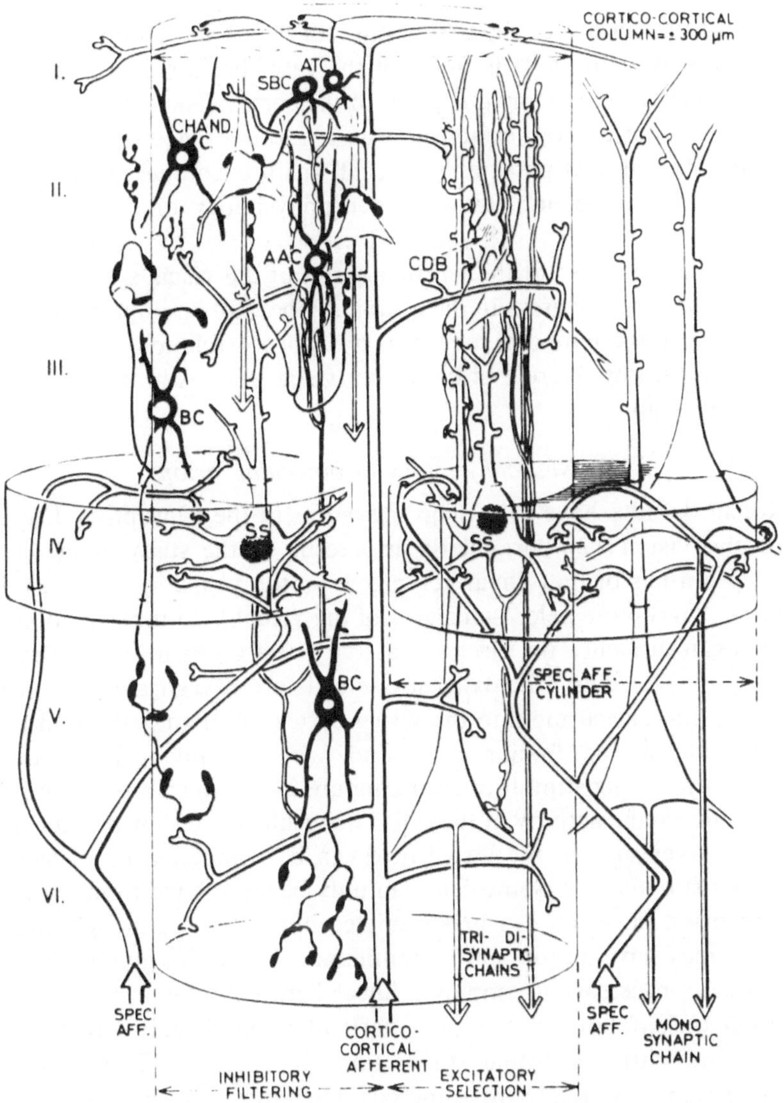

Fig. 10. — Diagram illustrating a single cortico-cortical column and two specific subcortical afferent arborization cylinders. Lamination is indicated on the left margin. The right half of the diagram indicates impulse processing over excitatory neurone chains, while the left half shows various types of inhibitory interneurones (full black). (From Szentágothai).

angles to the surface of the cortex (fig. 10) (11). Each module contains thousands of neurons. It is thus not the case that a single retinal element is represented at any one point in the cortex. The columnar structure of the cortex was established as a result of neurophysiological research. In the next paragraph we shall again encounter the columns, this time in connection with the neurophysiology of depth perception.

The area striata is not the terminal point of the visual system. There are secondary visual areas in the occipital lobe, and an important visual area exists in the temporal lobe. It is not yet possible to express a firm opinion regarding the role of the higher visual centres in the process of binocular vision.

IV. *Neurophysiology of binocular vision*

Recent decades have seen major advances in the neurophysiology of binocular vision (12), particularly as a result of the study of the electrical potentials of individual nerve cells in the visual system. In this, the term "receptive field"—the area of the visual field in which optical stimuli can influence the electrical activity of a given neuron—plays a central role. Receptive fields of striate cells are investigated by introducing a microelectrode into the visual cortex of an anaesthetized animal (usually a cat), finding a cell and, with the aid of a projection screen, introducing stimuli of such a nature and in such a position that they influence the activity of the cell. The results have shown that every cell in a given area of the visual field can be stimulated in a specific, characteristic manner. Some cells can only be stimulated monocularly; the majority, however, can be stimulated binocularly, although one of the eyes may have a pronounced dominance. For optimum stimulation it is usually necessary to employ a linear light stimulus in a particular position (orientation) and with a particular length and direction of movement. With monocular stimulation, the receptive fields of binocular cells have virtually the same characteristics in each eye.

The binocular cells are the physiological correlate of fusion, the merging of monocular image elements into a single image. If different stimuli are introduced into the receptive field of a binocular cell in each eye—e.g. a vertical strip of light for the right eye and a horizontal strip for the left eye—the cell is not activated. In this fact we recognize the neurophysiological correlate of rivalry, or suppression.

Here we have neurophysiological confirmation of the hypothesis that corresponding retinal elements converge towards a particular binocular

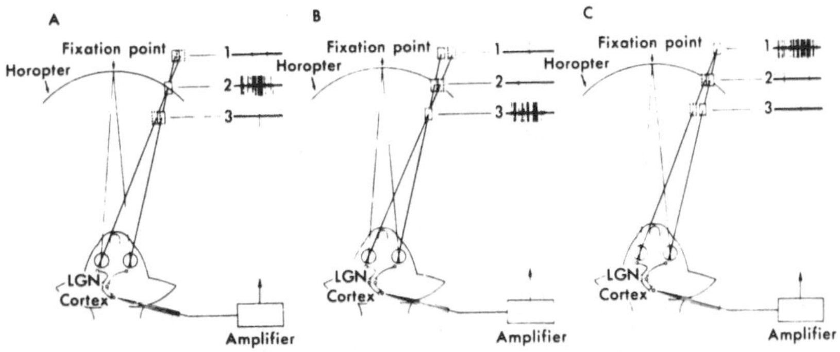

Fig. 11. — Scheme showing how binocular depth information can be coded by neurons in cat visual cortex. A. Maximal firing of binocularly activated neuron occurs when the two monocular receptive fields are in register and can be stimulated simultaneously, tracing 2. Being in register on horopter, this receptive field pair has zero disparity; that is, they are corresponding. B. Receptive field pair having convergent disparity; maximal firing, tracing 3. C. Receptive field pair having divergent disparity; maximal firing, tracing 1. (From Bishop).

cell. This implies that the receptive fields of many cortical cells lie on the horopter. Column A in figure 11 (Bishop 1, 2)) applies to these cells. Other cells, however, have a receptive field in front of, or behind, the horopter (B and C in fig. 11). These cells are referred to as "disparity detectors". They reflect our psychophysical experience of the fact that binocular vision can be achieved with both corresponding and disparate elements. The disparity detectors are extremely sensitive to a particular disparity. If a binocular stimulus with a slightly different disparity is presented, the cell is inhibited. In cats, binocular cells with a disparity sensitivity of only 10 minutes of arc have been found.

If the microelectrode penetrates the visual cortex at right angles, a number of cells which share a common characteristic of the receptive field are found in succession. Thus we find cell columns, all the cells of which can be better stimulated from one eye than from the other. Other columns are characterized by the fact that optimum stimulation of all cells occurs with a particular orientation of the linear light stimulus (fig. 12) (5).

Other columns might be of interest for the study of depth perception. According to recent studies, however, it appears that cells within a column show a random disparity scatter (2).

The facts described here reveal something of the neural mechanism of stereopsis. This mechanism imparts a quality of depth to minor characteristics of visual patterns, such as dots, and dashes with a particular orientation. Everything that has been written up to now, there-

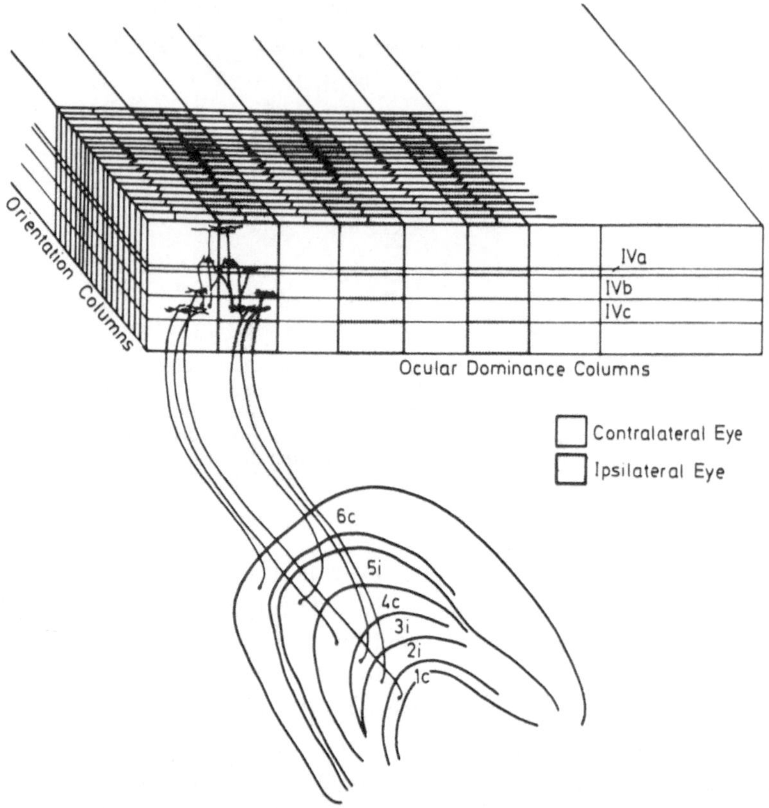

Fig. 12. — Idealized diagram showing for the monkey the projection from the lateral geniculate body to the visual cortex (area 17). The six layers of the lateral geniculate body are labelled according as they are associated with the ipsilateral (i) or contralateral (c) eye. These i and c layers project to specific areas so forming the ocular dominance columns for the ipsilateral and contralateral eyes. The stacked slab-like columns of the visual cortex are defined by the criteria of ocular dominance in one direction and orientation in the other direction (Hubel and Wiesel, 1974).

fore, relates to local stereopsis. As regards the mechanism of globality, i.e. depth perception in complex patterns, all has so far been conjecture. As stated earlier, globality was taken to mean the property of depth perception, with the aim of by-passing local success and ultimately, within a wider framework, reducing as many disparity stimuli as possible to a common denominator. This property assumes the storage and exchange of local information, with suppression of intrusive signals of a secondary nature. This demands a priori two mechanisms: binocular cells with neighbouring receptive fields must facilitate each other if their disparity tuning is virtually the same; conversely, they must inhibit each other if the disparity tuning differs significantly.

Here we find ourselves in the realm of hypothesis. It is clear that only now are we beginning to obtain a physiological insight into the most elementary aspects of stereopsis.

V. *Motor aspects of binocular vision*

Binocular vision imposes two demands on the motor system:

1. The movements of gaze must be of the same magnitude in both eyes in order to move the lines of gaze from a point on the horopter to another point. To meet this requirement, the two eyes are equally innervated during the movements of gaze.
2. If the fixation distance changes, or if the muscular balance is disturbed, the eye position must be adjusted by a disjunctive movement which is made in one direction in one eye and in the opposite direction in the other. This is described as "motor fusion" to distinguish it from the sensory fusion referred to on page 59. The eyes can perform horizontal, vertical and torsional fusion movements. The amplitude of these movements is only a few degrees, except in the convergent direction, in which it may be as much as 30°. Fusional movements are slow; in the vertical direction the rate may be less than half a degree per second.

Convergence is a disjunctive movement which occupies a place of its own, and not only by reason of its large amplitude: it is the only disjunctive movement which can be effected voluntarily; moreover, it forms part of the "proximity synkinesis", which comprises convergence, miosis and accommodation. If one regards convergence as a phenomenon separate from fusional movements in the strict sense of the term, one must allow for the possibility that there are two types of disjunctive movement in the convergent direction—a fusional convergence sensu strictiori and a "synkinetic convergence". The stimulus to disjunctive movements is disparity. Bitemporal disparity of the retinal stimuli produces convergence; binasal disparity results in divergence (fig. 13). In general, fusional movements do not cancel out the whole of the disparity; a small residue (fixation disparity) remains, the magnitude of which increases with the fusional effort required. The space within which fixation disparity can exist without diplopia is the amplitude of sensory fusion. Figure 14 shows the fixation disparity produced by burdening the fusion by the interposition of prisms. In this diagram, the amplitude of the sensory fusion is 30 minutes of arc.

Little is yet known about the neurology of the -versions and the -vergences. As these are eye movements induced by binocular stimuli,

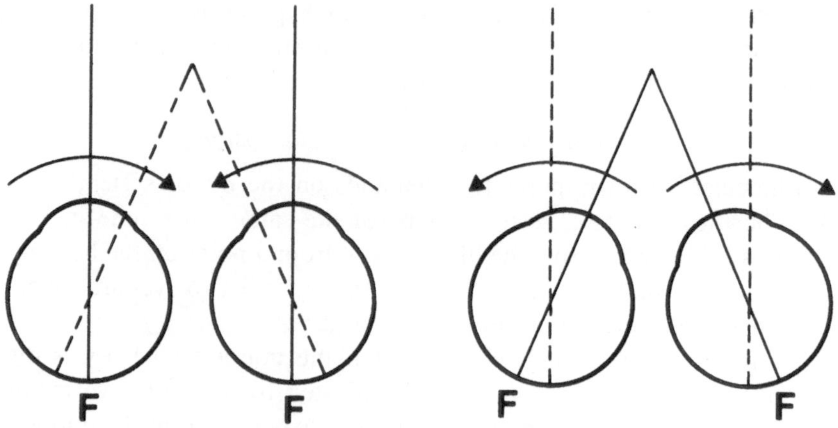

Fig. 13. — Bitemporal (exo-) disparity causes convergence; binasal (eso-) disparity, divergence.

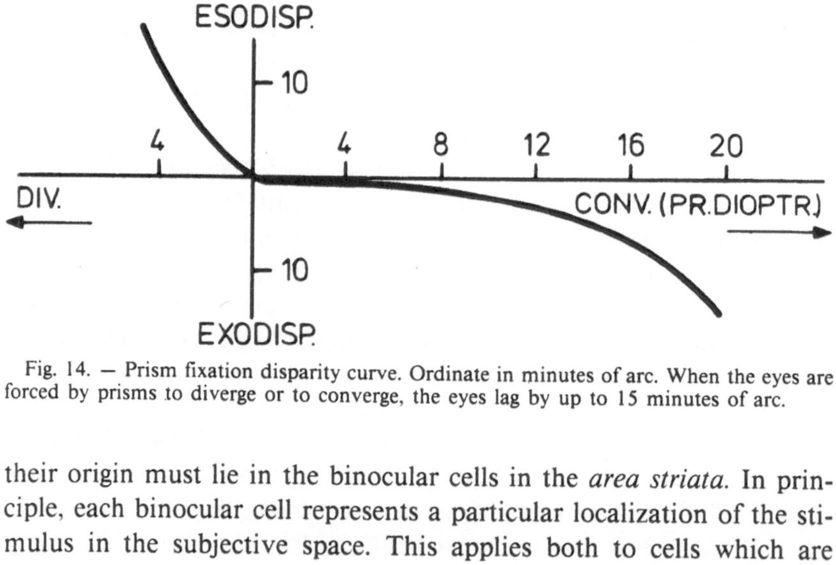

Fig. 14. — Prism fixation disparity curve. Ordinate in minutes of arc. When the eyes are forced by prisms to diverge or to converge, the eyes lag by up to 15 minutes of arc.

their origin must lie in the binocular cells in the *area striata*. In principle, each binocular cell represents a particular localization of the stimulus in the subjective space. This applies both to cells which are innervated by corresponding retinal elements and to the disparity detectors. It is therefore not surprising that the localization of stimuli in front of, or behind, the horopter is binocular (cyclopean) and independent of the monocular localization of the stimuli. Cells whose receptive fields lie at different places on the horopter differ in their directional localization and can—somehow—cause the gaze to move from one receptive field to another. In this, the difference of localization between the receptive fields regulates the degree of movement of the gaze. Cells with differing disparity tuning but identical directional tuning generate pure fusional movements, the magnitude of which again is regulated according to the difference in disparity tuning. Beyond this, the mechanism is not well understood. It is, however, certain that a subtle control mechanism is required for the binocular movements. As far as the nature of the fusion control system and the role of fixation disparity in this are concerned, the last word has not yet been spoken. At the neurological level, too, convergence occupies a separate place. Although the existence of a "centre of motor fusion" has never been demonstrated, it is known that, in the ape, the parieto-occipital lobe of the left hemisphere contains a centre from which, upon stimulation, convergence, accommodation and miosis can be induced (6).

VI. *Diagrammatic representation of binocular vision*

On the basis of the facts set out in the preceding paragraphs, we can now prepare a simple diagram representing normal binocular vision (3). This diagram (fig. 15) can serve as the starting point for others showing disturbances of binocular vision. Shown in the diagram, in descending order, are points in the objective space, the eyes, the optic chiasma, the binocular centre in the visual cortex and, finally, the subjective space with the subjective median plane in the centre.

In the binocular centre, the central representations of the retinae are shown as two layers, represented in cross-section by the lines 0D and 0S. Corresponding points lie directly above one another. F represents the foveae. To the right is the representation of the right half of the retinae, to the left that of the left half. The arrows L (0D) and R (0D) indicate the monocular localization of stimuli which reach the right eye. The line between the representations of the two retinae contains the "binocular cells" which determine the binocular localization, regulate the movements of gaze and, in the case of disparity detectors, generate the fusional movements. In the binocular plane between the two representations, numerous cells are simultaneously concentrated in one place. The point midway between F,F is a binocular cell with zero disparity and a receptive field "straight ahead". Also situated there is the binocular cell 1,1, of which the receptive field is also "straight ahead", but nearer. In motor terms, the binocular cell 1,1 causes a fusional movement, or at least is capable of doing so. The binocular cell 3,3 has its receptive field to the right of the subjective median plane and, because the disparity of 3,3 is zero, this is on the horopter. In motor terms, the cell can produce a movement of gaze to the right. The

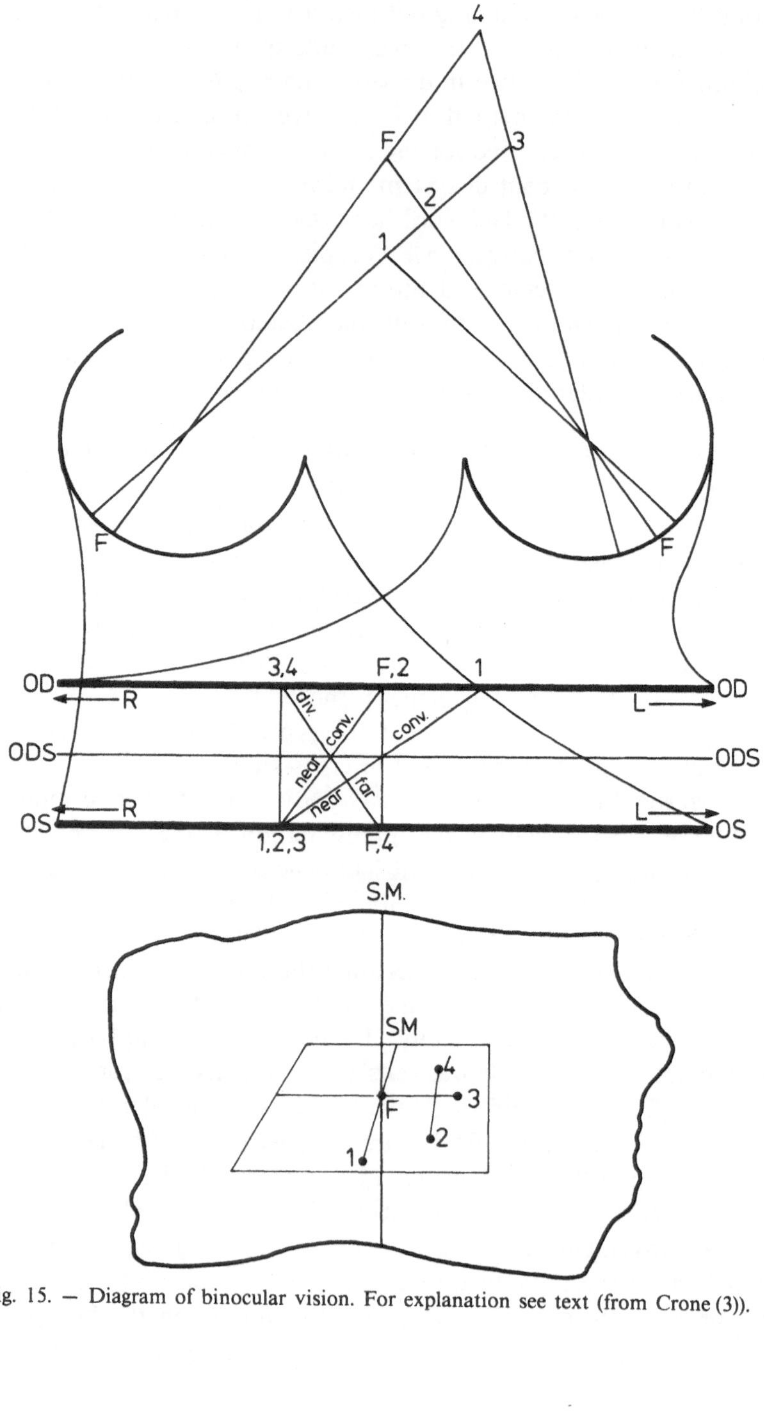

Fig. 15. — Diagram of binocular vision. For explanation see text (from Crone (3)).

receptive field of cell 2,2 lies in front of the horopter and to the right of the fixation point. In motor terms, this cell can produce a convergent movement and, at the same time, a movement of gaze to the right. The convergent movement is less pronounced than that produced by cell 1,1 (the line in the diagram is less oblique) and the movement of gaze is smaller than in the case of cell 3,3 (in the diagram 2,2 is closer to F,F than is 3,3). The localization is accordingly less far to the right than point 3 (cyclopean localization). Cell 4,4 provides the same directional information as cell 2,2 but its receptive field lies behind the horopter and the cell can give rise to a divergent fusional movement. The attention of the reader is drawn to the fact that the diagram is isomorphic in the frontal plane: points which are farther away than F in the horopter plane are farther away than F in the "cortical" diagram. In the depth dimension, however, there is no isomorphism. The degree of disparity is represented by the degree of slope of the binocular connections and not by a linear distance. The situation in the human cerebrum appears to be analogous: the visual cortex contains a retinotopic chart of directions, but no three-dimensional map of the visual space, in which cells with receptive fields behind the horopter would lie deeper in the cortex, or cells with receptive fields in front of the horopter more superficially.

BIBLIOGRAPHY

(1) BISHOP, P.O. — Binocular vision. In: Adler's physiology of the eye: clinical application. 7th ed. (Ed. Moses, R.A.), 575-649, St. Louis, C.V. Mosby, 1981.

(2) BISHOP, P.O. — Stereopsis and the random element in the organization of the striate cortex. *Proc. R. Soc. Lond. B 204*, 1979, 415-434.

(3) CRONE, R.A. — Diplopia. Amsterdam, Excerpta Medica, 1973.

(4) CRONE, R.A., LEURIDAN, O. — Tolerance for aniseikonia I. Diplopia thresholds in the vertical and horizontal meridians of the visual field. *Albrecht v. Graefes Arch. klin. exp. Ophthal.*, 1973, *188*, 1-16.

(5) HUBEL, D.H., WIESEL, T.N. — Sequence regularity and geometry of orientation columns in the monkey striate cortex. *J. Compar. Neurol.*, 1974, *158*, 267-294.

(6) JAMPEL, R.S. — Representation of the near response on the cerebral cortex of the macaque. *Amer. J. Ophthal.*, 1959, *48*, 573-581.

(7) JULESZ, B. — Foundations of cyclopean perception. Chicago, University of Chicago Press, 1971.

(8) MAILLETTE DE BUY WENNIGER-PRICK, L.J.J.M. — Binoculair zien bij microstrabismus. Thesis, Amsterdam, 1981.

(9) OGLE, K.N. — Researches in binocular vision. Philadelphia, W.B. Saunders Comp., 1950.

(10) SHIPLEY, T., RAWLINGS, S.C. — The nonius horopter. *Vision Res.*, 1970, *10*, 1225-1299.

(11) SZENTÁGOTHAI, J. — The local neuronal apparatus of the cerebral cortex. In: Cerebral correlates of conscious experience. Buser, P., Buser, A. (eds.), 131-138. Amsterdam, Elsevier Press, 1978.

(12) WHITTERIDGE, D. — The Bowman lecture 1977: The cortical contribution to binocular vision. *Trans. Ophthal. Soc. U.K.*, 1977, *97*, 39-47.

Bull. Soc. belge Ophtal., **195**, 75-123, 1981.

CHAPTER IV

NEUROMECHANICS OF THE HUMAN PERIPHERAL OCULOMOTOR SYSTEM

H. DE CORTE (*)

Electroneurophysiology, bioengineering and the application of control theory have increased markedly the knowledge of the oculomotor system and have put its study in the realm of exact sciences. As clinicians, interested in the treatment of strabismus and oculomotor disturbances, we have to consider the results of that fundamental research.

The oculomotor system is a control system, the function of which is to acquire visual targets rapidly and, once acquired, to stabilize their images on the retina in spite of relative movements between target and observer (39). There are five types of oculomotor activity: fixation (static condition) and saccades, smooth pursuit, vergence and vestibular eye movements (dynamic conditions).

This chapter deals with the mechanics and neurophysiology of that part of the oculomotor system which is made up by the ocular motor nuclei, their cranial nerves, the oculorotary muscles, the globe and the orbital tissues and which constitutes the final common path for all types of oculomotor activity.

The notion of control (command) implies relationship between two quantities, input and output, realized by a material system, the plant. The plant is controlled by the input which it transforms to output. The input-output relationship is the system's transfer function.

I. *Mechanical elements of the peripheral oculomotor system*

The peripheral oculomotor system is a neuromuscular system having a transfer function between neural activity in the ocular motor nuclei and eye position. The neural activity is transformed into activity of the oculorotary muscles, i.e. contraction which brings eye position about through the mediation of the viscoelastic elements of the oculomotor plant, i.e. the mechanical system suspended and rotated within the

Dr. H. De Corte, Verenigingstraat 39, 1000 Brussel, Belgium.

orbit (globe, extraocular muscles, orbital tissues). The functioning of the peripheral oculomotor system can be expressed in terms of innervation, tension, elasticity, viscosity and hysteresis. The interactions of the forces which mediate the static and dynamic oculomotor performances are represented in mechanical models. Figure 1 shows the model proposed by Collins (1975) (10-12).

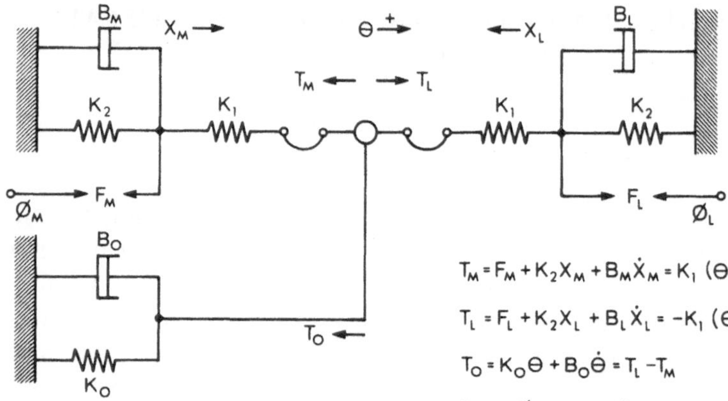

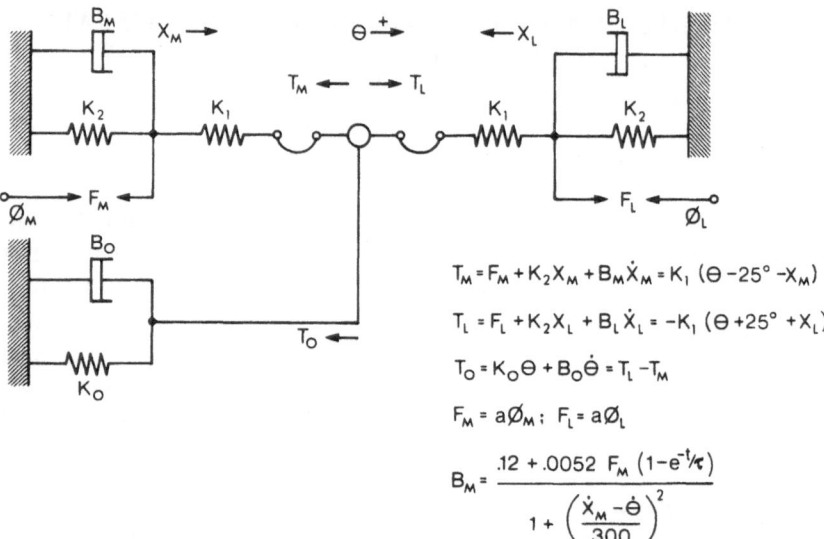

$$T_M = F_M + K_2 X_M + B_M \dot{X}_M = K_1 (\theta - 25^\circ - X_M)$$

$$T_L = F_L + K_2 X_L + B_L \dot{X}_L = -K_1 (\theta + 25^\circ + X_L)$$

$$T_O = K_O \theta + B_O \dot{\theta} = T_L - T_M$$

$$F_M = a\varnothing_M; \quad F_L = a\varnothing_L$$

$$B_M = \frac{.12 + .0052\, F_M (1 - e^{-t/\tau})}{1 + \left(\frac{\dot{X}_M - \dot{\theta}}{300}\right)^2}$$

Fig. 1. — Neuromechanical model of the human peripheral oculomotor system involving the pair of horizontal rectus muscles, and differential equations of motion. From Collins, 1975 (11).

The mass of the globe plays a negligible mechanical role (36-38, 18, 19, 7, 44); this is concluded from the time course of high inertial saccades (fig. 22) (36).

Elasticity (length-tension relationship) enables tissues to develop an amount of tension dependent upon the magnitude of extension, i.e. tissue length, and thus to resist extension (elastic resistance, force). It is represented by a length-tension (LT) curve, the slope $\Delta T/\Delta L$ of which determines, at a given point, the elastic coefficient K or stiffness. A tissue follows Hooke's law when its elasticity is linear (LT curve is a straight line, K is constant). The elasticities to be considered in the oculomotor system are K_1 of the series elastic element of muscle, K_2 of the parallel elastic element of muscle, and Ko (and its elements Ko_1 and Ko_2) of the globe restraining tissues (passive orbital component). An elastic element is represented by a spring with coefficient K expressed in g/deg (degrees of eye rotation as equivalent of tissue length).

Viscosity (force-velocity relationship) enables tissues to develop an amount of shearing stress dependent upon the velocity of internal motion and thus to resist motion (viscous resistance, force). The viscous coefficient B is the ratio of the tangential shearing force per unit area to the velocity gradient perpendicular to the direction of motion. Viscosity has a damping effect; it slows motion in a system, thus minimizing or absorbing shock, and brings the system to rest with minimal or no oscillation. The oculomotor system is heavily damped (36, 6); this is proven by the sluggish return motion of the globe after quick release from passive abduction or adduction (fig. 21). Many characteristics of the dynamic oculomotor performances, especially the very fast (saccades), are based upon viscosity. Two viscosities are to be considered in the oculomotor system: B of the muscle's contractile element,and Bo (and its elements Bo_1 and Bo_2) of the globe restraining tissues. A viscous element is represented by a dashpot with coefficient B expressed in g/deg/sec. A viscoelastic element with conjoint viscous and elastic properties is represented by a Voigt element, i.e. a dashpot in parallel with a spring.

Hysteresis is the retardation of an effect when its causative factor is changed. Plotting the output as a function of the input yields two curves forming a hysteresis loop. The loop of the common forms of physical hysteresis (for instance in magnetism) usually progresses in a counterclockwise direction. The mechanical (LT) characteristics of a rubber band show a clockwise directed hysteresis loop (13). The hysteresis discrepancy which has been demonstrated in the human oculomotor system (11, 13-15) also shows a clockwise progressing loop (fig. 11, 14, 15, 18) and has been described with the term anti- or counterhysteresis (11).

An oculorotary muscle is composed of a contractile element (CE) in series with a series elastic element (SEE). The contractile element consists of two mechanical elements in parallel: the developed tension F (active-state tension) and the viscosity B of the contractile element. In the model of figure 1 the parallel elastic element (PEE) is in parallel with the contractile element and in series with the series elastic element (9, 11, 12). For a long time the PEE was placed, as passive muscle component, in parallel with the CE and the SEE, both latter elements composing the active muscle component (36-39, 18, 7). In the model of figure 1 the globe restraining tissues (passive orbital component, POC) are represented by a Voigt element with elasticity Ko and viscosity Bo; in more detailed models of the POC two Voigt elements (Ko_1, Bo_1 and Ko_2, Bo_2) are in series (8, 9). The elasticities K_1, K_2 and Ko and the viscosities B and Bo are passive forces; the developed tension F is the active force, i.e. induced by innervation.

The input for the oculomotor plant is ϕ, the neural control signal for eye muscle activity. ϕ is a measurable quantity.

ϕ is composed of the action potentials produced by the neurons of an ocular motor nucleus and conducted to the fibers of the corresponding eye muscle. The magnitude of the neural activity of a single motoneuron is determined by the frequency R of its action potentials. R has been measured from electrophysiological recording of single neurons in the ocular motor nuclei of intact, alert, behaving monkeys (23, 47, 40, 32, 33, 52). At the myoneural junction, the neural action potential brings about depolarization which propagates, as muscular action potential, along the sarcolemma and from there into the inner of the muscle fiber. The electrical activity of single fibers of human eye muscles has been recorded by single fiber EMG (50). In the oculomotor system there is an anatomical and functional correspondence between the single motoneurons of a nucleus and the single fibers of the muscle, in a one to one relationship (9, 11). Therefore, single fiber EMG reflects the neural activity of the corresponding motoneuron, and the innervation of the whole muscle, i.e. the neural control signal ϕ, is composed of the neural activity of the simultaneously active single motoneurons of the nucleus. Thus, monitoring the electrical activity of a large statistically valid sample of single fibers in an eye muscle, as made by multiple electrode EMG (16, 9-12), permits sampling of the neural activity in a cross section of the ocular motor nerve and enables to quantify and qualify ϕ (16). Non-invasive measurement of single muscle innervation is possible by measuring the extended isometric muscle force with the LT forceps method (13, 14).

The muscle innervation signal ϕ induces contraction through which active-state tension F is developed. The transformation of ϕ to F occurs with a 8 msec delay due to the excitation—contraction coupling process (40, 45). Contraction is the state of activity of a muscle irrespective of shortening, lengthening or length constancy of the muscle. Contraction takes place in the myofibrils which contain the contractile structures. The contraction mechanism is dealt with in the sliding filament theory and the ratchet theory (28, 29, 25). The contractile element of an eye muscle is considered by most authors as a length-dependent force generator (36-39, 18, 19, 7, 5) in accordance to the well known LT diagrams obtained in classical muscle physiology by experiments in vitro on tetanized striated muscles (e.g. 53, 35, 3); many features of this LT relationship are simply explained by the sliding filament theory (25). Some authors (17, 11) consider the contractile element as primarily length changer rather than tension generator and consider the developed tension F to be determined only by innervation.

In figure 1, X = displacement of CE, $\dot{X}$ = velocity of CE, $\dot{\theta}$ = eye velocity.

The mechanical function of F, the active-state tension developed by the contraction mechanism, is to hold the eye in fixation position and to move it during the various dynamic oculomotor performances. But F acts not directly upon the globe because it is filtered through the elastic and viscous elements of the muscle (K_1, B). Therefore, F can never be measured (36, 11) but only evaluated by calculation and computer analysis (see time course of net active-state tension F_0 of the horizontal recti in saccades, smooth pursuit, vergences; figures 23, 39, 46).

Total muscle tension T is the filtered version of F and thus smaller than F (36, 11). T has been measured in situ in human eye muscles with miniature force transducers implanted in series between muscle tendon and its insertion on the globe; the miniature transducer, consisting of a 2 mm-diameter split ring in which a foil resistance strain gauge is cemented opposite the slit, permits the eye to move normally (8-12,

15). It is the tension T which, pulling on the globe at the scleral tendon insertion, produces the oculomotor effect of the muscle; this is a rotation effect the magnitude of which is given by $M = T \times d$, wherein M is the moment of rotation (torque) of the force T and d is the lever arm (the perpendicular, in the muscle plane, from the globe's rotation center C to the direction of the vector of T).

The total muscle elasticity, the coefficient of which is indicated with Kc, is made up by the elasticities of the series and parallel elastic elements. Kc is the series combination of K_1 and K_2. The relation between Kc, K_1 and K_2 is given by $Kc = K_1 \times K_2/K_1+K_2$ (8, 11).

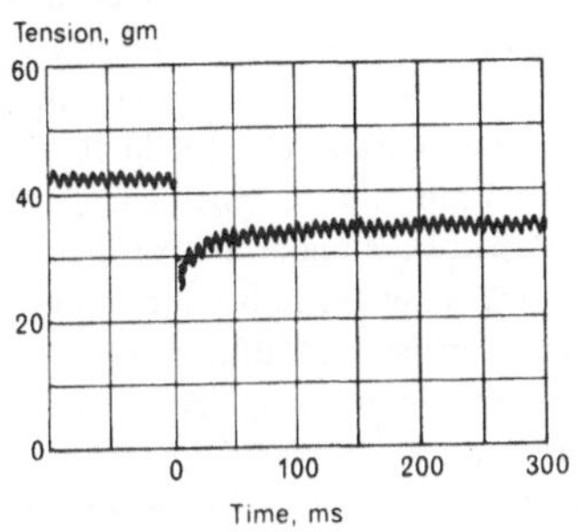

Fig. 2.

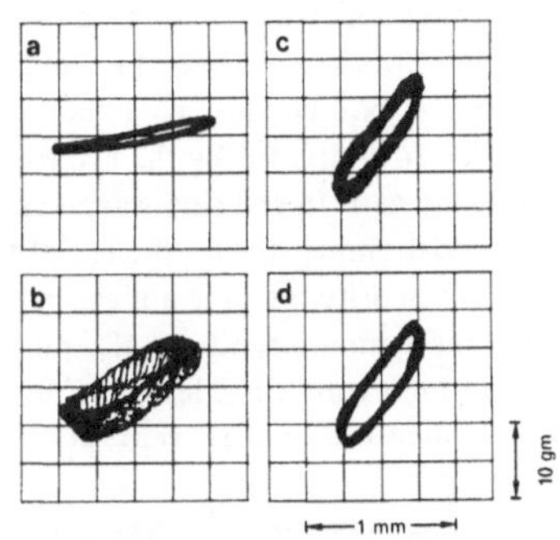

Fig. 3.

Fig. 2. — Time course of tension change in a cat lateral rectus muscle, initially held isometrically at 34 mm and then quickly released by 1 mm to 33 mm and held isometrically.

Fig. 3. — Dynamic LT curves of a cat lateral rectus muscle for various innervation levels. Sinusoidal mechanical oscillations are applied in the length of the muscle, with a fixed frequency of 20 Hz, an amplitude of approximately 1 mm peak to peak centered around primary length, and peak velocity of 300°-600°/sec.

Both experiments in vivo under general anesthesia. The muscle is activated by supramaximal (0.2 ms, 5 V) electrical stimulation of its nerve. In figure 2 the frequency is 150 pulses/sec, in figure 3 the innervation is varied; a: 0 pps (passive muscle); b: 50 pps.; c: 100 pps.; d: 200 pps. (maximal tension). Both figures from Collins, 1971 (8).

The series elastic element (Levin & Wyman, 1927; Hill, 1938; Katz, 1939; Wilkie, 1950) (2, 54) is made up by passive muscular structures which are in spatial succession with the contractile structures and thus stretch during contraction. They reside in part, but probably not entirely, in the tendons (tendon fibers and sarcolemmal endings of the muscle fibers where they attach in the tendons) (53, 54). The SEE is a stiff spring, linear in the physiologic portion of tension changes, and (53, 2, 3) not viscous. It plays an important role as mechanical filter for the tension F developed by the contractile element; it slows the development of total muscle tension T and reduces it (31, 53), thus smoothing out rapid changes in muscle tension (53). During the development of isometric contraction the total muscle length remains constant; nevertheless, length changes occur within the muscle: contraction extends the SEE (internal lengthening) which in turn allows the CE to shorten (internal shortening) (31, 53, 2).

From experiments in vivo on anesthetized cats, K_l of eye muscle was found to be a nonlinear function of innervation and muscle length, and a linear function of muscle tension (8).

This was concluded from 1 mm step quick release and sine wave experiments on lateral rectus muscles at primary length and various innervation magnitudes obtained by graded N VI-stimulation. The initial tension fall in the 1 mm quick release procedure (fig. 2) is due to shortening of the stretched SEE; this tension fall is instantaneous and very fast, proving that the SEE is not viscous. K_l is compiled, as $\Delta T/\Delta L$, from this tension change (in fig. 2; $42-28=14$ g) divided by the eye rotation equivalent of the 1 mm muscle length change (6 deg in the cat). In the sine wave experiment (fig. 3) the slope of the major axis of the LT ellipses determines the coefficient of the elastic element which is not encumbered by a large parallel viscosity, i.e. it is a measure of K_l of the SEE. One sees that this stiffness increases with innervation magnitude. K_l, plotted as a function of nerve stimulus frequency, increases with innervation but levels off to saturation beyond 150 pps. K_l increases linearly with muscle tension and is zero at zero tension. K_l increases nonlinearly with muscle length (8).

It is to be noted that the classical stress-strain curves of the SEE obtained by quick release experiments in vitro on striated muscles from a state of maximum isometric tetanic contraction (53, 54, 2, 3), are not linear in the higher portion of tension range where the SEE stiffness increases and the extensibility decreases (31). Physiologically, however, only the lower portion of the tension range is used and the SEE behaves like a linear spring.

Initially, 1.8 g/deg was used as model parameter value for K_l of human eye muscle (36, 38, 18, 19, 7). Measurements based on the quick stretch technique applied to horizontal recti at surgery, gave a value of approximately 2.5 g/deg for K_l (11).

Tension-time records were made from the detached muscle subjected to 1 mm step quick stretch and held isometrically at the new length. The measurements were done at different initial lengths and innervation magnitudes (performed by fixation with the contralateral eye). An instantaneous and very fast initial tension increase is followed by a slow tension decay to the final isometric value. K_l is calculated, as $\Delta T/\Delta L$, from the initial tension change divided by the eye rotation equivalent of the 1 mm muscle length change (11).

The parallel elastic element is made up by passive muscular structures which parallel the contractile structures: perimysium, endomysium, sarcolemma, sarcoplasmic reticulum, the nerves and blood vessels within the muscle (39). The PEE structures shorten with muscle shortening; they stretch with muscle stretching beyond a certain length, then exerting force upon the globe.

From experiments in vivo on anesthetized cats, K_2 of eye muscle was found to be a nonlinear function of innervation and muscle length, and a linear function of muscle tension (8).

K_2 can be computed from $K_2 = K_1 \times Kc/K_1 - Kc$ when K_1 and Kc are known. K_1 can be calculated from quick release, quick stretch and sine wave experiments. Kc is given by the slope of the static isometric LT curves (see below) and can also be compiled from quick stretch and quick release procedures. For instance, in figure 2 where the initial tension fall is followed by a slow tension rise to the final isometric value, the difference between initial and final tension is determined by the series combination of the SEE and PEE; thus, Kc is given by this final tension difference (in fig. 2; 42 − 34 = 8 g) divided by the eye rotation equivalent of the 1 mm muscle length change. K_2, plotted as a function of nerve stimulus frequency, increases with innervation but levels off to saturation beyond 150 pps. K_2 increases linearly with muscle tension and is zero at zero tension. K_2 increases nonlinearly with muscle length (8).

The value of K_2 of human eye muscle has been compiled as about 1.2 g/deg from $K_2 = K_1 \times Kc/K_1 - Kc$ where K_1 is about 2.5 g/deg (value obtained by quick stretch technique at surgery) and Kc is about 0.8 g/deg (given by the slope of the static isometric length-tension curves above 10 g; see below) (11).

Kc can also be compiled from the 1 mm quick stretch procedure; it is given, as $\Delta T/\Delta L$, by the final tension difference divided by the eye rotation equivalent of the 1 mm muscle length change (11).

Previously, 0.75 g/deg (19) and 0.36 g/deg (7) have been used as model parameter value for K_2 of human eye muscle.

The length-tension-innervation relationship of the human oculorotary muscle is exactly known (46, 17, 8, 15, 11). Fig. 4 and 5 represent a family of static isometric length-tension curves for various gaze innervation magnitudes. One sees that the static isometric tension varies from zero to 120 g, depending on muscle length and innervation. The fully innervated muscle has a tension of 40 g when it is under physiologically full contraction length and 120 g under physiologically full extension length (15,11). Below about 10 g the LT curves are nonlinear; they bend to zero tension indicating muscle slack (17, 8, 15, 11). Physiologically, in the awake condition, an oculorotary muscle never slacks (see: operational envelope); its tension never falls below the level at which the LT curves become nonlinear (8-12, 15-16). Above about 10 g the LT curves are parallel straight lines; the human eye muscle, under constant innervation, behaves like a linear spring (46, 17, 8, 15), following Hooke's law. Innervation change simply shifts the LT curves horizontally in a parallel manner along the length axis of the diagram (17, 11). The slope of the straight lines determines the value of Kc, the total muscle elasticity above about 10 g tension; Kc is constant and approxi-

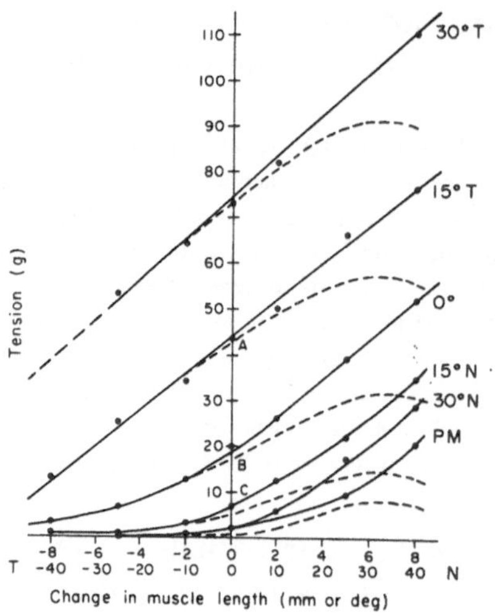

Fig. 4.

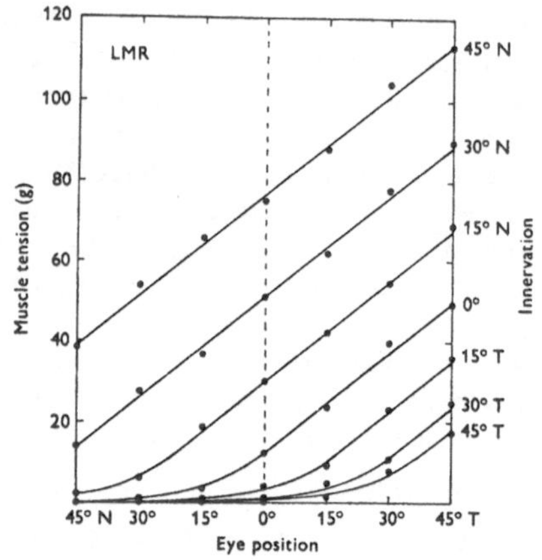

Fig. 5.

Fig. 4. — Family of static isometric length-tension curves of a lateral rectus muscle for various innervation levels. Tension measured with strain gauge force transducer connected to the detached muscle. From Robinson, O'Meara, Scott, Collins, 1969 (46).

Fig. 5. — Family of static isometric length-tension curves of a medial rectus muscle under various innervation. Tension measured with both implanted miniature force transducer and external strain gauge. The curves are means from measurements on 4 subjects (2 medial recti, 2 lateral recti). From Collins, O'Meara, Scott, 1975 (15).

The measurements were made under topical anesthesia on awake adult strabismus patients (most having intermittent exotropia) as an addition to required surgery. The eye under experiment is occluded. The studied muscle is fixed isometrically: in figure 4 the muscle is held by the strain gauge force transducer, in figure 5 the eye is held fixed by a restraining suture attached between the globe and the external strain gauge. The subject is requested to fixate with his unrestrained eye successively, for 4 sec, each of 7 targets spaced 15° apart between 45° L and 45° R. This is repeated for each of 7 fixed muscle lengths between 9 mm longer and 9 mm shorter than primary length (in figure 5 for each of the 7 positions in which the examined eye is to be held isometrically). Isometric tension is continuously recorded. Its mean value at the end of each of the 4 sec fixation periods constitutes, with the corresponding muscle length (or the equivalent eye position), a LT point of the diagram. On the right ordinate the innervation level is indicated by the position of the fixating contralateral eye temporal (T) or nasal (N) with respect to the tested eye. Below the graph, muscle length change from primary length (0) is given in mm and the equivalent eye position in degrees.

mately 0.8 g/deg at each point of the LT diagram above 10 g (15, 11). The bottom curve of the diagram, obtained when the contralateral eye fixates maximally out of the action field of the tested muscle, is considered as the LT curve of the passive muscle; it is the same curve as the one obtained from the muscle in general anesthesia (46, 17, 8, 48, 51, 15).

By subtracting this passive LT curve from each of the active-state LT curves, one obtains the LT curves of the active muscle component for various innervation levels (dashed lines in fig. 4). These curves rise to a peak and then fall, as expected from sliding filament theory.

The peak of each curve corresponds to the same muscle length Lp+6.5 mm. This is the value of Lo, the muscle length at which the contractile element produces maximum (i.e. peak) active-state tension F for any innervation level. Lo is inherently determined by the sliding filament mechanism (touching of the ends of the actin filaments at the sarcomere center, maximum actin-myosin overlap, maximal number of adequately acting cross-bridges). Lo = Lp+6.5 mm means that Lo of a human eye muscle corresponds to about 32 degrees out of its action field (46, 15). This implies that the muscle works over a length range from 1.07 Lo to 0.65 Lo, i.e. at lengths less than Lo for the greatest part of eye movement range (46).

Collins explained the configuration of the LT diagram by placing the parallel elastic element in parallel only with the contractile element, considering the muscle elasticity as the series combination of K_1 and K_2 (11), and by the notion that the contractile element is primarily length changer rather than tension generator (the CE varying its length upon innervation, as the square of linear innervation magnitude) (17, 11), and by the notion that the developed tension F is determined only by innervation (11).

In this way, Collins' analog computer model (fig. 1) duplicates the experimentally observed family of LT curves. With increasing levels of constant innervation producing constant levels of developed tension F, the model translates the passive-state LT curve, which reflects the series addition $K_1 \times K_2/K_1 + K_2$, leftwards along the diagram's length axis (11); the separation between two different innervated LT curves is determined by the contractile element length change corresponding to the innervation change (17). With increasing levels of constant innervation the PEE shortens and the LT curves start from shorter lengths. The nonlinearity in the LT diagram is due to the nonlinear PEE (K_2 becomes zero with muscle shortening and increases with lengthening).

Muscle viscosity B, due to the properties of the contractile proteins (53), constitutes a resistance to motion, in both directions, whithin the contractile structures, thus limiting the shortening and lengthening velocity of the contractile element. With the series elastic element, B plays a role in the gradual rise of total muscle tension T. B determines the force-velocity relationship of the muscle. In classical muscle physiology this relation has been investigated by isotonic experiments in vitro on striated muscles from a state of maximum isometric tetanic contraction (e.g. 31, 53, 35, 3). The well known hyperbolic form of the force-velocity function (Fenn and Marsh, 1935; Hill, 1938) shows that muscle viscosity is nonlinear. Muscle viscosity was found to be inconstant, varying nonlinearly with velocity, being proportional to tension, and decreasing with increasing velocity (Hill, 1938) (18, 19, 8, 7). Muscle viscosity is asymmetrical, depending upon the direction of motion in the contractile structures; lengthening velocities are smaller than shortening velocities (31).

Eye muscle viscosity, investigated by experiments in vivo on anesthetized cats, was found to be a nonlinear function of innervation and muscle length, and a linear function of muscle tension; it was found to be Newtonian for low velocities of motion, and to present the phenomenon of thixotropy (8).

B was compiled from 1 mm quick release and sine wave experiments on lateral rectus muscles. In figure 3 the area within the LT ellipses is a measurement of the energy dissipated per cycle of sinusoidal oscillation due to the muscle's viscous resistance; B is also given by half the minor ellipse axis (the vertical separation of the two curves of the LT ellipse at its center) divided by the peak velocity of the sinusoidal oscillation. One sees from the ellipse area and minor axis that the viscosity increases with innervation magnitude. In the 1 mm step quick release experiments (fig. 2) B is calculated from $\tau = B/K$ where τ is the time constant (to 63% of the final value) of the slow tension rise to the final isometric value; the stiffness Kc is calculated as $\Delta T/\Delta L$ from the final tension difference. B, plotted as a function of nerve stimulus frequency, increases with innervation but levels off to saturation above 100 pps. B increases linearly with muscle tension and is zero at zero tension. B increases nonlinearly with muscle length (8).

B can also be compiled from the dynamic LT curves obtained by muscle stretch at various ramp (i.e. constant) velocities from 0.2 to 100 mm/sec under various constant innervation levels obtained by graded nerve stimulation (8). The tension required to extend a muscle at higher velocities is greater due to muscle viscosity. Subtracting static tension (0.2 mm/sec velocity) from dynamic tension gives the viscous force; B is derived by dividing the viscous force by the corresponding velocity. Plotting viscous force and B as a function of extension velocity shows that for low velocities up to 30°/sec (range of following movements) the muscle's viscosity is Newtonian (8), i.e. the viscous resistance varies linearly with velocity and B remains constant, independent of velocity; this is found for any constant innervation level. Above 30°/sec the viscous force and B decrease progressively with increased velocity, B falling off to 20% of its static value at 600°/sec (saccadic velocity). This decrease of viscosity with increased velocity is thixotropy which facilitates fast movements (saccades) with less energy expenditure (8).

Human eye muscle viscosity has been measured at surgery with the quick stretch method applied to horizontal recti at various length and innervation (11).

In the 1 mm step quick stretch procedure B is compiled from $\tau = B/K$ where τ is the time constant of the slow tension decay to the final isometric value and the stiffness Kc is calculated as $\Delta T/\Delta L$ from the final tension difference. Least spread of all data was obtained by plotting B against muscle tension (0 to 55 g), whether derived from innervation or stretch. This plot shows a value of B of 0.03, 0.13 and 0.4 g/deg/sec for a muscle tension value of zero, 10 and 55 g respectively (11). Previously, 0.036 g.sec/deg was used as model parameter value of B (36, 38), Some models (19, 7) include the nonlinear asymmetric characteristics of B. See in fig. 1 an equation for B (11).

The ratio B/K of viscosity to elasticity has a time dimension and is a mechanical time constant: $\tau = B/K$. Although both B and K vary widely with muscle length and tension over the normal range of eye movements, τ remains constant since B and K vary in parallel fashion, linearly with tension (8).

A time constant characterizes the velocity and duration of a transient state and is usually expressed by the time at which the response obtains 2/3 of its final value; the response time (duration of the transient state) is about 3 times the time constant.

Oculomotor model performance plays a valuable role in the quantitative study of the variation of human eye muscle viscosity during the various dynamic conditions, for example during saccades (11).

The passive orbital component (POC) is the mechanical component due to the passive tissues of the orbit, except those of the oculorotary muscles, which viscoelastically exert force upon the globe (globe restraining tissues). The checkligaments, the intermuscular membrane and annular ligament, the connections of the outer layers of Tenon's capsule with the meshwork of the surrounding fat tissue, have a restraining action upon the globe; the optic nerve and the shear in Tenon's capsule are considered to be major factors of POC viscosity (39).

To investigate the mechanical properties of the globe restraining tissues in the horizontal plane, both horizontal rectus muscles are detached from the globe (horizontally isolated eye). The static length-tension relationship of the globe restraining tissues is shown in figure 6. One sees that the elasticity of the POC is linear up to 30° of eye rotation with an elastic coefficient Ko of about 0.5 g/deg; beyond 30° Ko increases, the elasticity becomes slightly nonlinear (46, 17, 48, 51, 8).

Step quick release experiments demonstrate that the POC is not a single viscoelastic element but consists of a fast and slow element which can be represented by two Voigt elements (Ko_1, Bo_1 and Ko_2, Bo_2) in series (8, 9, 48).

An isolated globe, pulled into an eccentric position and then suddenly released, returns towards the primary position due to the viscoelastic force of the extended passive orbital tissues (39, 8). The time course of this movement consists of two phases which differ in time constant and amplitude (fig. 7). Ko_1 and Ko_2 are calculated as $\Delta T/\Delta L$. Bo_1 and Bo_2 are calculated from $\tau o_1 = Bo_1/Ko_1$ and $\tau o_2 = Bo_2/Ko_2$. The stiffness Ko of the POC, given by the LT slope (fig. 6), is the series addition of Ko_1 and Ko_2. $Ko = Ko_1 \times Ko_2/Ko_1 + Ko_2$ (8).

In the model of figure 1 the globe restraining tissues are represented by a single (Ko, Bo) instead of two Voigt elements. Ko, about 0.5 g/deg, is predominantly linear and therefore expressed in simple linear terms. The value of τ_0, the mean time constant, is taken as 120 msec. Bo, calculated from $\tau_0 = Bo/Ko$, is about 0.06 g/deg/sec (11). (Previously,

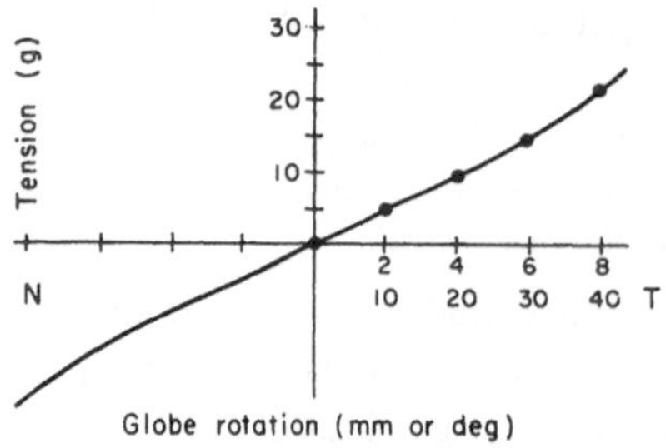

Fig. 6.

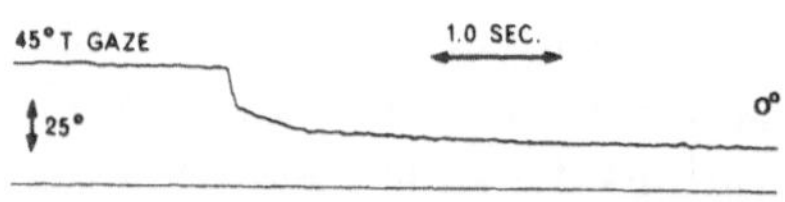

Fig. 7.

Fig. 6. — Static length-tension relationship of the globe restraining tissues. The upper right quadrant contains experimental data for temporal rotation, the curve in the lower left quadrant assumes symmetry of elasticity for nasal rotation. Measurement on patient with intermittent exotropia under general anesthesia. Both horizontal recti are detached from the globe. A force measuring strain gauge (attached to a micromanipulator to permit controlled displacement of strain gauge and tissue) is connected to the globe at the insertion of the detached muscle via a suture running tangentially to the globe. The eye is pulled temporally in increments up to 40° and the pulling force is recorded as a function of displacement. From Robinson, O'Meara, Scott, Collins, 1969 (46).

Fig. 7. — Time course of the return movement of a horizontally isolated eye towards primary position, as response to quick release from 45° temporal rotation. Measurement under general anesthesia. Time course of eye movement recorded by means of a photoelectric eye position indicator. The 45° temporal rotation required 30 g force. The fast phase with 0.02 sec time constant and 27° amplitude is followed by a slow phase of 1 sec time constant and 18° amplitude. From Collins, 1971 (8).

0.018 g . sec/deg was used as model parameter value for Bo (18, 19, 7)).

From sine wave, quick release and ramp displacement experiments on the horizontally isolated globe of anesthetized cats, it was found that Ko, Ko_1, Ko_2 and Bo are nonlinear functions of eye rotation (and orbital tissue length) and linear functions of To, the tension of the globe restraining tissues (8).

II. *Fixation*

Fixation is the oculomotor activity which holds the eye steadily directed upon a stationary visual target in order to ensure maximal vision of it.

Recording of the neural activity of single ocular motoneurons of monkeys (23, 40, 47, 32, 45, 33) reveals that for any fixation position θ the discharge frequency R of a motoneuron is quite constant and repeatable by refixation; the variability of R is only about 6% of the mean rate (40, 45, 33, 42, 44). Each motoneuron has a constant R (θ) relationship which is linear (23, 32, 33, 40-45, 47, 52) and determined by a threshold θ_T and a position parameter k (fig. 8). The motoneurons of a nucleus differ greatly in θ_T and k. About 16% of the units have no

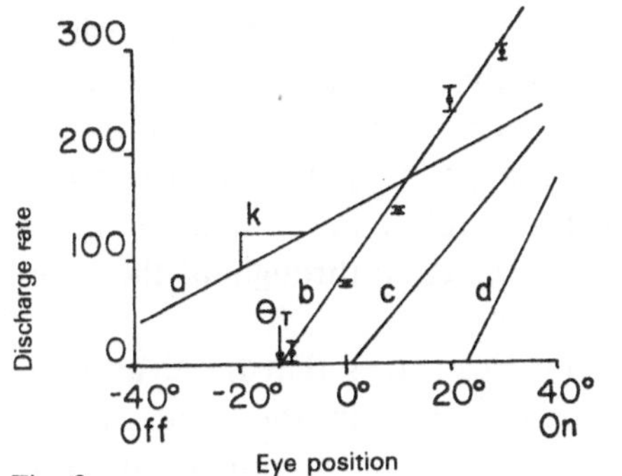

Fig. 8.

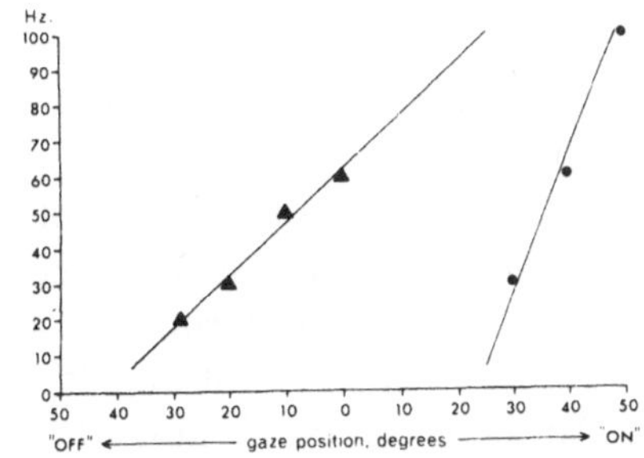

Fig. 9.

Fig. 8. — Discharge frequency — eye position relationship of single motoneurons of monkeys. The intersection of the R(θ) line with the zero frequency axis determines the threshold, i.e. the eye position at which the motoneuron is first recruited into activity. The slope of R(θ) determines the position parameter k expressing, in (spikes/sec)/deg, the rate of change in discharge frequency with change in eye position. From Robinson and Keller, 1972 (45).

Fig. 9. — Discharge frequency — eye position relationship of two single fibers of a human left lateral rectus muscle (single fiber EMG). From Scott and Collins, 1973 (50).

threshold ($\theta_T < -45°$) and thus never cease firing in the awake condition (40, 45). The θ_T values of the remaining units are quite uniformly distributed between $-45°$ and $+25°$ (40, 47, 24, 45). No motoneurons were found with a threshold value beyond $+25°$ (40, 47, 45, 33). The coefficient k has a unimodal and broad distribution ranging from 1.1 to 14.5 (spikes/sec)/deg with a population mean of 4 (45, 33, 44). By their difference in threshold the motoneurons of a nucleus form a spectrum which is continuous (41). Generally high threshold units appear to have steeper slopes k (40,24). The lower threshold neurons are assumed to be of smaller diameter (40).

The increase of neural activity in a motor nucleus as fixation moves in the on-direction from $-45°$ to $+45°$, occurs by increase of the number of simultaneously active neurons, i.e. by recruitment of the neurons into activity, and by increase of the discharge frequency in each recruited neuron (47, 40, 32, 33, 45), in order to produce increasing muscle force needed to hold the eye at successively larger gaze deviations against the elastic restraining forces of the oculomotor plant (45). The motoneurons are always recruited in a fixed, rank order (44). At the extreme off-position the neural activity is due to the neurons with $\theta_T < -45°$. The recruitment of the other units into the active pool is more or less uniform (40, 24); for each 10° eye position change in the on-direction an additional 11% of the neuron population is recruited (40, 45). Recruitment ceases at +25°; beyond this eye position, increase of muscle force must occur only by further increase of the discharge rate of the neurons (40, 45), especially of the high threshold neurons which, having high k values, change fastly their discharge rate. It is to be noted that a unit, although not active during fixation at eye positions below threshold, is nevertheless active throughout the entire eye position range during saccades (23, 47).

Single fiber EMG of human eye muscles shows that the neuromuscular units of the oculomotor system behave in the same way in humans as in monkeys, except that the discharge rate is lower in humans (50). Each muscle fiber has a constant discharge frequency-eye position relationship (fig. 9) which is linear and characterized by a threshold and a position parameter. The fibers differ widely in both parameters;they form a continuous spectrum. Low threshold fibers which recruit earlier are situated in the superficial muscle layers and increase slowly their activity with gaze change in the on-direction (low slope); high threshold fibers which recruit later are in the deeper muscle layers and increase their activity more rapidly (steep slope) (50).

The neural control signal for fixation to single eye muscles has been recorded by multiple electrode EMG (16, 9-12). The relationship between fixation innervation and fixation position is nonlinear (11); the static $\phi(\theta)$ transfer function is a power function, predominantly parabolic (fig. 10 and 11). This nonlinearity, observed in both small and large fiber populations, is due to the fact that during recruitment motoneurons with increasing values of θ_T and k come into action and that the units, after completion of recruitment, continue to increase their discharge rate as fixation moves further in the on-direction.

The relative contribution of the small (superficial, outer) fibers and the large (deeper) fibers to fixation is seen in figures 10 and 12 (11, 16).

In fixation activity the small fibers play the predominant role. The large fibers have no fixation activity in the off-field, whereas the small fiber group exhibit activity even at extreme off-position. In the extreme on-position the contribution of the small fibers, being maximally active (having their maximal activity as in saccades) (fig. 10), is 1/3 of the potential maximal (saccadic) activity of the total muscle (fig. 12); the contribution of the large fibers, having about half their maximal (saccadic) activity, is also 1/3 of the potential maximal activity of the total muscle. Thus, in fixation at extreme on-position 1/3 of the muscle's capability remains unused. It is to be noted (fig. 10) that near extreme

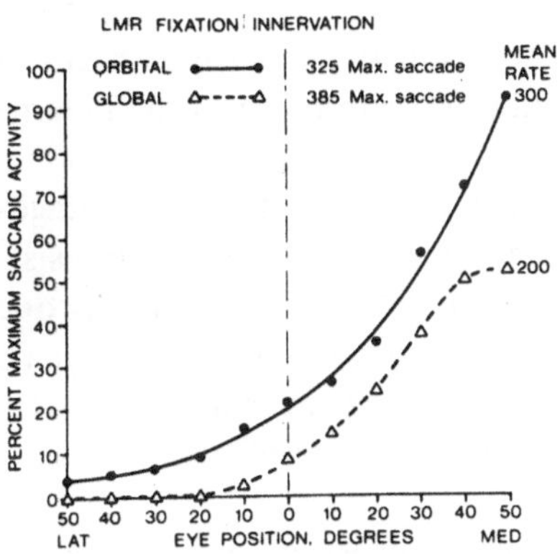

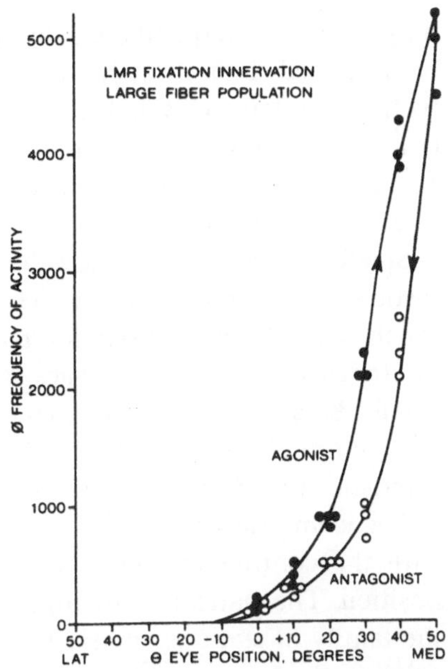

Fig. 10.

Fig. 11.

Fig. 10. — Fixation innervation of the small (orbital) and large (global) fiber population of a left medial rectus muscle, as a function of eye position. Multiple electrode EMG. The activity of each fiber group is expressed in % of maximum saccadic activity (the mean EMG frequency of each fiber type is compared to the maximum frequency of the type during saccades).

Fig. 11. — Fixation innervation of the large fiber population of a left medial rectus muscle acting first as agonist and then as antagonist, as a function of eye position. Multiple electrode EMG. Innervation is expressed in EMG frequency. Note the neural antihysteresis. Both figures from Collins, 1975 (11).

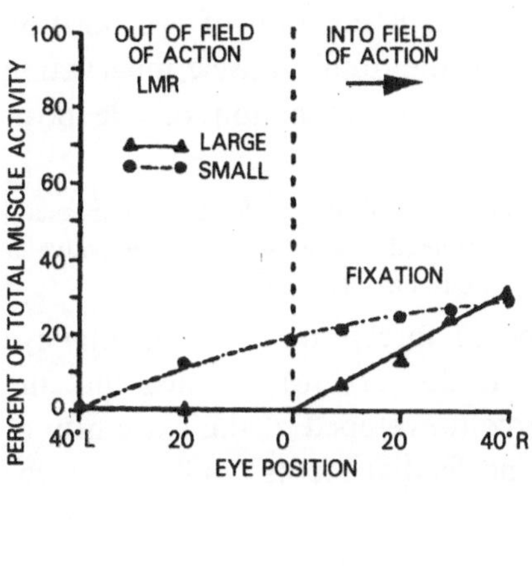

Fig. 12. — Fixation innervation of the small and large fiber population of a left medial rectus muscle, as a function of eye position. Multiple electrode EMG. The activity of each fiber group is expressed in % of total muscle activity (EMG activity of each group is compared to the potential maximal EMG activity of the total muscle during saccades). From Collins and Scott, 1973 (16).

on-position the large fibers exhibit saturation suggesting their fatiguing by sustained fixation at the extremity of the muscle's action field. In fixation the large to small fiber activity ratio varies progressively from 0:1 at extreme gaze out of the muscle's action field to a maximum of 1:1 at extreme gaze into the action field (there are twice as many large fibers as small) (16, 11).

Small fiber activity outside the muscle's action field has an antagonistic and tonic effect (16, 11). The antagonistic effect consists in resisting the agonist muscle; fixation tension of an antagonist is not only due to stretch of its passive tissues but also to contraction activity of its small fibers. The tonic effect consists in avoiding mechanical slack of the eye muscles so that they work in the linear region of their LT characteristics (fig. 4, 5) (8-12, 15, 16).

The isometric force of a single eye muscle, measured during fixation with the contralateral eye, is a nonlinear, parabolic function of eye position. The static T isom. (θ) transfer function has been derived from the family of static isometric LT curves obtained with invasive measuring methods at surgery (fig. 13) (17, 8). The more recent method with the LT forceps permits automatic graphical display of the T isom. (θ) function of single eye muscles of the intact eye (fig. 14, 15) (11, 13, 14).

During fixation of a target at extreme gaze out of the action field of the studied muscle, the studied eye is grasped with the LT forceps and held rigidly at that extreme position. The subject fixates with his contralateral eye a series of targets of known positions (or tracks a target moving at slow, 10°/sec velocity) from the extremity of the out-field to the extremity of the action field of the studied muscle. In this test the studied muscle is fully stretched and its antagonist is relaxed to slack length and zero tension level. Thus, the forceps measures the isometric tension of a fully extended single muscle. This tension is displayed on a XY oscilloscope or XY plotter as a function of the EOG recorded contralateral eye position (13, 14).

The extended isometric muscle force as a function of eye position (fig. 14) is quantitatively proportional to the (total) muscle innervation determined by multiple electrode EMG as a function of eye position (11, 13, 14).

Therefore, the extended isometric force measurement with the LT forceps is a measurement of single muscle innervation and has been proposed as a non-invasive alternative or supplement and even substitute for multiple electrode EMG (13, 14).

Active force measurements with the LT forceps on the horizontal eye muscles of 29 orthophoric subjects (18-33 yrs) (14) revealed that the mean of the maximum isometric force (developed at the extremity of the action field) is 26% greater for the medial rectus (74.8 g) than for

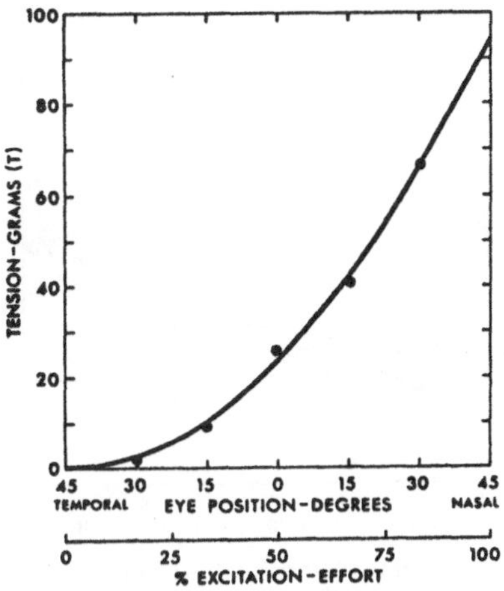

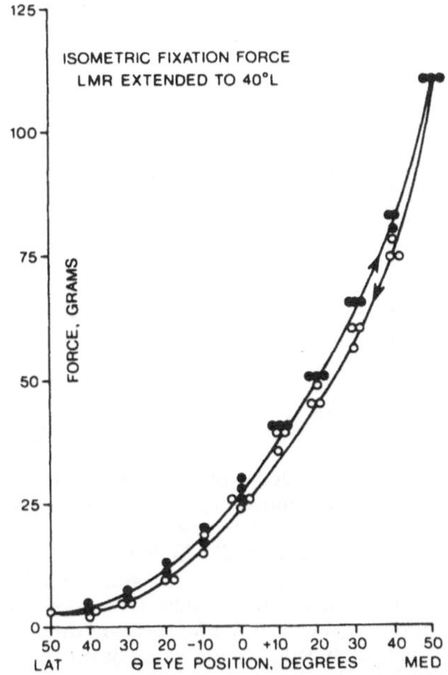

Fig. 13.

Fig. 14.

Fig. 13. — Transfer function relating isometric muscle force to its corresponding gaze innervation (i.e. to the contralateral eye fixation position) for a right medial rectus muscle extended at Lp+2 mm. Derived from the muscle's family of static isometric LT curves obtained with invasive measurement method (strain gauge force transducer connected to the detached muscle). The intersection of the vertical line at a given muscle length (here Lp+2 mm) with the different LT curves indicates the isometric tensions produced by different innervation magnitudes corresponding to the contralateral eye fixation positions (Hering's law). Plotting the obtained tensions against these fixation positions gives the static T isom. (θ) transfer function. The innervation is expressed as linear innervation (gaze innervation in % of its maximum) given by the fixation position (here of the contralateral eye) in degrees from the extreme position out of the muscle's action field divided by the total extent of eye position range. From Collins, Scott, O'Meara, 1969 (17).

Fig. 14. — Record of the isometric force of a 40° extended left medial rectus muscle as a function of the contralateral eye position. Measurement with the LT forceps method, the RE tracking smoothly a target from 50° L to 50° R and return. The difference between the two curves is due to residual antihysteresis. From Collins, 1975 (11).

the lateral rectus (59.1 g). The individual variation of the maximum isometric force was 2 to 1 (45-103 g; 48-103 g for MR, 45-92 g for LR). A maximum isometric tension less than 45 g suggests paresis. An eye muscle exerts up to 25% of its maximum isometric tension outside its action field and only 25-30% in the primary position. The zero net force position at which the active isometric forces of the medial and lateral rectus are equally balanced was found to be not the primary position but 12°-15° temporally (14).

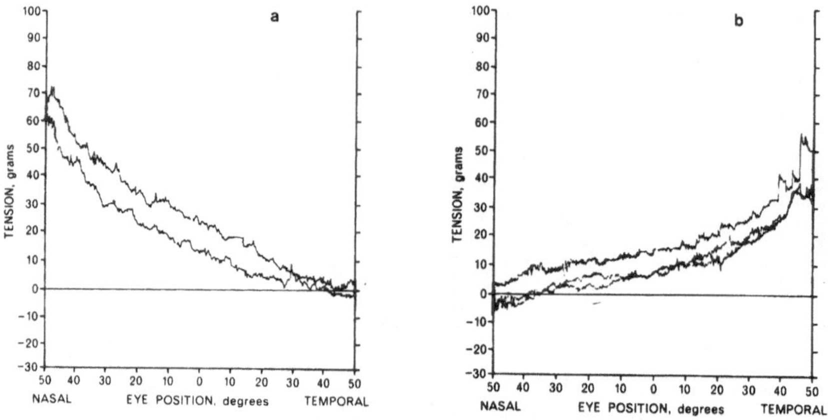

Fig. 15. — Record of the isometric force of a 50° extended left medial (a) and lateral (b) rectus muscle during agonist (upper curves) and antagonist (lower curves) activity, as a function of contralateral eye position. Measurement with the LT forceps method on an orthophoric subject; the RE is tracking a target at 10°/sec ramp velocity. In (a) one cycle of activity is recorded, in (b) one and one half cycle. The transient peaks to 73 g (a) and 55 g (b) are associated with saccadic refixation. The tension difference between upper and lower curves is related to the innervation direction and becomes greater with increased velocity; at very slow velocity the value of muscle force antihysteresis, applied by neural antihysteresis, can be determined. From Collins, Carlson, Scott, Jampolsky, 1981 (14).

The relationship between fixation tension of a single eye muscle and fixation position of the eye, T fix. (θ), is a nonlinear function, the roughly parabolic shape of which is called static locus (fixation tension curve) (8-12, 15). The static locus has been derived from the family of static isometric LT curves obtained by isometric measurements with a strain gauge attached to the muscle (8) (fig. 16) or with implanted miniature force transducers (15) (fig. 17). The actual fixation tensions measured in unrestrained muscles of freely moving eyes by means of implanted miniature force transducers and graphically displayed as a function of the position of the fixating measured eye (15), are the same as the isometrically measured fixation tensions (fig. 17). Despite individual variation the same parabolic characteristic of T fix. (θ) was found. Maximum fixation tension, at the extremity of the action field, ranged from 28 to 44 g; the minimum fixation tension, occuring at 15° out of the action field, ranged from 8 to 12 g; at the extremity out of the action field the tension ranged from 15 to 19 g, being about 7 g higher than at 15° out of the action field. The upward slope in the muscle's action field mirrors the T isom. (θ) function; the lesser upward slope from 15° out of the action field to the extremity of this field is due to stretch of the passive tissues in the maximally extended muscle (15, 11).

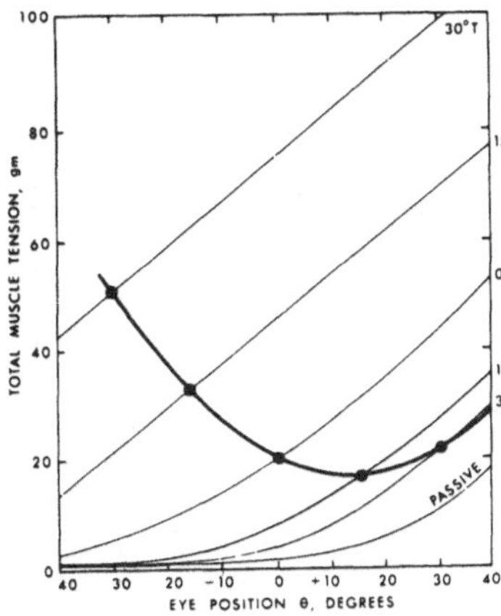

Fig. 16.

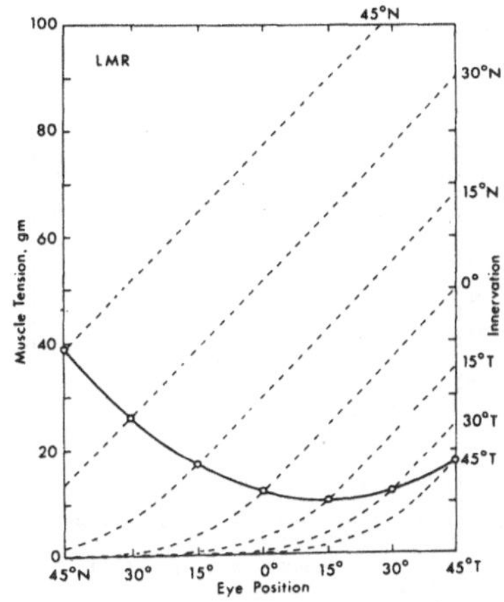

Fig. 17.

Fig. 16. — Static locus of a lateral rectus muscle, derived from the family of static isometric LT curves (lines in the background) obtained with invasive measurement method (strain gauge force transducer attached to the desinserted muscle). The intersection of the vertical line at a given eye position (the latter being the rotation equivalent of the muscle length at which the measurement is made) with the LT curve of corresponding innervation (noted, at the right ordinate, as fixation position of the contralateral eye) determines the static tension utilized to hold the eye steady at the given eye position. The line joining the LT points thus determined for various eye positions, constitutes the static locus. From Collins, 1971 (8).

Fig. 17. — Static locus for a typical medial rectus muscle. The dashed lines constitute the family of LT curves obtained by isometric measurements with both implanted miniature force transducer and external strain gauge attached to the globe by a restraining suture. The data are the means from measurements on 4 subjects (2 medial recti, 2 lateral recti). The static locus derived from this LT diagram corresponds to the actual fixation tensions (circles on the static locus) measured with implanted miniature force transducers in unrestrained muscles of the freely moving fixating eye and recorded as a function of the position of that eye. From Collins, 1975 (11).

A muscle has to overcome resisting forces which constitute the muscle load. An oculorotary muscle is loaded by its antagonist and associated passive orbital tissues.

Because the eye is protected by the bony orbit, its rotary muscles, unlike most skeletal muscles, are not subjected to external mechanical forces (40, 32, 45, 44); their load is only due to forces inherent to the oculomotor plant. The mass of the globe plays a negligible role as element of muscle load. Since the passive orbital tissue elasticity is predominantly linear (fig. 6) the major nonlinearity of the load of a single eye muscle is due to the nonlinear characteristic of the antagonist (15, 11).

The orbital load (passive load) is made up by the combined passive tissues, i.e. the passive tissues of muscle and associated globe restraining orbital tissues. It is the load to be overcome by the net active (isometric) muscle force, i.e. the active force difference between both mus-

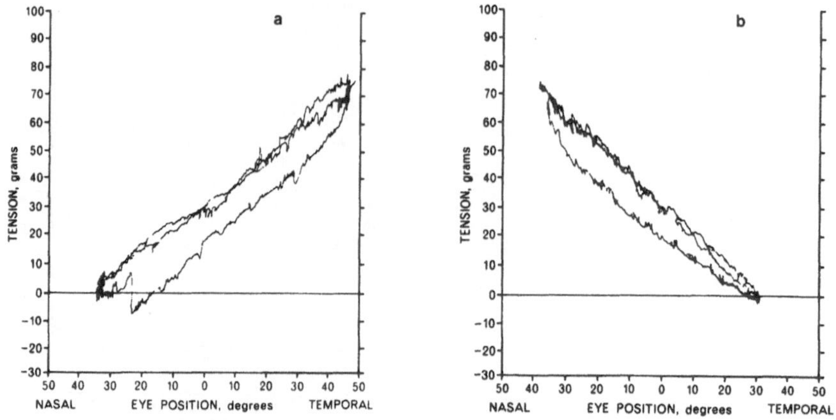

Fig. 18. — Length-tension relationship of the temporal (a) and nasal (b) orbital load, recorded on the left eye of an orthophoric subject during extension (upper curves) and relaxation (lower curves) at 10°/sec. Measurements with microsonar LT forceps method. a: The LE is passively rotated from 30° N to 45° T (extension), then returned to 30° N (relaxation) and again rotated to 45° T, the RE maintaining fixation on a 30° R target. b: the LE is rotated from 30° T to 40° N (extension), returned to 30° T (relaxation) and again rotated to 40° N, the RE maintaining fixation at a 30° L target. Position of the rotated LE is measured with microsonar device. In this subject the average orbital load stiffness for temporal pull (K_T) is 0.86 g/deg, for nasal pull (K_N) 1.1 g/deg. In (a), during the release phase near 20° N, a saccade to the right was attempted. The 10-15 g difference between extension and relaxation phase is due to viscosity and antihysteresis. From Collins, Carlson, Scott, Jampolsky, 1981 (14).

cles of a pair acting in reciprocal innervation, producing a torque reponsible for eye rotation.

The mechanical characteristics of the orbital load have been studied recently in orthophoric subjects with the microsonar-LT forceps method (fig. 18) (13, 14).

The studied eye is rotated passively under constant innervation (the contralateral eye fixates steadily), and the force needed to pull the eye is recorded as a function of eye position measured with the microsonar device. For measuring the temporal load (load for temporal rotation) the subject has to fixate with the contralateral eye a target 30° temporal to that eye such that the studied eye has a 30° nasal position; the studied eye, grasped with the LT forceps at the nasal limbus, is rotated slowly from its initial 30° nasal position to 30° temporal or more, and then returned to the starting position (fig. 18a). Measurement of the nasal load is done in a similar fashion but in mirror imagery (fig. 18b). The measured force changes occur under constant innervation and therefore are essentially elastic in nature which is shown by the constant slope of the LT curves (13, 14).

The slope of the obtained LT curves determines the elastic coefficient or stiffness of the orbital load. K_T, temporal load stiffness, is composed of the elasticity of the medial rectus muscle and associated orbital tissues restraining globe movement in temporal direction. K_N, nasal load stiffness, is the sum of the stiffness of the lateral rectus and the stiffness of the orbital tissues restraining globe movement in nasal direction (14). It is to be noted that orbital load stiffness is independent of active muscle force; the load LT curves for various constant innervations (determined by various fixation positions of the contralateral eye) are parallel, they have the same slope; innervation change simply shifts the LT curves horizontally (48, 51, 13, 14).

Passive force measurements with the microsonar LT forceps method on 29 orthophoric subjects (18-33 yrs) (14) revealed that the LT curves of the orbital load are for the most part linear. In most subjects the load stiffness was asymmetrical; the mean of K_N (1.05 g/deg) was 11% greater than the mean of K_T (0.94 g/deg) suggesting that the medial rectus muscle is stronger than the lateral rectus because it has to overcome a greater orbital load. Individual variation of the load stiffness was 2 to 1 (0.8-1.7 g/deg for K_N; 0.77-1.2 g/deg for K_T). Large load stiffness may be normal if it is balanced by large active muscle force. The mean load stiffness for all the examined subjects was found to be 1 g/deg (14).

Previous measurements with the suction contact lens method yielded a globe stiffness value of 1.2 g/deg for temporal rotation (37, 38, 44), 1.25 g/deg for nasal rotation from 0° to 5° and 0.65 g/deg from 5° to 10° (6), 1.5-1.8 g/deg for temporal rotation from 0° to 30° (51, 48).

Horizontal globe rotation implies motion of the orbital load by the net active force of the horizontal recti.

The temporal load $K_T \times \theta$ (K_T from upper curve fig. 18a) is moved by a net active force, the curve of which is calculated by subtracting the antagonist medial rectus muscle force (lower curve fig. 15a) from the agonist lateral rectus force (upper curve fig. 15b). When the net active force curve coincides exactly with the load LT curve orthophoria exists (14).

Generally the passive muscular tissues contribute about 2/3 and the globe restraining orbital tissues about 1/3 to the orbital load stiffness; the determination of this relative contribution necessitates passive stiffness measurement at surgery before and after horizontal muscle detachment (14).

Fixation innervation, static isometric force and fixational force of single oculorotary muscles are nonlinear functions of the fixational eye position. Nevertheless, the oculomotor system, observed from the outside, is linear; eye position varies linearly with linear innervation. This linearization occurs because each eye muscle pair functions as a reciprocally innervated push-pull unit employing class A mode of operation which cancels out the second degree nonlinearities in each muscle (8, 15, 10-12).

The mutually corresponding and inversely related innervation of the two muscles of a pair makes that, as the force of one muscle increases, the force of its antagonist decreases. So the nonlinearity of one muscle is balanced off by the opposed inverse nonlinearity of its antagonist (8, 15). The resulting force difference between both muscles of a pair (net isometric force, net fixational force) which is responsible for globe displacement, becomes a linear function of eye position. The linear net fixational muscle force acts on the predominantly linear elasticity of the globe restraining tissues (10-12) (fig. 6: only at extreme gaze the LT curve of these tissues presents a small nonlinearity); the linear net isometric muscle force acts on the linear elasticity of the orbital load (fig. 18). The endresult is linear eye positioning. Push-pull class A mode of operation, as employed in fixation and tracking, automatically eliminates second harmonic (in fact all even harmonic) distortions (8, 15, 11).

Antihysteresis has been demonstrated in the human oculomotor system (11, 13-15), namely in the LT relationship of eye muscle (mechanical antihysteresis), in the LT relationship of the orbital load (passive or load antihysteresis: fig. 18), in the T isom. (θ) transfer function (muscle force antihysteresis: fig. 14, 15) and in the $\phi(\theta)$ transfer function (neural antihysteresis: fig. 11). Hysteresis discrepancy has also been reported in ocular motoneurons of monkeys (21).

The LT characteristics of eye muscle and orbital load (fig. 18) present two distinct curves forming a clockwise progressing loop. The tension depends upon the direction of motion, being higher during extension than during relaxation; on reversing the pull a rapid tension change occurs. This tension difference is due to viscosity and hysteresis caused by internal friction of the studied tissues (13, 14). It becomes greater with increased extension-relaxation velocity due to viscosity. If the tension difference is due to viscosity only, the latter can be determined from the area within the loop or as half the tension difference divided by the extension-relaxation velocity. The value of hysteresis can be determined at extremely slow velocity reducing to about zero the effect of viscosity (13, 14). In fig. 18 the total force due to viscosity and hysteresis is plus 6 g during the pull and minus 6 g during the release; for 10°/sec velocity both forces are considered to be equal, i.e. 3 g each in each direction, the orbital load viscosity being 0.3 g/deg/sec (14). Orbital load viscosity was previously evaluated to be 0.22 g/deg/sec (40, 37).

Figures 11, 14, 15 show that innervation and isometric force depend upon the innervation direction, i.e. upon whether the activity is agonistic or antagonistic. The $\phi(\theta)$ and T isom. (θ) functions show two distinct curves forming a clockwise loop; on reversing the direction of innervation a rapid innervation and tension change occurs (11, 14).

It was concluded (11, 10) that the central nervous system employs antihysteresis in innervating the eye muscles. Neural antihysteresis applies muscle force antihysteresis having the same magnitude as the orbital load antihysteresis. Neural activity leads the desired eye position; more innervation is supplied to the muscle when it needs more force to extend the antagonist, less innervation is supplied when less force is needed in permitting the antagonist to become shorter. Neural antihysteresis increases the effective innervational gain of the oculomotor system (11, 10).

III. *Saccades*

Saccades are very fast conjugate eye movements produced by a pulse-step (36, 42, 43) neural command.

This section deals with saccades as voluntary movements used to scan the visual field, i.e. to direct rapidly the eyes, from one fixation point to another, upon the visual target such that its image becomes centered on the retina, in the central fovea. Apart from this deliberate scanning activity the saccadic system is also called into action during fixation (microsaccades), tracking (following saccades) and vergences; the quick phases of vestibular and optokinetic nystagmus are also saccades (39, 42, 43). Eccentric retinal stimulation by a visual target (retinal error) is a stimulus for saccadic activity (20). Nevertheless, saccades need not per se a retinal input; they can be performed without reference to a visual target, the eyes being open or closed (20, 43). Saccadic latency is about 200 msec (39, 42). Although the saccadic refractory period has been established as 200 msec, it was found to be much smaller under certain conditions (80 msec; see following saccades) (37, 39); moreover, the notion that two saccades must be spaced apart by some minimum refractory period seems to be destroyed (43) by the results of experiments involving saccadic reactions to double-step stimuli (4). Saccades obey the laws of equal and reciprocal innervation. In saccades the push-pull employs class B or C mode of operation realizing larger power output with loss of output fidelity (8). During saccades the vision is very low (saccadic suppression).

It is to be noted that in normal viewing 85% of the saccades have a size of less than 15 degrees (1, 22). Fig. 19 shows a family of different sized saccades of the same subject.

Slight overshoot or undershoot at the saccade end, presenting great individual and occasional variation, is thought to be due to a slight mismatch between pulse duration and step height in the saccadic control signal (42, 5); overshoot is not due to mechanical oscillation.

Saccades are the fastest activity of all striated muscles. Saccadic velocity is seldom lower than 200°/sec. In monkeys it is found to be higher (typical value 800°/sec, maximal value 1000°/sec) than in humans (600°/sec; 800°/sec) (Fuchs, 1967) (40, 45). More recently this difference has been questioned, the limit for human saccadic velocity being found to be around 1100°/sec (7). It is not possible to influence saccadic velocity by voluntary effort (20). In saccades the eye accelerates, reaching peak velocity nearly halfway the movement, and then decelerates. The deceleration phase has been found to be longer than the acceleration (30, 7). Saccadic peak velocity increases with saccadic size but levels off to saturation (20, 30, 7). Saccadic duration increases linearly with saccadic size (20, 30, 36, 7).

Initially, saccadic muscle tension has been measured as net isometric tension of the horizontal recti in suction contact lens experiments (36). The tension was found to rise rapidly (870 g/sec) to a peak, reached near the end of the saccadic movement, then to drop quickly at first

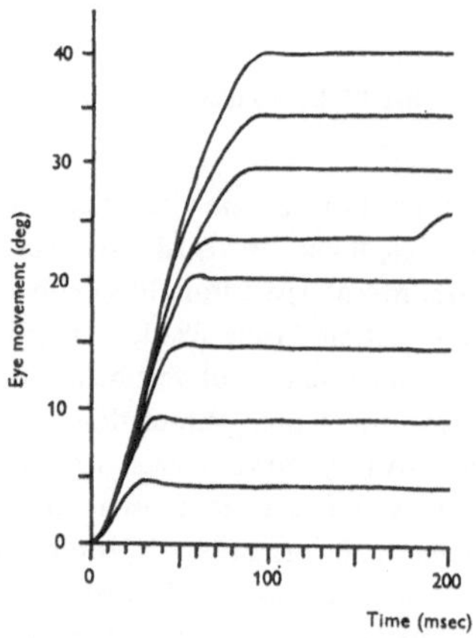

Fig. 19.

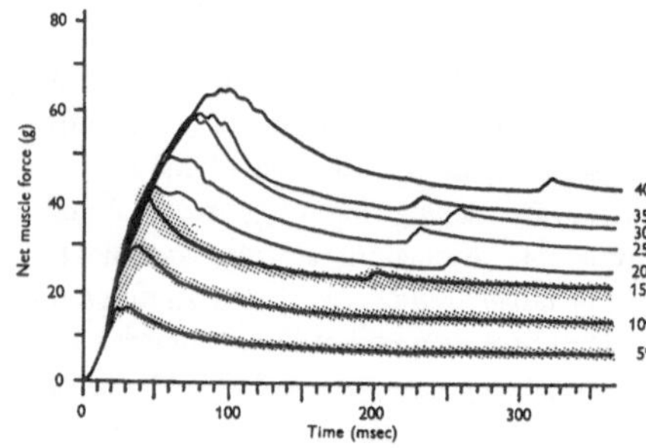

Fig. 20.

Fig. 19. — Superimposed records of the time course of different sized horizontal saccades.

Fig. 20. — Superimposed records of the time course of the net isometric tension change in the horizontal recti during different sized saccades.

Suction contact lens experiments. Eye position measured with scleral search coil in a magnetic field. Tension recorded from a rod restraining movement of the tested (isometric) eye during saccadic movements of the unrestrained contralateral eye. Both figures from Robinson, 1964 (36).

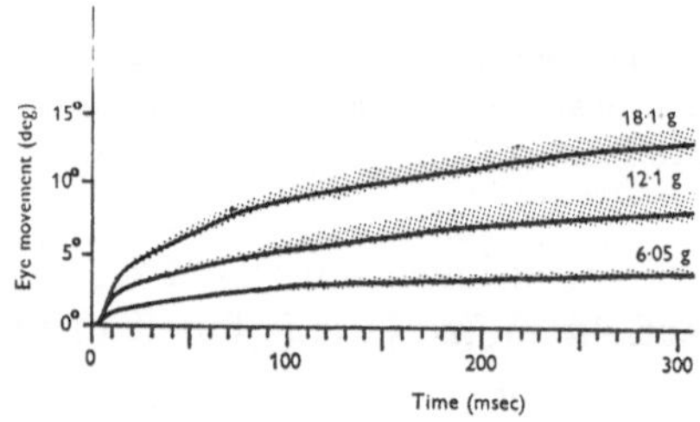

Fig. 21.

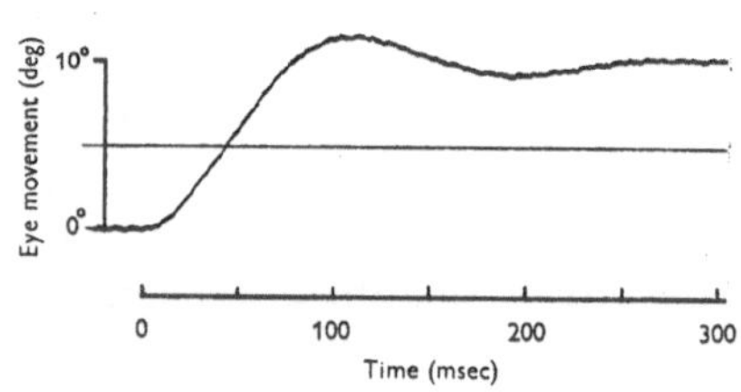

Fig. 22.

Fig. 21. — Superimposed records of the time course of the return motion of a globe after quick release from passive abduction performed by application of various forces. Suction contact lens experiments. The contralateral eye fixates in primary position.

Fig. 22. — Record of the time course of a horizontal 10° saccadic movement of a globe loaded by a moment of inertia 9750% greater than the globe's own inertia. Suction contact lens experiment.

Both figures from Robinson, 1964 (36).

and finally to decay approximately exponentially to the new steady-state fixation level (fig. 20). This tension behavior is interpreted (36) on the basis of the high viscosity of the oculomotor plant which is demonstrated (36, 6) by the sluggish response of the globe on quick release from passive rotation into an eccentric position (fig. 21). Viscosity, dependent upon velocity, is the greatest impedance to fast eye movements (36, 46). Most of the viscosity of the oculomotor plant is internal muscle viscosity (18, 19, 46). The viscous load for an agonist muscle during an on-saccade resides in the antagonist muscle (predominantly) and associated globe restraining orbital tissues (15, 11).

The mass of the globe plays a negligible mechanical role (fig. 22) (36-38, 18, 19, 7, 44).

A saccade of an eye loaded with a moment of inertia 9750% greater than the eye's own inertia, presents merely a slight transient oscillation with an overshoot of only 18%. The time course of such high inertial saccades indicates the hihgly overdamped nature of the oculomotor plant preventing mechanical resonance (36).

The initial tension excess (the extra force much greater than the force needed to hold the eye in the new fixation position; "pre-emphasis") serves to overcome the viscosity of the oculomotor plant. The exponential tension decay is interpreted as a counterbalance for the stress relaxation of the slow element of the orbital load at the saccade end (36, 46).

The return motion of the eye towards primary position after quick release from an eccentric position (fig. 21) comprises at least two exponentials, a fast one followed by a slow one (36, 6). The passive tissues corresponding to the slow component are thought to stress relieve at the saccade end. If the agonist muscle tension would fall abruptly to the new fixation level, stress release of these tissues, stretched at high saccadic velocity, would cause a drift of the eye beyond the desired goal. This is avoided by the agonist muscle decreasing its force gradually at a rate matching the slow stress relaxation (36, 46).

The time course of the net active-state muscle tension needed to drive the eye during different sized saccades was evaluated on the analog computer (36). It takes the form of a pulse-step (fig. 23). The step (i.e. difference between final and initial tension) serves to hold the eye at its new fixation position against elastic forces. The pulse (burst), added to the step at its beginning and producing an initial tension excess (difference between burst or peak tension and final tension: "pre-emphasis"), is rectangular and has the same duration as the saccadic movement; it overcomes viscous forces. The pulse ceases abruptly a few milliseconds before movement completion but is followed by a tail of slow tension decay matching the stress relaxation of the slow component of the orbital load (36).

For the 10° saccade the burst of net active-state tension of the horizontal recti was evaluated as 43.4 g lasting about 40 msec, the tension excess (258%) was 24.6 g, the step 15 g, and the slow decay component 3.9 g (36).

The magnitude of the active-state tension excess (25 g) was found to be independent of saccadic size (36).

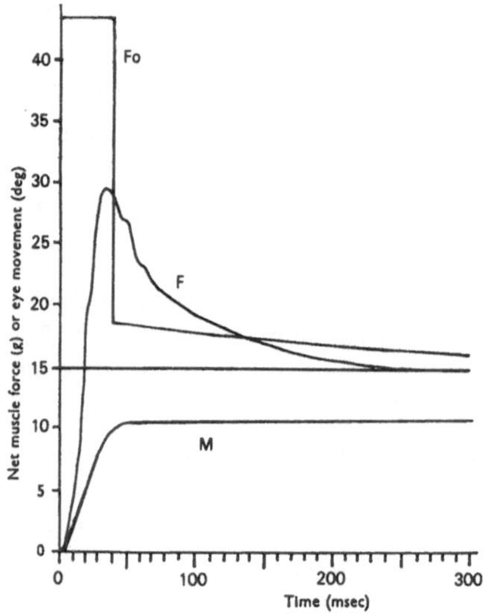

Fig. 23. — Record of the time course of a horizontal 10° saccadic movement (M) and corresponding net isometric tension change in the horizontal recti (F), from suction contact lens experiments. F_0 is the computed time course of the net active-state tension of the horizontal recti required to produce the experimental curves M and F. After Robinson, 1964 (36).

This suggested the existence of a pulse generator acting in an all or none fashion, working only when a saccade is to be made, and being able to vary only the duration of its activity but not the magnitude of its force which is no more or less than about 25 g, such that larger saccades are produced by a larger duration of a nearly constant force (36).

Saccadic tension of single eye muscles has been recorded as a function of time (46, 8, 48, 51, 15, 11).

Isometric measurements were done on the muscle connected to a strain gauge force transducer and held at primary length, while the contralateral eye performed saccadic movements in and out the studied muscle's action field (46, 8, 48, 51). More recently saccadic tensions were measured simultaneously in both horizontal recti with implanted miniature force transducers, not only in isometric conditions (the studied eye held in primary position by means of a restraining suture) but also during unrestrained saccades of both free eyes (15, 11). The figures 24-27 are records of saccadic muscle tension measured in situ as a function of time.

In a muscle acting as agonist during unrestrained saccades (upper curve fig. 24, lower curve fig. 25, tracing b upper part fig. 26, top curve upper part fig. 27) the tension initially rises rapidly, nearly isometrically, before the eye moves. As the eye performs a significant movement with shortening of the agonist, a break occurs in the tension curve. The tension increases further, but slower, to a peak value which is followed by an approximately exponential decrease to the new fixation level (15, 11). These characteristics are best seen in faster speed records There are several differences between isometric and unrestrained saccadic tension of the agonist. Isometric tension presents no break during the initial rise, the peak tension is greater and the tension decay leads to a

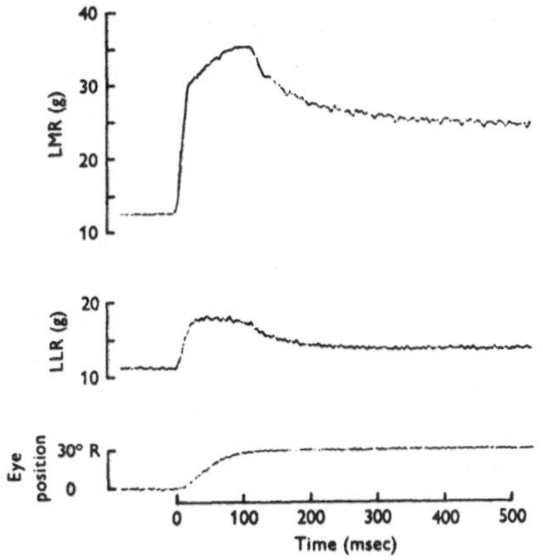

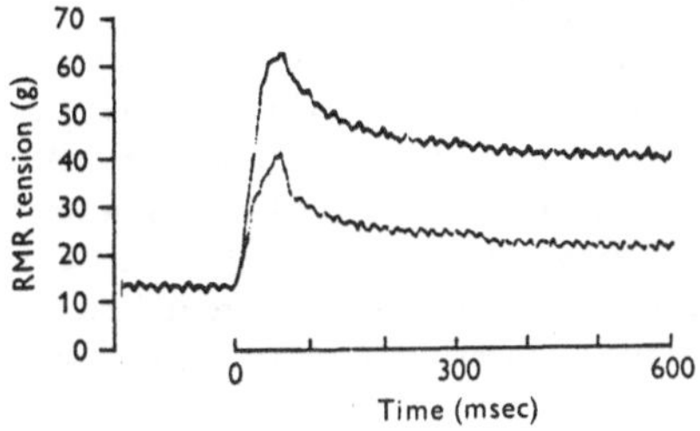

Fig. 24. Fig. 25.

Fig. 24. — Recorded time course of tension change in an agonist left medial rectus (upper curve) and antagonist left lateral rectus muscle (middle curve) during unrestrained saccade from primary position to 30° R.

Fig. 25. — Superimposed recorded time courses of tension change in an agonist right medial rectus muscle during isometrically restrained (upper curve) and unrestrained (lower curve) saccade from 15° L to 30° L.

In situ measurements with implanted miniature force transducers; for isometric measurement the eye is restrained by sutures. EOG recording of eye movement. Both figures from Collins, O'Meara, Scott, 1975 (15).

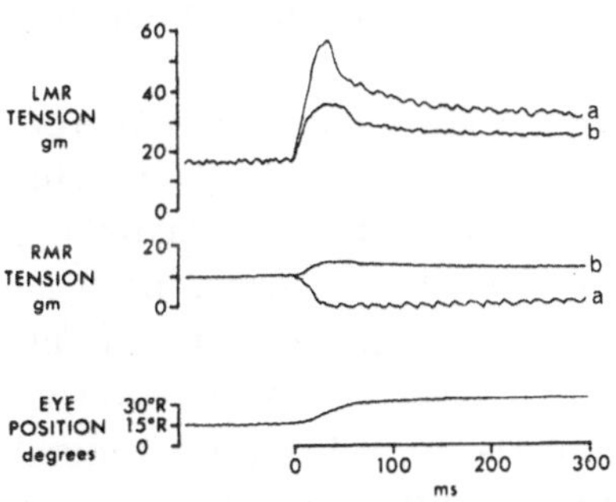

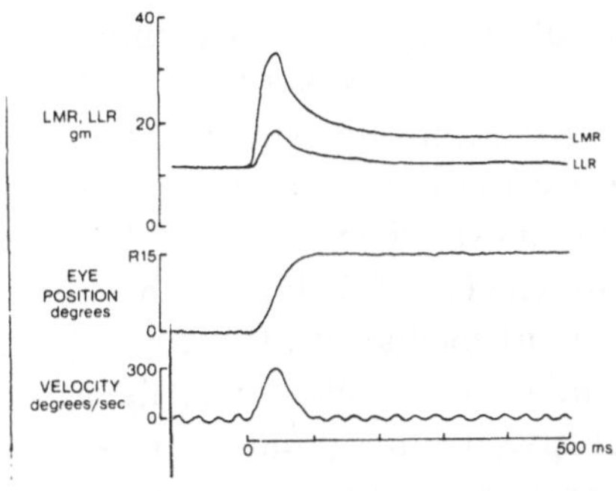

Fig. 26. Fig. 27.

Fig. 26. — Superimposed recorded time courses of tension change in an agonist left medial rectus (upper grouping) and antagonist right medial rectus muscle (middle grouping) during a saccade from 15° R to 30° R. a: isometric saccade. b: unrestrained saccade.

Fig. 27. — Superimposed recorded time courses of tension change in an agonist left medial rectus and antagonist left lateral rectus muscle during an unrestrained saccade from primary position to 15° R. Lower curve: time course of eye velocity.

Tension measured with implanted miniature force transducers; for isometric measurement the eye is restrained by sutures. EOG recording of eye movement. Both figures from Collins, 1975 (11).

higher final fixation level than in free saccades (upper curve fig. 25; tracing a, upper part fig. 26). These differences have been accounted for by foreshortening of the contractile element and series elastic element (15, 11).

During the initial roughly isometric tension rise, the CE shortens (internal shortening) which stretches the SEE (internal lengthening). When the muscle tendon force has increased sufficiently to move the unrestrained eye a small amount, the muscle length reduces and the stretched SEE structures shorten. The release of this stiff spring decreases significantly the muscle tension and a break occurs in the curve. The slower tension rise after the break is due to the resulting shortening of the CE. In isometric saccades, on the contrary, the initial tension rise cannot move the restrained eye, the SEE is not released and the muscle tension continues to rise to a greater peak value than in the unrestrained saccades (15,11).

It has been found (15, 9-12) that in unrestrained saccades the antagonist presents an initial tension rise before the new fixation level is attained (mid curve fig. 24, curve b mid part fig. 26, lower curve top part fig. 27); this tension rise is much less and slower than the initial agonist tension rise. It is due to the agonist tension stretching the neuropassive antagonist at a rate faster than it can relax due to its viscosity. On the contrary, tension rise in the antagonist is not seen during isometric saccades because muscle stretch is prevented. In this condition the antagonist tension falls to zero before attaining the final fixational value (curve a, midpart fig. 26) due to complete inhibition (antagonist innervation is completely turned off for saccades greater than 10° (15, 11)) (15, 9-12).

Recording unrestrained muscle tension with implanted miniature force transducers as a function of the position of the freely moving tested eye, yields dynamic LT records of contracting and relaxing eye muscles (15, 11). Figure 28 represents a dynamic LT record from an agonist medial rectus muscle during unrestrained saccadic refixations. The LT path followed by the agonist muscle tension between two successive fixation points, consists of three parts (15, 9-12). (1) An initial approximately isometric rise of tension with little change of muscle length; this part is roughly isometric due to the large viscosity to be overcome by the agonist. (2) During the eye movement the saccadic tension is higher than the static fixation tension for the corresponding eye position; this tension increment (15-25 g) above the static locus, which is said to be approximately isotonic, is the product of load viscosity and equilibrium velocity of eye movement. (3) At the end of the movement the tension falls roughly isometrically to the new fixation level due to innervation decrease and velocity drop. The plateaus of

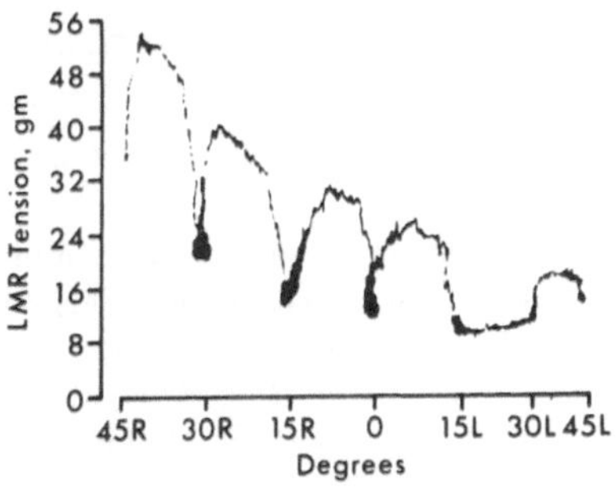

Fig. 28.

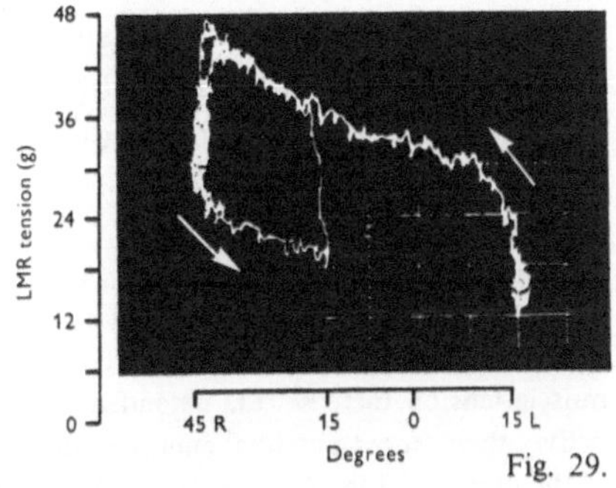

Fig. 29.

Fig. 28. — Dynamic length-tension record from an agonist left medial rectus muscle during successive unrestrained 15° saccadic refixations from 45° L to 45° R. From Collins, 1975 (11).

Fig. 29. — Dynamic length-tension record from an agonist left medial rectus muscle. The eye makes a 60° saccade from 15° L to 45° R, then a slow return movement from 45° R back to 15° R, finally a 30° saccade from 15° R to 45° R. Both saccades follow the same LT path in their common operational range. Tension measurement with implanted force transducer. EOG recording of eye position. From Collins, O'Meara, Scott, 1975 (15).

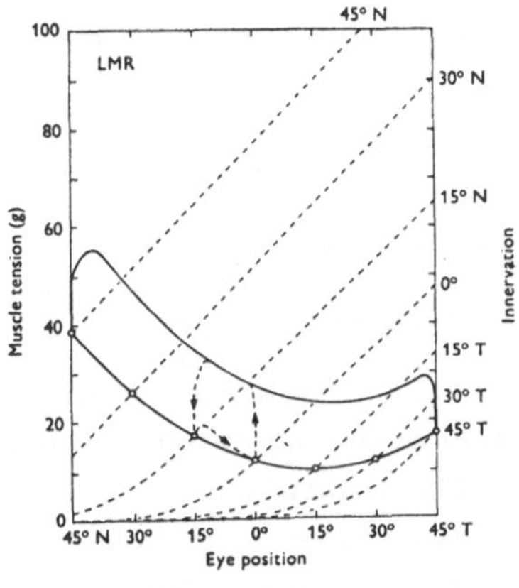

Fig. 30. — Family of static isometric length-tension curves and operational envelope of the normal ranges of muscle tension for a typical medial rectus muscle. The counterclockwise LT loop from 0° to 15° N on the static locus represents the muscle's agonistic activity, the smaller flattened clockwise loop from 15° N to 0° represents the antagonistic activity. From Collins, O'Meara, Scott, 1975 (15).

saccadic tensions constitute the so called dynamic locus (15, 11). The steady-state tension values during the fixation periods at different eye positions lie on the parabolic static locus. Saccadic LT loops follow a unique fixed path (15, 11); this stereotype behavior is shown in fig. 29 by two saccades of 30° and 60° having coinciding LT paths in their common operational region.

Some energy considerations have been made from the saccadic LT loops. In fig. 30 the counterclockwise LT loop from 0° to 15° N on the static locus concerns a muscle acting as agonist during a saccade into its action field. The initial tension increase preceeds muscle shortening and eye movement; thus the LT loop progresses counterclockwise, indicating that the muscle is delivering energy to the globe and acts as a motor (15, 9-12).

During the initial tension rise, the CE shortens which stretches the series elastic structures, thus storing potential energy in them. This occurs in an isometric muscle undergoing no external shortening, the eye does not move, no external work is done by the muscle, no or negligible external energy is dissipated. When the eye moves significantly owing to the muscle tension increase, the extended series elastic structures are allowed to shorten and deliver their stored potential energy in the form of kinetic energy of movement. At the end of the movement the CE relaxes which again occurs isometrically with respect to the external world. This working mode minimizes energy dissipation; least work is demanded from the contractile element (15, 11, 10).

The smaller flattened clockwise LT loop from 15° N to 0° in fig. 30 concerns the muscle as antagonist during a saccade out of its action field. It shows, as a function of eye position, the tension changes in the neuropassive antagonist due to stretching of its passive tissues by the agonist force (fig. 24, 26, 27). The passive tension increase preceeds relaxation of the muscle; thus the LT loop progresses clockwise, indicating that energy is absorbed by the muscle which is acting as a brake (15, 11, 9, 12).

The area within the boundaries of the saccadic loops for the muscle as agonist and antagonist, represents the mechanical work done by the muscle during a full cycle of motion, i.e. the energy delivered minus the energy absorbed by the muscle (net energy) during an on-and off-saccade between two given fixation positions. The isometric phase of the agonist muscle behavior is analog to the adiabatic (isoenergetic) condition of the Carnot cycle of a heat engine, the "isotonic" phase is analog to the isothermal condition (15, 11, 9).

Recording the neural activity of single ocular motoneurons of monkeys (23, 47, 40, 24, 32, 33, 45) revealed that during an on-saccade the neurons exhibit a rapid intense burst of firing frequency much greater than required to maintain the eye in the new fixation position. The time course of the instantaneous firing frequency shows that an on-saccade is created by a pulse-step of R (fig. 31). The burst starts and stops rather abruptly; the change of R can be found less sharp at the saccade end. The pulse duration equals the saccadic movement duration. The burst preceeds the start and stop of the saccadic movement by a time interval of about 8 msec due to the excitation-contraction coupling process (40, 45). Following the burst end, the firing frequency falls not at once to the new steady-state fixation level but decreases gradually; this slow decay of R is thought to compensate for the stress relaxation of the slow component of the combined passive tissues at the saccade end (40).

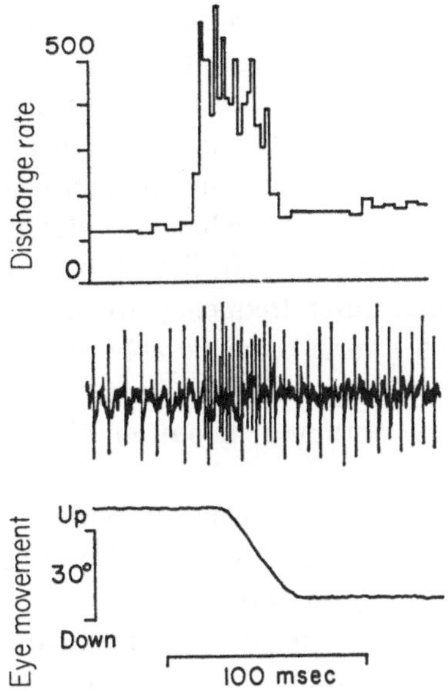

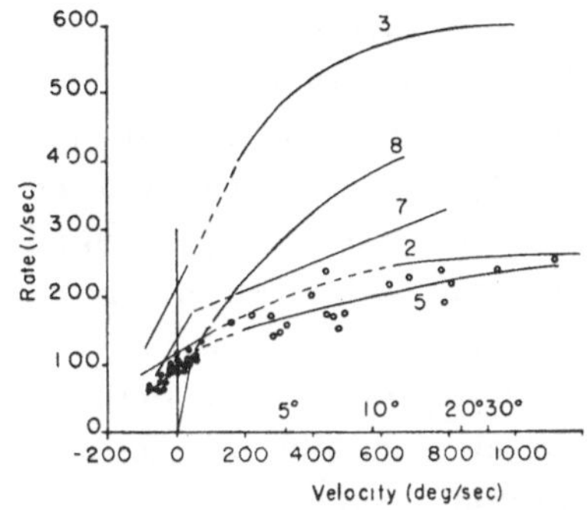

Fig. 31.

Fig. 32.

Fig. 31. — Neural activity of a single ocular motoneuron (nucleus III, inferior rectus) of a monkey during an on-saccade. Upper curve: time course of instantaneous discharge frequency (reciprocal of interspike interval). From Robinson and Keller, 1972 (45).

Fig. 32. — Discharge frequency — eye velocity relationship of different single ocular motoneurons of monkeys for pursuit (0°-50°/sec) and saccadic (200°-1200°/sec) velocities in the on-direction. Selection of different sized on-saccades crossing a given fixed position about halfway the saccadic movement. From Robinson, 1970 (40).

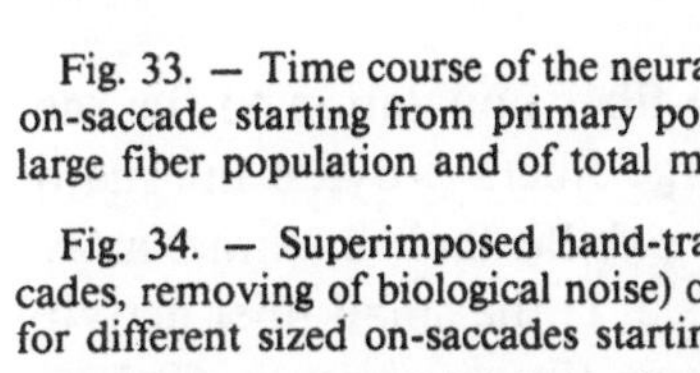

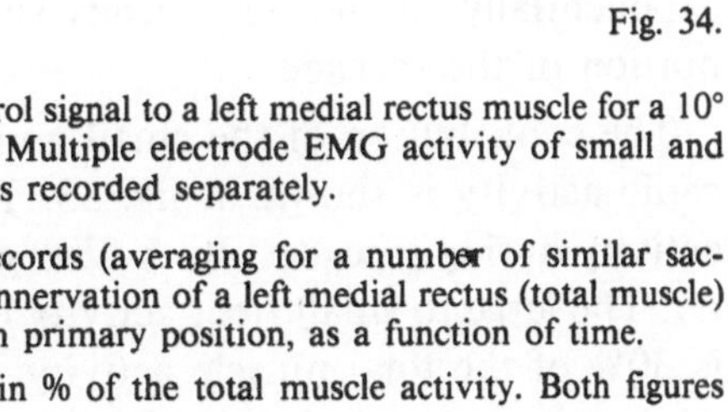

Fig. 33.

Fig. 34.

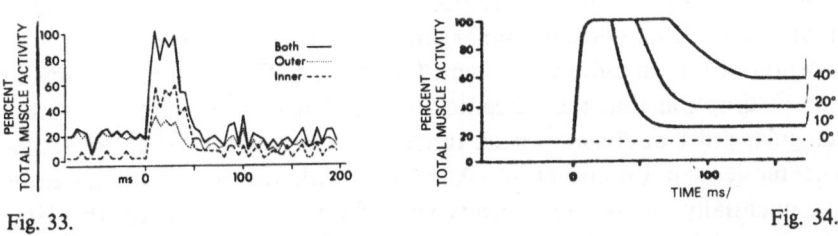

Fig. 33. — Time course of the neural control signal to a left medial rectus muscle for a 10° on-saccade starting from primary position. Multiple electrode EMG activity of small and large fiber population and of total muscle is recorded separately.

Fig. 34. — Superimposed hand-traced records (averaging for a number of similar saccades, removing of biological noise) of the innervation of a left medial rectus (total muscle) for different sized on-saccades starting from primary position, as a function of time.

In both figures the activity is expressed in % of the total muscle activity. Both figures from Collins and Scott, 1973 (16).

The burst frequency of a motoneuron increases with saccadic velocity but the neurons exhibit saturation of R with increasing velocity (23, 24, 40, 44). Fig. 32 shows the discharge frequency-velocity relationship of different single motoneurons for saccadic velocities in the on-direction. Saccadic R (dθ/dt) curves differ among motoneurons by their slope and saturation shape. Motoneurons with higher values of velocity parameter r for smooth pursuit present larger change in R with change in saccadic velocity (40). The maximum burst frequency (observed during very large saccades, i.e. of 40°-45°) varies considerably among motoneurons; it ranges from 150-200 to 800 sp/sec with a mean value of about 400 sp/sec and shows a relatively normal distribution (40, 47, 23, 32, 33, 45).

During saccades in the off-direction there is complete inhibition of the motoneurons; the activity falls to zero, at the saccade end it rises abruptly to the new fixation level (47, 32, 33, 45, 43).

The end of a saccade is simply due to the stop of the pulse in the motoneurons of the agonist and of the inhibition in the antagonist (40, 47, 23, 24). There is no evidence of nor need for active control of the saccade end; the high viscosity of the oculomotor plant brings the eye rapidly at rest in the new fixation position (36, 38).

It is to be noted that the motoneurons' discharge rate does not change during saccades perpendicular to the on-direction (40).

The saccadic innervation signal to single eye muscles has been recorded by multiple electrode EMG (16, 9-12). The innervation pattern is the same for the small and large fiber population (fig. 33) and for all saccadic sizes (fig. 34). Complete depolarization of the muscle is obtained within about 10 msec (rise time to peak activity). It was found that the peak of constant innervation is maintained during the first portion of the saccadic movement (16, 10-12). This is in opposition to the assumption that the saccadic control signal to an agonist is a rectangular pulse of constant peak innervation lasting for the entire saccadic movement duration (16). After the peak the innervation decays exponentially to the new steady-state fixation level during the later portion of the saccade.

The contribution of the small and large fiber population to the saccadic activity is shown in fig. 35. The large fibers provide the major activity during saccades. Both fiber groups exhibit their maximal activity. The large to small fiber activity ratio is 2:1; the small fiber activity is 30% of the total muscle activity, the large fiber activity is 60-70%. This ratio, being the ratio of the number of large to small fibers in an

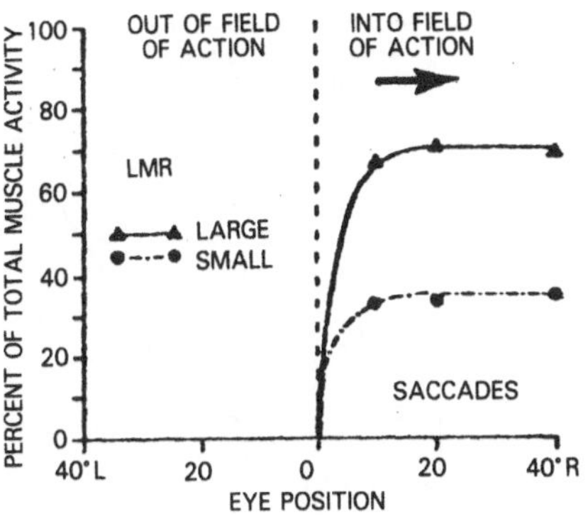

Fig. 35. — Innervation of the small and large fiber population of a left medial rectus muscle for on-saccades of 10° and more starting from primary position, as a function of eye position. Multiple electrode EMG data. Activity is expressed in % of total muscle activity. From Collins and Scott, 1973 (16).

eye muscle, remains constant during the saccadic burst because all fibers are "on" during on-saccades (16).

It was found that with increasing saccadic size both amplitude and duration of the saccadic peak innervation vary (fig. 36) but not in a similar fashion; the burst amplitude increases rapidly at first and then saturates for larger saccades thus following a logarithmic relationship, while the burst duration follows a power function, increasing slowly at first and more rapidly for larger saccades (fig. 37). From these findings it was stated that saccadic size is determined by impulse modulation (11).

The saccadic impulse (product of amplitude times duration of the burst or peak innervation) represents the innervational energy required to move the eye saccadically to a given position. It is proportional to the force required to hold the eye at the final fixation position. It is a square function of the saccadic size (11).

In the large fiber group the difference between saccadic burst innervation and final fixation innervation, i.e. the innervation overshoot, as a function of saccadic size, increases up to about 20° saccadic size and then decreases. Most of the overshoot activity is contributed by the large fibers (11).

From fig. 38, representing the time course of innervation of the large fiber group of a medial rectus muscle for 10° on-saccades starting from different eye positions, one sees that the amplitude of the saccadic peak innervation, the magnitude of the innervation overshoot and the shape of the innervation signal depend upon the starting eye position (11).

Robinson's model (1975) shows the saccadic system as a bang-bang control system consisting of a simple negative feedback system whose forward path contains the saccadic pulse generator PG followed by the common neural integrator NI. This model rejects the concept that the

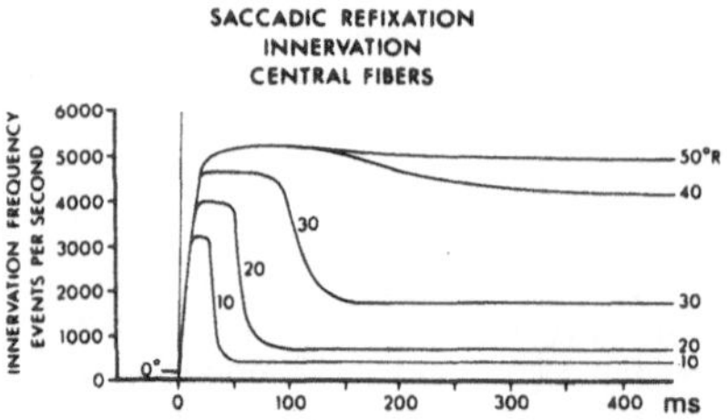

Fig. 36.

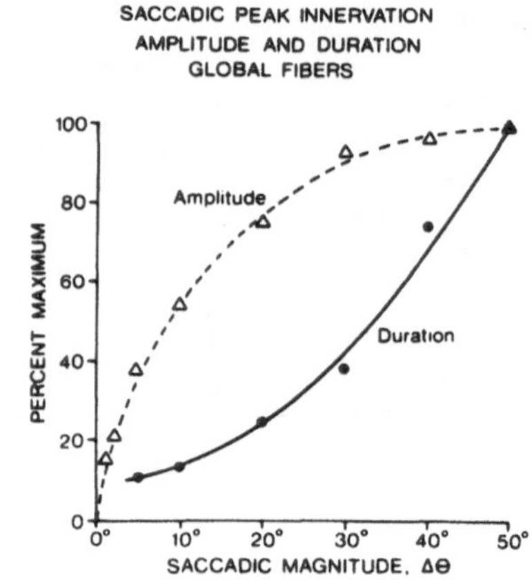

Fig. 37.

Fig. 36. — Superimposed hand-traced averaged records of the innervation, expressed in multiple electrode EMG frequency, of the large fiber population of a left medial rectus muscle for different sized on-saccades starting from primary position, as a function of time.

Fig. 37. — Amplitude and duration of saccadic peak innervation of the large fiber population, both expressed in % of maximum (% of their value during large 50° saccades), as a function of saccadic size. Functions derived from fig. 36 data.
Both figures from Collins, 1975 (11).

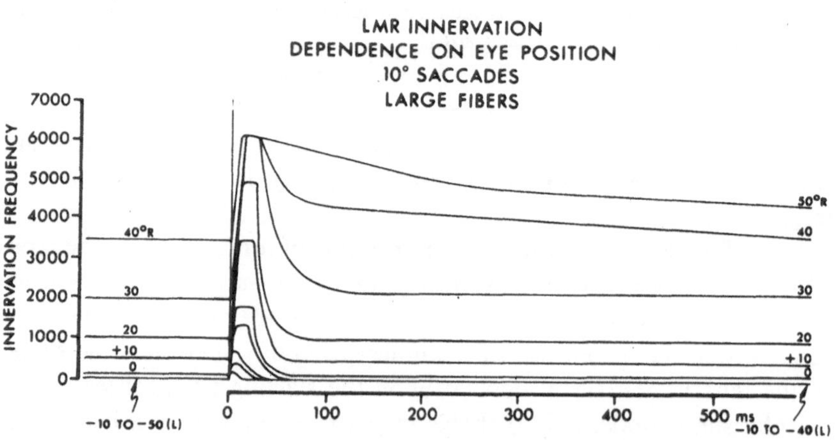

Fig. 38. — Superimposed hand-traced time records of the innervation, expressed in multiple electrode EMG frequency, of the large fiber population of a left medial rectus muscle for 10° on-saccades starting from different eye positions over the complete range from 50° L to 50° R. From Collins, 1975 (11).

brain samples visual data before processing it (42, 43) (4) and also the concept that saccades are ballistic movements (preprogrammed movements, calculated in advance from the retinal input and which cannot be modified in midflight) (4, 43); the model adopts the notion of parallel processing of saccades (42, 4, 43). Robinson's model explains saccade stop and the velocity-duration-amplitude relationship of saccades (43).

The pulse generator PG, a high-gain saturating amplifier with a dead zone, is either off or on, driving maximally in one direction or the other. It is built up by the burst cells (Cohen and Henn, 1972; Keller, 1974) in the PPRF (paramedian pontine reticular formation). A saccade is created by a burst of synchronized high-frequency activity of a subpopulation of burst cells which lasts as long as the saccadic movement. The PG pulse, being an eye velocity command, is conducted to the motoneurons but also to the neural integrator which creates its integral, i.e. the eye position command which is a step. The neural integrator is built up by the tonic or eye position cells (Keller, 1974) in the PPRF. The addition of pulse and step is presented, as saccadic control signal, to the motoneurons (43).

In Robinson's model eye position and target position are coded in a head-coordinate system as signals $\hat{\theta}$ and $\hat{\theta}_T$ respectively. This permits the oculomotor system to make orienting responses in a body-image reference frame, as do many skeletal motor systems (43).

The efference copy of the integrator output, i.e. the copy of the eye position command to the motoneurons, is fed back into the visual processing and constitutes the signal $\hat{\theta}$. This signal is the internal representation of eye position with respect to the head, it is the neural event determining the perception of the spatial location of the eye; from it the brain knows where the eye is (43).

In the visual processing, $\hat{\theta}$ is added to the retinal error e to create the signal $\hat{\theta}_T$ which is the internal representation of target position with respect to the head; $\hat{\theta}_T$ determines the perception of the spatial location of the visual target, from it the brain knows where the target is (43).

At the beginning of the bang-bang system, $\hat{\theta}$ is subtracted from $\hat{\theta}_T$ to create the signal ê, the difference between eye position and target position in head-coordinates. The signal ê drives the eye saccadically. ê makes the PG going "on" at a moment that it equals the retinal error (ê=e). Thus, the retinal error determines the PG output. During the saccadic movement ê guides the eye. The PG output, being an eye velocity command, causes the NI to produce the eye position command, the (efference) copy $\hat{\theta}$ of which is fed back and reduces ê in the course of the eye movement. When ê becomes zero, i.e. when $\hat{\theta}$ matches $\hat{\theta}_T$, the PG is going off. Thus, in a saccade the eye is driven by the error between eye position and desired eye position; when this error is zero, i.e. when the eye is there where it is desired to be, namely at the desired target position, the eye stops automatically (43).

Saccadic velocity is determined by the height of the PG pulse, saccadic duration by the duration of the PG pulse. The shape of the velocity-amplitude relationship of saccades (velocity increasing with amplitude but leveling off to saturation) is considered to be determined by the shape of the PG-function relating the magnitude of the PG output to saccadic amplitude, the PG being a high-gain saturating amplifier (the burst cells fire at high rates very near saturation) and its outputs being eye velocity commands. The increase of saccadic duration, in proportion to saccadic amplitude, is due to the PG output having exactly the same duration as the saccadic movement. Digital simulation of Robinson's bang-bang system, when the nonlinear PG-function is given a 0.25° dead zone and begins saturating between 200 and 575°/sec, produces a family of different sized saccades, the time courses of which are quite similar to the actual measured ones (fig. 19). The shape of this nonlinear function in PG determines the saccadic velocity-amplitude relationship, so that larger saccades have higher peak velocities and longer durations, as seen in fig. 19 (43).

IV. *Smooth pursuit*

Smooth pursuit movements are slow conjugate eye movements produced by a step-ramp (43, 44) neural command. This section deals only with smooth pursuit in tracking of a moving target.

The purpose of this following activity is to ensure clear vision of the moving target by stabilizing its image upon the central fovea. The smooth pursuit system operates in a continuous manner (20, 37, 39) and employs visual negative feedback (37, 39, 42, 43). The visual system appreciates not only the retinal error but also its rate of change (velocity of retinal image slip) (37, 42, 43). The latter is done by means of direction-selective visual neurons (retinal ganglion cells whose discharge frequency is proportional to the retinal-image velocity), the output of which constitutes the signal which drives the smooth pursuit system (37, 42, 43); these units saturate with target velocity, ceasing their response for velocities greater than about 30°/sec (42). Smooth pursuit has a 125 msec latency, a refractory period less than 75 msec, a response time of about 133 msec (37, 39) and a velocity up to 30°/sec in humans. Smooth pursuit obeys the laws of equal and reciprocal innervation.

In tracking both saccadic and smooth pursuit systems are called into action (20) and work independently (37). Smooth pursuit lags behind the moving target and, consequently, is interrupted by small saccades in the following direction which are corrective movements for the smooth pursuit error (following saccades) (20). Pure smooth pursuit can be elicited by a step-ramp target motion.

Ramp target motion (initially stationary target beginning a movement of constant velocity) elicits combined following activity (fig. 40). In a step-ramp target motion (devised by Rashbass, 1961) the target initially jumps in one direction and then immediately begins a motion of constant velocity in the opposite direction (fig. 39). If the step amplitude, expressed in degreees, is about 0.2 times the ramp velocity, expressed in deg/sec, such that the target recrosses its initial position 200 msec after its starting, the eye responds with a smooth pursuit movement without corrective saccades. At the beginning the eye moves away from the target (in order to match its velocity), indicating that the stimulus for the smooth pursuit system is target velocity rather than—and even regardless of—target position (37, 39, 42).

The time course of the pure smooth pursuit eye movement and associated net isometric tension change in the horizontal recti, in response to a (2°, 10°/sec) step-ramp target motion, is represented in figure 39 (37). The eye movement is devoid of following saccades. After an

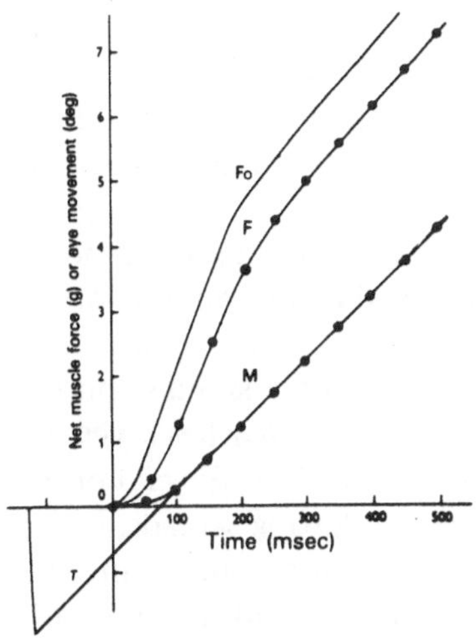

Fig. 39.

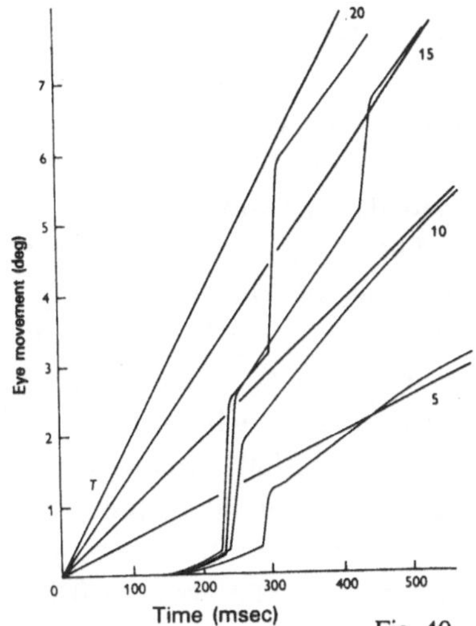

Fig. 40.

Fig. 39. — Mean time course of eye movement (M) and net isometric tension change in the horizontal recti (F), in response to a 2°, 10°/sec step-ramp target motion (T). Suction contact lens experiments. Eye movement measured, in one eye, by scleral search coil in magnetic field. Net isometric muscle tension recorded from the other isometrically restrained eye. M and F are averaged from six measurements. F_0 represents the computed time course of the net active-state tension of the horizontal recti. After Robinson, 1965 (37).

Fig. 40. — Time course of eye movement, in response to ramp target motion (T) of 5, 10, 15, 20°/sec. Suction contact lens experiments. Each response is the segmental mean of 10 responses of the most common type. From Robinson, 1965 (37).

initial acceleration the eye moves at a constant velocity matching the 10°/sec ramp velocity of the target. Associated to the eye acceleration there is an initial excess of the rate of net isometric muscle tension change (during the first 200 msec) reaching a peak (20.8 g/sec); then the rate sinks to a steady-state value (12 g/sec) accompanying the 10°/sec ramp eye movement. The computed time course of the net active-state tension change of the horizontal recti shows an initial excess (150%) of rate reaching a peak (30 g/sec) before the rate takes its steady-state value (12 g/sec). The initial excess rate of muscle tension change serves to overcome the viscosity of the oculomotor plant (37). It was calculated that without this smooth pursuit "pre-emphasis" the desired 10°/sec ramp eye velocity would not be reached before 500 msec. With the initial excess the 10°/sec velocity change is compressed to about 130 msec (taken as working value for the smooth pursuit response time, i.e. the time required to accelerate the eye from one constant velocity to another; it is slightly longer for larger velocity changes) (37). Smooth pursuit activity exhibits saturation with increasing target velocity; the initial rate of muscle tension change and the final smooth pursuit velocity of the eye were found to saturate at 20°/sec. Larger velocity changes are performed with relatively smaller initial excess rate of muscle tension change, take slightly longer time and exhibit less or no velocity overshoot (37).

The time course of eye movements in response to ramp target motions of various velocity (fig. 40) shows the interruption of the smooth pursuit by following saccades (37). The 10°/sec ramp target motion elicits, after a 125 msec latency, an initial smooth pursuit movement by which the eye accelerates 60°/sec^2 and reaches a velocity of 6.1°/sec after a displacement of 0.38° in 112 msec; at the end of this movement the lag of the eye is about 2°. The following saccade, occurring 237 msec after the target motion start, has an amplitude of 1.42° and reduces the error to 0.7°. The post-saccadic smooth pursuit has a constant velocity of 12.2°/sec thus presenting velocity overshoot (velocity greater than the target ramp velocity) and lasts 200 msec whereafter the velocity slackens off to 10°/sec (37).

There is a variability in temporal spacing between smooth pursuit and following saccades, and in post-saccadic velocity overshoot. The curves of fig. 40 concern the most common type of response.

With increased target velocity the following saccades appear earlier and with larger amplitude. One sees in fig. 40 that the 15°/sec target motion elicits two saccades, the second occuring 200 msec after the first. In the 20°/sec target motion, however, the two saccades are only 70 msec apart which is much less than 200 msec, the established value for saccadic refractory period (37, 39).

In a model of Robinson (1973) following saccades are responses to the error that will exist one reaction time in the future, i.e. they are made to where the target will be in 200 msec. The predicted error E is given by $E = e + \lambda \dot{e}$, where e is the retinal error, $\dot{e}$ is the rate of error change, and λ is about 0.2 (42). The anticipated error E determines the decision to make a correcting saccade and the magnitude of the saccade (37, 42). In this way the brain leads the target as a hunter leads a moving target with his gun (42).

Recording from single ocular motoneurons of monkeys (23, 47, 40, 32, 45, 33, 52) shows a progressive increase of discharge frequency during smooth pursuit into the on-direction and progressive decrease into the off-direction, indicating smooth modulation of R by the central nervous system (fig. 41). R varies linearly with eye position θ, it varies also with eye velocity dθ/dt; at any given eye position, R is greater or less than its fixational value by an amount proportional to the velocity with which the eye traverses that position in the on- or off-direction. Each neuron has a constant R(dθ/dt) relationship which, for smooth pursuit, is approximately linear and determined by the velocity parameter r (coefficient relating discharge frequency to smooth

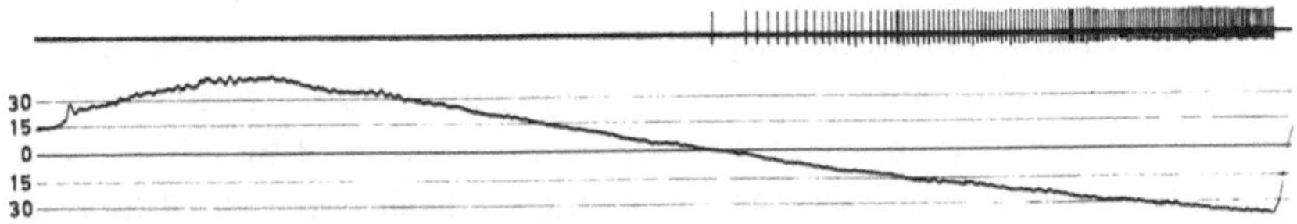

Fig. 41. — Upper trace: neural activity of a single motoneuron of nucleus III (inferior rectus) of a monkey during downward smooth pursuit. Lower trace: vertical eye movement (upward deflection = elevation, downward deflection = depression). In this particular unit firing does not commence during tracking until the eye is near primary position. From Schiller, 1970 (47).

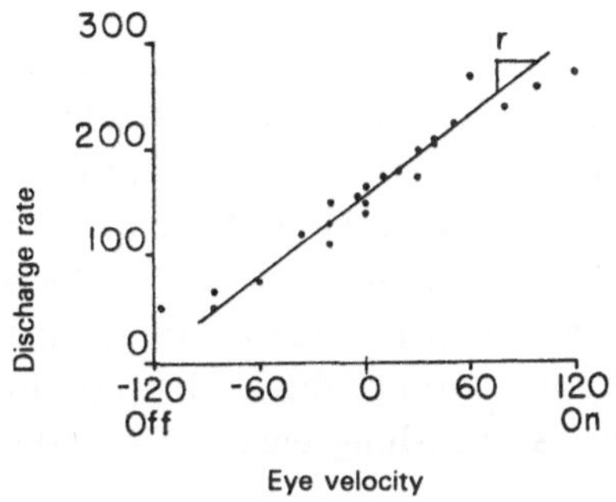

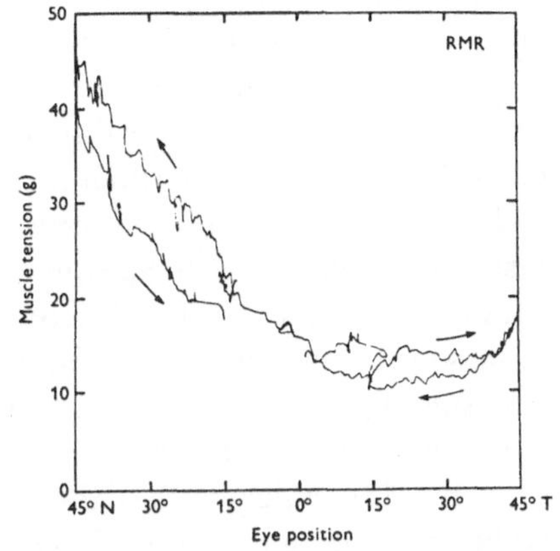

Fig. 42.

Fig. 43.

Fig. 42. — Discharge frequency — eye velocity relationship of a single motoneuron of a monkey. The instantaneous frequency is plotted against the pursuit velocity with which the eye passes through a given fixed position going in the on- or off-direction. The slope of the R(dθ/dt) line determines the motoneuron's velocity parameter r. From Robinson and Keller, 1972 (45).

Fig. 43. — Dynamic length-tension record of a right medial rectus muscle during 10°/sec smooth pursuit starting at primary position, moving to 45° R (T), then to 45° L (N) and returning to 15° L (N). Made with implanted miniature force transducer in a freely moving eye. The continuous lower right and upper left curves concern the agonistic activity out and in the action field; the continuous lower left and upper right curves concern the antagonistic activity in and out the action field (gap from 15° N to primary). From Collins, O'Meara, Scott, 1975 (15).

pursuit velocity) (fig. 42) (40-42, 32, 33, 44, 45, 52). The motoneurons differ greatly in r (40, 32, 45, 33, 44) which has a unimodal and broad distribution ranging from 0.25 to 3.7 (sp/sec)/(deg/sec) with a population mean of 0.9 (44).

Single fiber EMG of human horizontal eye muscles (50) revealed in each examined unit a progressive activity change during smooth pursuit. By multiple electrode EMG it was found (16, 11) that the muscle innervation during slow following movements is quite similar to fixation innervation (it closely approximates the pattern of fig. 10, presenting only a slight increase); the small fiber population contributes the greater part of activity; the large to small fiber activity ratio varies progressively from 0:1 to 1:1 between the extreme eye positions (16, 11).

Dynamic LT records from single eye muscles during following activity (15, 11) (fig. 43) show that in its action field the muscle as agonist has a higher tension (lying between static and dynamic locus) than as antagonist (the tension then closely approximates the static locus). This tension increment in excess of the static locus overcomes the viscosity of the oculomotor plant residing predominantly in the extending antagonist (11); it is generally small (6 g for 10°/sec velocity in fig. 43, but up to 10 g for faster pursuit). Outside its action field the muscle as antagonist has a slightly higher tension than as agonist (then the tension matches the static locus); this difference is due to extension of the passive tissues in the relaxing antagonist muscle. The counterclockwise LT loop (left side, fig. 43) indicates that the muscle is delivering energy to the globe and acts as a motor; the clockwise direction of the LT loop (right side, fig. 43) indicates that the muscle is absorbing energy from the globe and thus acts as a brake (15, 11).

V. *Vergences*

Vergences are slow disjunctive eye movements produced by a step (33, 43-45) neural command. This section deals only with horizontal vergence.

The vergence system is a continuous system (20, 37, 39, 42). The stimuli for vergence are binocular retinal disparity (produced by change in target distance, prisms, cover-uncover test in heterophoria), accommodation (produced by changes in target distance, hyperopia, negative lenses) and also (5) high-level clues (perspective, visual size of known objects, overlap of contours etc.) causing awareness of nearness and fartherness and thus contributing to accommodation and vergence. Fusional or disparity vergence is the motor response of the vergence system to binocular disparity; it brings the target's image upon the fovea of each eye (binocular fixation or fusion). In this kind of vergence the vergence system works intrinsically with visual negative feedback; the visual system appreciates the difference between the retinal errors in the two eyes rather than the retinal error in each eye (39). Accommodation vergence does not need binocularity and is intrinsically an open-loop performance of the vergence system. Disparity vergence latency is 160 msec, accommodation vergence latency 150-200 msec (38). During vergences the vision is more or less clear (20). Vergences obey the law of reciprocal innervation. Classically, they are said to be of equal amount in each eye (39, 7). Nevertheless, unequal contribution of the two eyes to vergence has been found and has been attributed to eccentric position of the binoculus (visual egocenter) on the base line (34). The binoculus position would depend upon eye dominance, tending to be closer to the dominant eye (34, 5). Thus, it was stated that Hering's law of equal innervation is applicable to vergence only if the position of the binoculus is taken into account (34).

Many investigations have demonstrated that, under normal viewing conditions, fixation changes between targets at different distances are performed by combinations of vergences and versions (saccades), and that the vergence and saccadic systems act independently (39, 33). Pure vergence has been studied neuromechanically (38, 33) in the classical experimental condition inducing pure accommodation vergence (asymmetric accommodation vergence). This is elicited by a step change of fixation between a far target A and a near target B when both are aligned on the visual axis of one eye (for example the right eye) being the seeing eye, the other (left) eye being occluded. In changing fixation between A and B, the right eye, performing the visual task, changes its accommodation but does not move; the occluded left eye makes a vergence movement which is purely accommodative and devoid of saccades.

If in this experiment the two eyes are open, both vergence and saccadic systems are activated (fig. 44). Fixation change from A to B constitutes not only an accommodative but also a disparity stimulus due to the binocular condition. After a 160 msec latency both eyes make a vergence movement on which, shortly after its beginning, a saccade is superimposed. This saccade, which obeys the law of equal innervation, brings the eyes to a point lying on the line joining the near target to the binoculus (34, 5). Then the vergence achieves bifoveal fixation of the near target. Thus, the right eye makes a saccade to the right followed by a vergence to the left to end at its starting angular position; the left eye makes a saccade to the right followed by a vergence to the right. If the binoculus lies on the midpoint of the base line, then, at the end of the saccade, the near target lies on the bisector of the convergence angle; thus the (temporal) disparity is equal in each eye and induces equal vergence in the two eyes (34, 5). If the binoculus has an eccentric position (lying to the side of the

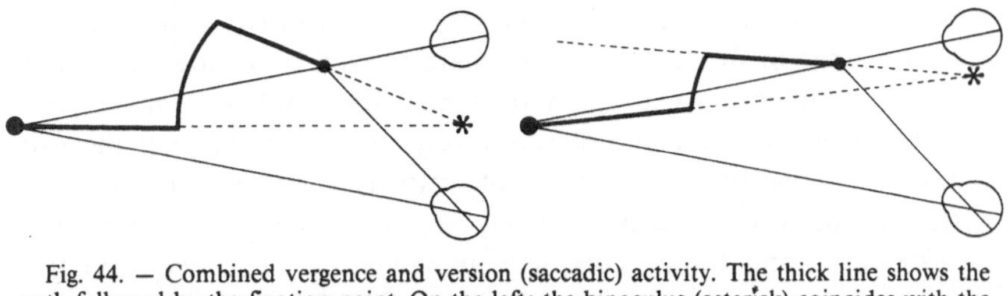

Fig. 44. — Combined vergence and version (saccadic) activity. The thick line shows the path followed by the fixation point. On the left: the binoculus (asterisk) coincides with the midpoint of the base line, both eyes contribute equally to vergence. On the right: the binoculus is closer to the dominant right eye which contributes less to vergence. In each case the saccade is equal in the two eyes. After Carpenter, 1977 (5).

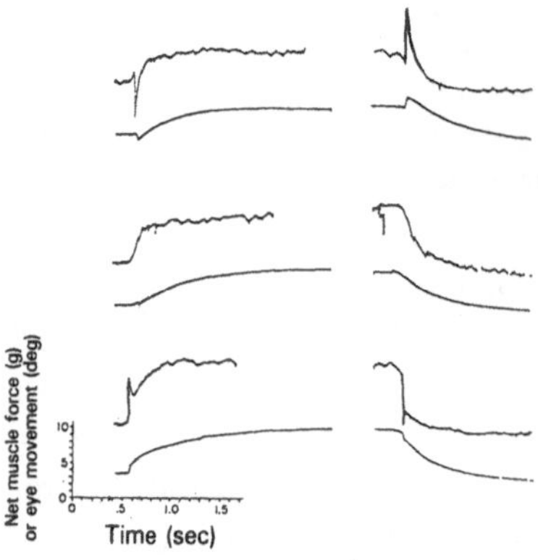

Fig. 45.

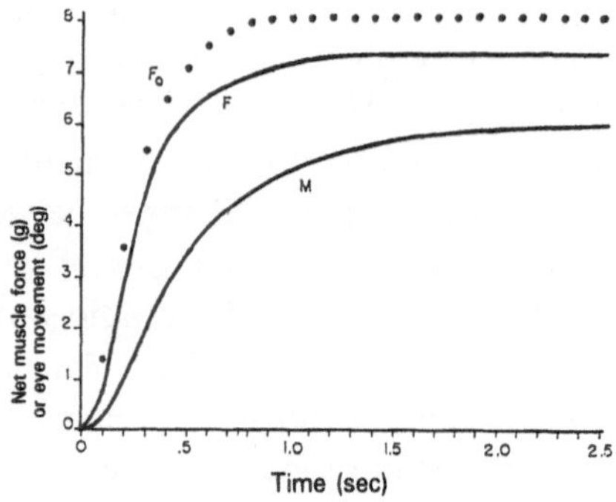

Fig. 46.

Fig. 45. — Time course of convergence (left) and divergence (right) movement of the left eye, and associated net isometric tension change of the horizontal recti, in response to step fixation change between a far (183.5 cm) and near (45.8 cm) target constituting a 1.63 Δ accommodation stimulus inducing left eye vergence of about 6°. Suction contact lens experiments on a subject with an orthophoric stimulus AC/A ratio. The R.E. performs the visual task. The L.E., occluded by the black contact lens, is used for separate measurement of movement (L.E. unrestrained) and net isometric muscle tension (L.E. restrained). Middle grouping: pure accommodation vergence (near and far target aligned with the right eye's visual axis). Upper and lower groupings: combined vergence and saccadic activity (horizontal offset of near target 1 cm to the left and right respect. of the in line position, inducing a 1.25° saccade added to the vergence).

Fig. 46. — Mean time course of accommodation divergence movement of 6° (M) and associated net isometric tension change in the horizontal recti (F), in response to a 1.63 Δ accommodation stimulus; means of 8 measurements with suction contact lens as described under figure 45. F_0 is the computed time course of the net active-state muscle tension.

Both figures from Robinson, 1966 (38).

dominant eye) the near target, after completion of the saccade, does not lie on the bisector of the convergence angle; the disparity presents an error difference and the resulting vergence is not equal in the two eyes (34); the error being less in the dominant eye, this eye contributes less to vergence (5).

Vergences are slow, approximately exponential movements. The comitant change of muscle tension is characterized by a slow onset and the absence of initial excess (there is no "pre-emphasis" in vergence) (38). In a pure (accommodation) vergence of 6° (fig. 46) the eye accelerates sluggishly reaching a peak velocity of 10°/sec in 200 msec whereafter the velocity declines slowly; the movement is 90% complete in 1200 msec and totally complete in 2500 msec. The net isometric muscle tension rises at a rate of about 10 g/sec reaching a peak of 24 g/sec in 100 msec whereafter the tension rise is roughly exponential with a 275 msec time constant (to 63.2% of the final value); the final tension value (7.4 g) is 90% established in 550 msec and totally established in 1100 msec (38). The dynamics of the disparity and accommodation vergence does not differ markedly; accommodation vergence has a longer latency and its time course is somewhat slower.

The time relationship between vergence and saccadic activity has been studied by placing the near target B in an outline position in the described experimental condition of pure accommodation vergence; a slight horizontal offset of B to the left or right of the visual line of the seeing (right) eye to the far target A, induces a conjugate saccadic movement of both eyes. In figure 45 (upper and lower groupings) the time course of the movement and net isometric muscle tension change of the left eye shows a saccade added to the accommodation vergence shortly after its beginning; the saccadic component is directed with or against the vergence, depending on the direction of the near target's outline position, and always occurs after vergence initiation (38).

Recording of the neural activity of single motoneurons in an abducens nucleus of monkeys during pure accommodation vergence of the ipsilateral eye (33, 45), revealed that convergence is associated with a decrease in R of the abducens motoneurons; divergence is associated with an increase in R, indicating that divergence ("convergence relaxation") is an active process (fig. 47 and 48).

The neural command for vergence is a step change in discharge frequency of the horizontal recti motoneurons (step increase in the agonist, step decrease in the antagonist); at the beginning of each vergence movement, R changes abruptly to a new level and remains at that level during and after the movement (fig. 48) (33, 45). During fixation at a given eye position, R is the same in the presence or absence of convergence; it depends only upon the angular eye position (33, 45). The combined vergence and saccadic activity of an abducens motoneuron when the near target has an outline position, is shown in figure 47B (left abducens unit, offset of target B to the right); at the beginning of the convergence the saccade to the right occurs with an abrupt total inhibition of the neuron, at the beginning of the divergence the saccade to the left is associated with a high-frequency burst of discharge frequency (33). Recording from single neurons of the abducens nucleus ipsilateral to the stationary seeing eye during asymmetric accommodation vergence, revealed no change in discharge frequency; this is a negative evidence for cocontraction of the horizontal recti of the stationary seeing eye (33).

Tensions recorded from a single medial rectus muscle during accom-

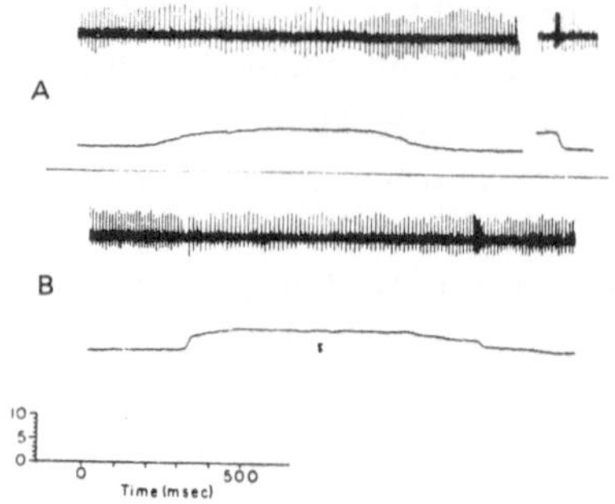

Fig. 47.

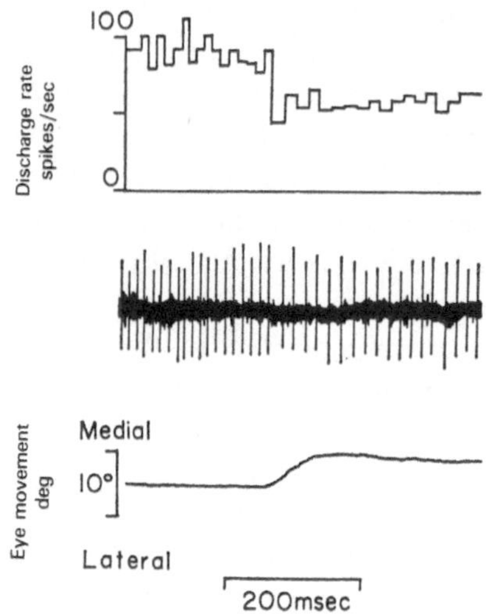

Fig. 48.

Fig. 47. — Neural activity of single left abducens motoneurons of monkeys during a 4° convergence (left) and divergence (right) of the left eye, in response to step fixation change between a far (2 m) and near (17 cm) target constituting a 5.4 Δ accommodation stimulus inducing left eye vergence of mean amplitude 4.1°. The RE performs the visual task. The occluded LE is used for movement measurement (implanted coil of wire, alternating magnetic field). A. Pure accommodation vergence (both targets in line with the right eye's visual axis). On the far right: activity of the same neuron during subsequent lateral saccade between the same two angular positions. B. Combined vergence and saccadic activity (small horizontal offset of the near target to the right of the in line position). From Keller and Robinson, 1972 (33).

Fig. 48. — Neural activity (middle trace) of a single left abducens motoneuron of a monkey during a pure 4° accommodation convergence of the left eye, in response to a 5.4 Δ accommodation stimulus (as described under figure 47). Top trace: time course of the instantaneous discharge rate (reciprocal of interspike interval). From Robinson and Keller, 1972 (45).

modation vergence follow the same pattern as those of fixation in version (force measured isometrically with the LT forceps in a maximally extended muscle, as a function of the contralateral eye position; measurement of unrestrained muscle tension with implanted miniature force transducer) (11, 10).

Vergences are the slowest of all eye movements (20, 39); the classical values of vergence velocity are 6° to 22°. The vergence slowness is due to the fact that the neural signal is a step change in motoneuron discharge frequency resulting in a step change of muscle tension acting with slow onset and without initial excess upon a heavily damped oculomotor plant (38, 45, 39, 33, 44); the very low gain of the integrator in the forward path of the vergence system makes the performance only little better than the performance of the plant alone (39).

*
* *

The muscle tendon forces lie within an operational envelope (fig. 30), the upper limit of which is the dynamic locus of saccadic tensions and the lower limit the static locus of fixation tensions; this envelope comprises merely 20% of the LT diagram (15, 9-12).

Physiologically, muscle tendon forces never exceed the dynamic locus nor become less than the static locus. The latter is true for a muscle even during fixation out of its action field due to continuous antagonistic tonic activity of the small fibers. Even in an antagonist during off-saccades, despite complete innervation cut-off, the tension does not fall under the static locus, the contracting agonist keeping the antagonist on the stretch. The operational envelope's lower limit lying above about 10 g, eye muscles never slack in the awake condition, thus working in the linear region of their LT characteristics (8-12, 15, 16).

The peripheral oculomotor system is the final common path for all types of oculomotor activity. By recording from single ocular motoneurons of monkeys (23, 47, 40, 32, 33, 45, 52) and single fibers of human oculorotary muscles (50) it is established that all motor units participate in fixation, saccades, pursuit, vergences and vestibularly induced movements. Therefore, one may not attribute a specific motor activity to a given muscle fiber type (41, 44).

The morphological difference between oculorotary muscle fibers (there are 5 types) is not based upon the motor activity type, but upon metabolic demands and fatigability which are determined by the amount of labor done during the waking day time, and this is fundamentally related to the unit's threshold value (40, 45, 33, 50, 41, 52, 44).

The mechanical properties of the peripheral oculomotor plant are reflected in the neural activity of the ocular motoneurons. Robinson (40) approximated the relation between R, θ and $d\theta/dt$ in monkeys by the simple first-order linear differential equation $R = k(\theta - \theta_T) + r\, d\theta/dt$. R is directly translated into active-state tension F of the contractile element. Orbital load elasticity is overcome by an amount of neural activity $k(\theta - \theta_T)$, orbital load viscosity by $r\, d\theta/dt$. The coefficient k (4 sp/sec/deg population mean) reflects the elastic coefficient, r (0.9 sp/sec/deg/sec) reflects the viscous coefficient, and the ratio r/k (225 msec) reflects the mechanical time constant of the oculomotor plant. This was concluded from the similarity between the aforementioned equation and the equation, based upon mechanical experiments on the oculomotor plant, relating net muscle active-state tension to eye position and eye velocity (40, 45). Each motoneuron participates in each type of oculomotor activity according to its particular equation (θ_T, k and r are the motoneuron's characteristics). The simplicity of the equation, based upon the orbital load invariability, reflects the reproducible machinelike behavior of R and the stereotype nature of eye movements (40, 42-45, 52).

Robinson's equation says that in every type of eye movement the brain has to produce two signals, an eye position signal and an eye velocity signal. This notion plays a considerable role in the study of the central processing of oculomotor signals (52, 41-44).

According to Robinson, the central nervous system, for each dynamic oculomotor activity, starts with an eye velocity signal which is converted into an eye position signal by the common neural integrator (43). The velocity signal is conducted to the motor nuclei but also to the integrator which is thought to be in the PPRF (paramedian pontine reticular formation) and built up by the so-called tonic or eye position cells (Keller, 1974). These cells create the integral of the eye velocity signal, i.e. the eye position signal; they create desired eye position from desired eye velocity and hold the eye in place after movements (their activity is linear to eye position). The signal presented to the motoneurons is the addition of the velocity and position signals (43).

In saccades the eye velocity signal is a pulse generated by the pulse generator; it causes the neural integrator to create a step as position signal. The saccadic signal is a pulse-step. The pulse overcomes viscous forces and moves the eye rapidly; the step holds the eye in place against elastic forces (43, 44).

The signal for ramp movements (pursuit movements, vestibularly induced movements, slow phase of optokinetic and rotary nystagmus) is a step-ramp (43, 44).

Vergences are produced by a step change in R; the movement approaches exponentially the new position with a time constant which equals the mechanical time constant of the oculomotor plant; the movement is not finished until about 3 times this time constant (43, 44).

A fundamental controversy existed about the role of proprioception in oculomotor activity. Granit (26) postulated low and high-order proprioception in the oculomotor system like in the skeletal motor system; according to Robinson and others the oculomotor system comprises only high-order proprioception (32, 45, 41, 42, 44).

Like in most animals the eye muscles of man and macaque monkey contain muscle spindles which are length and velocity transducers in parallel with the extrafusal muscle fibers. Golgi tendon organs are tension receptors in series with the muscle fibers. In the skeletal motor system low-order proprioception is performed by the monosynaptic stretch reflex occuring in a negative feedback loop around the muscle and modulated by the γ system (α-γ coactivation). The stretch reflex is a servo-assist device used for load compensation, maintenance of body position (posture, antigravity function) and locomotion (control of contractions and movement coordination (27)).

Strong evidence against the existence of the classical stretch reflex in the oculomotor system is given by recording from single ocular motoneurons of the monkey (32).

Recording from single abducens motoneurons while the ipsilateral eye is abducted or adducted by means of a suction contact lens and the contralateral eye fixates steadily, reveals no change in R; this is true for all fixation positions even far in the studied muscle's action field (32). In the latter case, if there where low-order proprioception, the strong central innervation command, while accompanied by strong γ-activation of the muscle spindles (α-γ coactivation), certainly should have facilitated low-order proprioceptive change of R. During identical saccades the discharge pattern was found to be the same, irrespective of the fact that the saccadic movement was free or isometrically restrained, proving that the stretch reflex plays no role in eye movement control (32).

The neural activity of ocular motoneurons, therefore, seems to be determined only by central neural commands and not by changes of muscle length inducing low-order proprioceptive feedback (32).

The following oculomotor system characteristics, in contradistinction to those of the skeletal muscle system, were taken into account in the argumentation (44, 40, 32, 45) against the need for low-order proprioception in the oculomotor system: freedom from external mechanical forces and from load change and load nonlinearity, and relative freedom from muscle nonlinearity (straight and parallel fiber arrangement; linearization by push-pull with only two muscles in a given plane; the same moment arm during muscle shortening and lengthening since the muscles wrap around the globe like a pulley). Oculorotary muscles, therefore, have no load compensation nor antigravity function, they do not cocontract but obey rigourously the law of reciprocal innervation (44).

Eye muscle proprioceptors serve high-order proprioception; their information ascends polysynaptically to the brain (cerebellum) for more global integrative control functions (32, 45).

BIBLIOGRAPHY

(1) BAHILL, A.T., ADLER, D., STARK, L. — Most naturally occuring human saccades have magnitudes of 15 degrees or less. *Invest. Ophthal.*, 1975, *14*, 468-469.

(2) BAHLER, A.S. — Series elastic component of mammalian skeletal muscle. *Amer. J. Physiol.*, 1967, *213*, 1560-1564.

(3) BAHLER, A.S., FALES, J.T., ZIERLER, K.L. — The dynamic properties of mammalian skeletal muscle. *J. gen. Physiol.*, 1968, *51*, 369-384.

(4) BECKER, W., JÜRGENS, R. — Saccadic reactions to double-step stimuli: Evidence for model feedback and continuous information uptake. In: Basic mechanisms of ocular motility and their clinical implications. G. Lennerstrand, P. Bach-y-Rita (Eds). Pergamon Press, Oxford, 1975, pp. 519-524.

(5) CARPENTER, R.H.S. — Movements of the eyes. Pion Ltd., London, 1977.

(6) CHILDRESS, D.S., JONES, R.W. — Mechanics of horizontal movement of the human eye. *J. Physiol.*, 1967, *188*, 273-284.

(7) CLARK, M.R., STARK, L. — Control of human eye movements. I: Modelling of extraocular muscle. *Math. Biosci.*, 1974, *20*, 191-211. II: A model for the extraocular plant mechanism. *Math. Biosci.*, 1974, *20*, 213-238. III: Dynamic characteristics of the eye tracking mechanism. *Math. Biosci*, 1974, *20*, 239-265.

(8) COLLINS, C.C. — Orbital mechanics. In: The control of eye movements. P. Bach-y-Rita, C.C. Collins, J.E. Hyde (Eds). Academic Press, New York, 1971, pp. 283-325.

(9) COLLINS, C.C. — Force transducers in eye research. Proc. Western Regional Strain Gauge Committee, 1973, pp. 11-17.

(10) COLLINS, C.C. — Human eye movement control. Proc. IEEE Internat. Conf. on Cybernetics and Society, San Francisco, 1975, pp. 340-341.

(11) COLLINS, C.C. — The human oculomotor control system. In: Basic mechanisms of ocular motility and their clinical implications. G. Lennerstrand, P. Bach-y-Rita (Eds). Pergamon Press, Oxford, 1975, pp. 145-180.
(12) COLLINS, C.C. — Human oculomotor control simulation. Proc. 1975 Winter Computer Simulation Conference, Sacramento, California, 1976, pp. 69-76.
(13) COLLINS, C.C. — Length-tension recording strabismus forceps. In: Smith-Kettlewell symposium on basic sciences in strabismus. Mechanical and tonic factors on strabismus diagnosis and surgery. Proc. of the V Congress of the C.L.A.D.E., Oct. 16-17, 1976, Guaruja, Brasil. C. Souza-Dias (Ed.), São Paolo. Officinas das Edições Loyola, 1978, pp. 7-19.
(14) COLLINS, C.C., CARLSON, M.R., SCOTT, A.B., JAMPOLSKY, A. — Extraocular muscle forces in normal human subjects. *Invest. Ophthal.*, 1981, *20*, 652-664.
(15) COLLINS, C.C., O'MEARA, D., SCOTT, A.B. — Muscle tension during unrestrained human eye movements. *J. Physiol.*, 1975, *245, 351-369.*
(16) COLLINS, C.C., SCOTT, A.B. — The eye movement control signal. Proc. Second Bioengineering Conference, Ophthalmology Section, Milan, Italy, Nov. 1973, 4: 1-18.
(17) COLLINS, C.C., SCOTT, A.B., O'MEARA, D.M. — Elements of the peripheral oculomotor apparatus. *Amer. J. Optom.*, 1969, *46*, 510-515.
(18) COOK, G., STARK, L. — Derivation of a model for the human eye positioning mechanism. *Bull. Math. Biophys.*, 1967, *29*, 153-174.
(19) COOK, G., STARK, L. — Dynamic behavior of the human eye-positioning mechanism. *Comm. in Behavioral Biol.*, 1968, Part A, *1*, 197-204.
(20) DODGE, R. — Five types of eye movement in the horizontal meridian plane of the field of regard. *Amer. J. Physiol.*, 1903, *8*, 307-329.
(21) ECKMILLER, R. — Hysteresis in the static characteristics of eye position coded neurons in the alert monkey. *Pflügers Arch.*, 1974, *350*, 249.
(22) FISCHER, F.P. — Über die Verwendung von Kopfbewegungen beim Umhersehen. *A.v. Graefe's Arch. Ophth.*, 1924, *113*, 394-416.
(23) FUCHS, A.F., LUSCHEI, E.S. — Firing patterns of abducens neurons of alert monkeys in relationship to horizontal eye movement. *J. Neurophysiol.*, 1970, *33*, 382-392.
(24) FUCHS, A.F., LUSCHEI, E.S. — The activity of single trochlear nerve fibers during eye movements in the alert monkey. *Exp. Brain Res.*, 1971, *13*, 78-89.
(25) GORDON, A.M., HUXLEY, A.F., JULIAN, F.J. — The variation in isometric tension with sarcomere length in vertebrate muscle fibers. *J. Physiol.*, 1966, *184*, 170-192.
(26) GRANIT, R. — The probable role of muscle spindles and tendon organs in eye movement control. In: The control of eye movements. P. Bach-y-Rita, C.C. Collins, J.E. Hyde (Eds). Academic Press, New York, 1971, pp. 3-5.
(27) GRANIT, R. — The functional role of the muscle spindles. Facts and hypotheses. *Brain*, 1975, *98*, 531-556.
(28) HUXLEY, H.E. — Molecular basis of contraction in cross-striated muscles. In: The structure and function of muscle. G.H. Bourne (Ed). 2nd edit. Academic Press, New York, 1972, vol. 1, part 1, pp. 301-387.
(29) HUXLEY, H.E., HASELGROVE, J.C. — The structural basis of contraction in muscle and its study by rapid X-ray diffraction methods. In: Myocardial failure. G. Riecker et al. (Eds). Springer, Berlin, 1977, pp. 4-15.
(30) HYDE, J.E. — Some characteristics of voluntary human ocular movements in the horizontal plane. *Amer. J. Ophthal.*, 1959, *48*, 85-94.
(31) KATZ, B. — The relation between force and speed in muscular contraction. *J. Physiol.*, 1939, *96*, 45-64.
(32) KELLER, E.L., ROBINSON, D.A. — Absence of a stretch reflex in extraocular muscles of the monkey. *J. Neurophysiol.*, 1971, *34*, 908-919.
(33) KELLER, E.L., ROBINSON, D.A. — Abducens unit behavior in the monkey during vergence movements. *Vision Res.*, 1972, *12*, 369-382.
(34) PICKWELL, L.D. — Hering's law of equal innervation and the position of the binoculus. *Vision Res.*, 1972, *12*, 1499-1507.
(35) RITCHIE, J.M., WILKIE, D.R. — The dynamics of muscular contraction. *J. Physiol.*, 1958, *143*, 104-113.

(36) ROBINSON, D.A. — The mechanics of human saccadic eye movement. *J. Physiol.*, 1964, *174*, 245-264.
(37) ROBINSON, D.A. — The mechanics of human smooth pursuit eye movement. *J. Physiol.*, 1965, *180*, 569-591.
(38) ROBINSON, D.A. — The mechanics of human vergence eye movement. *J. Pediat. Ophthal.*, 1966, *3*, 31-37.
(39) ROBINSON, D.A. — The oculomotor control system: a review. *Proc. IEEE*, 1968, *56*, 1032-1049.
(40) ROBINSON, D.A. — Oculomotor unit behavior in the monkey. *J. Neurophysiol.*, 1970, *33*, 393-404.
(41) ROBINSON, D.A. — Oculomotor control system. *Invest. Ophthal.*, 1973, *12*, 164-166.
(42) ROBINSON, D.A. — Models of the saccadic eye movement control system. *Kybernetik*, 1973, *14*, 71-83.
(43) ROBINSON, D.A. — Oculomotor control signals. In: Basic mechanisms of ocular motility and their clinical implications. G. Lennerstrand, P. Bach-y-Rita (Eds). Pergamon Press, Oxford, 1975, pp. 337-374.
(44) ROBINSON, D.A. — The functional behavior of the peripheral oculomotor apparatus: a review. In: Disorders of ocular motility. Neurophysiological and clinical aspects. G. Kommerell (Ed). Bergmann Verlag, München, 1978, pp. 43-61.
(45) ROBINSON, D.A., KELLER, E.L. — The behavior of eye movement motoneurons in the alert monkey. In: Cerebral control of eye movements and motion perception. J. Dichgans, E. Bizzi (Eds). Bibl. Ophthal., vol. 82, pp. 7-16 (S. Karger, Basel, 1972).
(46) ROBINSON, D.A., O'MEARA, D.M., SCOTT, A.B. COLLINS, C.C. — Mechanical components of human eye movements. *J. Appl. Physiol.*, 1969, *26*, 548-553.
(47) SCHILLER, P.H. — The discharge characteristics of single units in the oculomotor and abducens nuclei of the unanesthetized monkey. *Exp. Brain Res.*, 1970, *10*, 347-362.
(48) SCOTT, A.B. — Extraocular muscle forces in strabismus. In: The control of eye movements. P. Bach-y-Rita, C.C. Collins, J.E. Hyde (Eds). Academic Press, New York, 1971, pp. 327-342.
(49) SCOTT, A.B. — Force and velocity tests in strabismus. *Trans. Amer. Acad. Ophthal. Otolaryng.*, 1975, *79*, 727-732.
(50) SCOTT, A.B., COLLINS, C.C. — Division of labor in human extraocular muscle. *Arch. Ophthalmol.*, 1973, *90*, 319-322.
(51) SCOTT, A.B., COLLINS, C.C., O'MEARA, D.M. Extra-ocular muscle forces in strabismus. Trans. First Congress of the I.S.A., Acapulco, Mexico, 1970. P. Fells (Ed). Henry Kimpton, London, 1971, pp. 125-133.
(52) SKAVENSKI, A.A., ROBINSON, D.A. — Role of abducens neurons in vestibulo-ocular reflex. *J. Neurophysiol.*, 1973, *36*, 724-738.
(53) WILKIE, D.R. — The mechanical properties of muscle. *Brit. Med. Bull.*, 1956, *12*, 177-182.
(54) WILKIE, D.R. — Measurement of the series elastic component at various times during a single muscle twitch. *J. Physiol.*, 1956, *134*, 527-530.

Bull. Soc. belge Ophtal., **195**, 125-177, 1981.

CHAPTER V

SYMPTOMATOLOGY

R.A. CRONE (*)

I. *Definitions and terminology*

A. *Definition of strabismus*

In strabismus there exists a pathological deviation of the position of one eye with respect to the other. For a closer definition, it is first necessary to describe the normal eye position.

The eye position is *normal* if a visual object is imaged on corresponding retinal elements in both eyes. Pre-eminently, the fixation point is imaged on the foveae, but in addition a line situated in the frontal plane is imaged on corresponding retinal meridians. When looking straight ahead and into the distance, the visual axes (the lines which pass through the central foveae and the nodal points of the eyes) are parallel, as are the corresponding (e.g. vertical) meridians. A further criterion for a normal eye position is that interruption of the rays of light entering one of the eyes must not influence the relative positions of the eyes.

The normal eye position has physiological limits:

1. The characteristics apply only from gaze at infinity to the physiological near point of convergence.
2. Minor deviations from the normal eye position following the interruption of binocular vision, especially during near vision, are held to be physiological.
3. The small, systematic inaccuracies in binocular vision caused by physiological fixation disparity are normal.

(*) Director of the Department of Ophthalmology, Academic Medical Center, Amsterdam, the Netherlands.

We speak of *strabismus* where a pathological deviation from the normal eye position exists. With the foregoing description of the normal eye position in mind, strabismus may be briefly defined as a situation in which the visual axes do not intersect at the fixation point and corresponding retinal meridians are not parallel.

B. *Classification of strabismus in accordance with various criteria*

Depending upon the eye position, a strabismus is said to be convergent if the visual axes intersect in front of the object of fixation, and divergent if they intersect behind it. Two further types of strabismus, vertical and torsional, are distinguished. In the former, one visual axis is higher than the other, while in the latter the vertical retinal meridians are not parallel.

The nature of strabismus is commonly indicated by the suffix "tropia". The following forms are distinguished:

- esotropia;
- exotropia;
- hypertropia;
- hypotropia;
- incyclotropia (vertical retinal meridians intersect at the top);
- excyclotropia (vertical retinal meridians intersect at the bottom).

Depending upon the manner of fixation, a distinction is made between alternating strabismus, in which the eyes squint alternately, and unilateral strabismus, in which one eye squints all the time. In alternating convergent strabismus, the right eye is usually employed in the left visual field and the left eye in the right visual field.

Depending upon the behaviour in terms of time, a distinction is made between *permanent* and *intermittent* squint. In many cases, intermittent squint eventually gives way to permanent squint. In intermittent squint the deviation frequently manifests itself during fatigue or nervousness. "Cyclic" strabismus is a particular form of nervous intermittent squint. The intermittent character may also be connected with the fixation distance. This is true of the various types of accommodative squint, in which the squint angle is greatest during near vision.

In the literature, intermittent squint is also classified on the basis of occurrence at various *fixation distances*. The last-named type, for example, is described as "convergence excess", while the term "divergence weakness" is used where a convergent squint occurs particularly during distant vision. The value of this classification is descriptive rather than pathophysiological.

Depending upon the magnitude of the squint angle in various directions of gaze, a distinction is made between *concomitant* and *incomitant* strabismus. In the concomitant type (comes = companion), the eyes accompany each other in the sense that the squint angle remains constant despite changes in the direction of gaze. This is not the case in incomitant squint. This type is best characterized by the squint which results from ocular muscle palsy. It is for this reason that incomitant strabismus is sometimes referred to as paralytic squint. There are, however, other causes of incomitant strabismus, among them orbital traumas and myopathies.

The convergent squint which occurs during the first years of life is the most important example of strabismus concomitans. This is not to say that the comitance is perfect in all cases. Frequently there are changes in the horizontal squint angle during upward and downward gazing, and so-called cyclovertical deviations which, somewhat paradoxically, may be described as "incomitances in concomitant strabismus".

In addition to the abovementioned manifest forms, there is *latent strabismus*, or *heterophoria*, in which a manifest squint occurs only after the interruption of binocular vision by occlusion. Depending upon the direction of the deviation following occlusion, the terms "esophoria", "hyperphoria", etc. are used. In manifest, small-angle convergent squint, occlusion may produce a significant increase in squint angle. A "phoric element" is then said to be present in the manifest squint. Heterophoria will not be dealt with thematically in this book and will be referred to only insofar as is necessary for the study of manifest convergent squint.

II. *Sensory anomalies I: Suppression and amblyopia*

A. *Suppression*

Practically all patients with convergent squint suppress the image in the squinting eye to a greater or lesser degree. Diplopia, the disturbance which one would initially expect to find in strabismus, is comparatively rare. Suppression is a sensory adaptation employed to eliminate the irritating double image. In some cases it is extensive and intense, in others cursory and local. In intermittent squint, suppression occurs only during periods of deviation. In alternating squint, the suppression switches with the change of fixating eye.

Suppression can in many cases be interrupted by artificial means—for example, by placing a red glass in front of one eye.

Suppression at two points in the visual field—one zone around the point of fixation and another which corresponds to the fovea of the squinting eye—is relatively difficult to disrupt. The two zones can merge to form a "suppression scotoma" (also known as a binocular scotoma), which in convergent squint is situated in the temporal half of the visual field of the non-fixating eye. The suppression scotoma may have a somewhat hemianopic border, and where this is so the term "hemiretinal suppression" (46) is used to describe it (fig. 1).

Suppression develops easily in young children, albeit the power to suppress varies greatly from one individual to another. In later life, suppression is more difficult to achieve. Yet there are adults who suppress—for example, after an ocular muscle palsy.

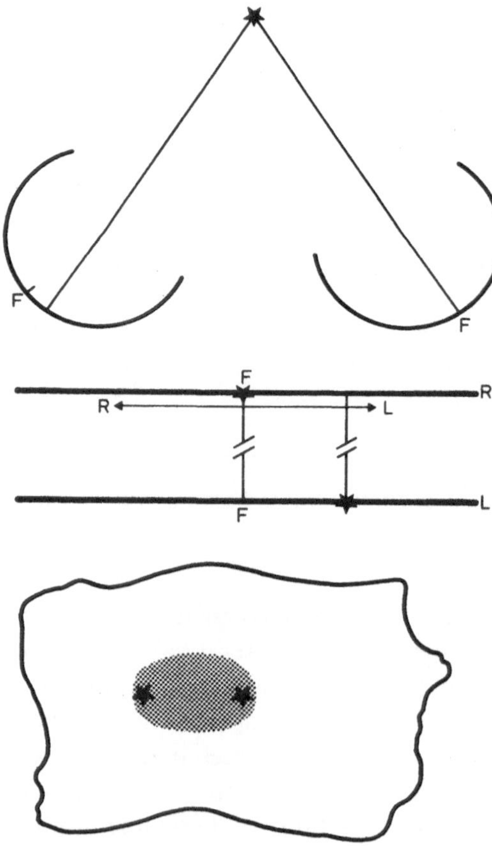

Fig. 1. — Suppression scotoma in strabismus convergens.

In many cases, suppression, once it has been interrupted by a particular course of action, will not return, even if the action is reversed. Measures and situations which adversely influence suppression include:

- Late operations for squint (after the age of 7), especially if overcorrection has occurred.
- Orthoptic exercises. The elimination of suppression should be part of the orthoptic programme.
- Treatment for amblyopia. From time to time one sees cases of diplopia following treatment for amblyopia.
- Post-operative incomitance. Experience has shown that suppression is interrupted—or at least occurs less easily—if the angle of squint varies with changes in the direction of gaze.

B. *Amblyopia*

In uniocular (non-alternating) squint, the visual acuity of the squinting eye declines. Moreover, a retinal area on the nasal side of the fovea is in many cases used as the fixation point. This phenomenon is known as eccentric fixation. Amblyopia is a process which is akin to suppression in some ways, but differs greatly from it in others. Suppression is the elimination of the image of the squinting eye, and is maintained while the other eye fixates. Amblyopia and eccentric fixation, in contrast, do not disappear as soon as the squinting eye is forced to fixate. Amblyopia is definitive, at least until such time as medical action is taken. While suppression may be regarded as a useful adaptation for the obviation of diplopia, amblyopia is a harmful loss of function. Such is the clinical significance of amblyopia that a separate chapter has been devoted to the subject. It is therefore superfluous to deal with it in detail here.

III. *Sensory anomalies II: Anomalous binocular vision*

The ability of a child with strabismus to obviate diplopia by means of suppression is in itself a great advantage. Still more benefit is obtained through "anomalous binocular vision" (5, 23), with which the squinting eye makes a fresh contribution to binocular vision. This contribution can consist of the restoration of the binocular field of vision, even of stereoscopic vision and motor fusion. Anomalous binocular vision is mainly observed in cases where the squint occurred early (before the age of two) and the angle is small. In late strabismus, and where the angle is large, suppression remains the principal means of adapting the vision to the pathological eye position. Generally speaking, anomalous binocular vision is a poorly developed form of binocular vision which can easily be disrupted by a wide variety of means, whereupon suppression recurs. For this reason, the existence of anomalous binocular vision (stereoscopic vision, fusional movements) is often difficult to prove.

A. *Anomalous retinal correspondence*

Because the existence of anomalous binocular vision can seldom be demonstrated directly from the presence of stereoscopic vision or fusional movements, one usually has to rely on indirect evidence. The principal proof lies in anomalous retinal correspondence. This phenomenon is explained in figure 2.

The fixating right eye sees a circle and a vertical line; the squinting eye sees the same circle and a horizontal line. The patient with anomalous retinal correspondence sees a circle with a cross. During fixation by the right eye, point P of the left retina—the "binocular pseudofovea"—evidently localizes in the same direction as the fovea of the right

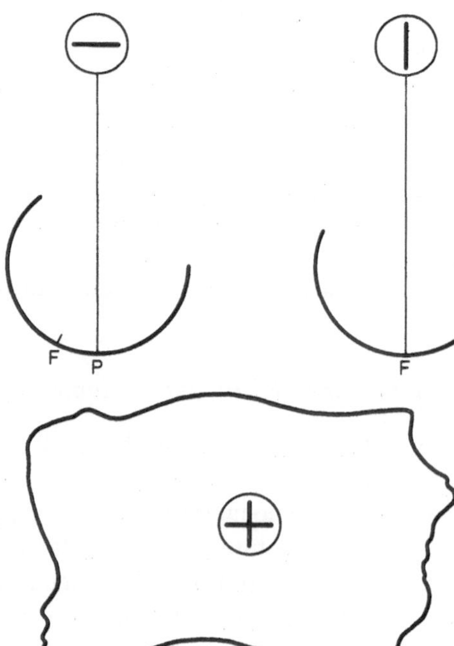

Fig. 2. — "Harmonious" anomalous retinal correspondence.

eye. This is known as anomalous retinal correspondence. The retinal correspondence has shifted through an angle—the "angle of anomaly"—which is equal to the angle of squint. The identity of the angle of anomaly and the angle of squint is expressed in the term "harmonious" anomalous retinal correspondence. In the situation reproduced in figure 2, it is assumed that the circle is anomalously localized by the left eye also, with the result that it is seen binocularly. This is obvious, but, strictly speaking, it has not been proved, for the circle may have been suppressed. In other words, when different symbols *which have a disparity corresponding to the angle of squint*, and which are presented haploscopically (to each eye separately), are localized in the same direction, it is indirectly concluded that anomalous binocular vision exists. Put another way, anomalous correspondence—the abnormal localization of "dissociated" stimuli which differ for the two eyes—suggests the presence of anomalous binocular vision, i.e. fusion of "associated" stimuli which are identical for both eyes.

The anomaly in the localization of haploscopically presented symbols in strabismus does not in all cases correspond to the angle of squint. The angle of anomaly may be smaller. It is then described as a sub-harmonious angle of anomaly. The symbols may even be localized by normal retinal correspondence. May one then conclude that anomalous binocular vision is not present? To do so would be wrong, for anomalous retinal correspondence is not a proper means by which to demonstrate anomalous binocular vision. One presents differing stimuli to the two eyes, thus actually interrupting binocular vision, and by doing so professes to demonstrate binocular vision itself! Despite this paradoxical fact—that we attempt to demonstrate a particular type of binocular vision by a method which interrupts binocular vision—in practice it is not easy to dispense with the monocular, "dissociated" symbols if we desire to distinguish between anomalous binocular vision and suppression. Retinal correspondence tests are most conclusive when they leave the anomalous binocular vision intact as far as possible and when the haploscopic, dissimilar stimuli cause minimal disturbance of the anomalous binocular vision. Such tests are described as "minimally dissociating". The one devised by Bagolini and employing striated lenses (fig. 3) is an excellent example.

These lenses, with parallel striations, produce a linear halo when the subject looks at a light source, but otherwise do not disturb the binocular image. Tests in which the monocular stimuli predominate (or are even presented entirely without binocular stimuli) are "highly dissociating". Experience has shown that minimally dissociating tests frequently reveal harmonious retinal correspondence, whereas with greater dissociation sub-harmonious, or even normal, retinal correspondence is observed. This constitutes a strong argument in favour of the existence of anomalous binocular vision in cases of anomalous retinal correspondence.

The best example of a highly dissociating test is the after-image test of Hering (fig. 4).

In this test, a vertical after-image is imprinted on the fovea of one eye, followed by a horizontal after-image on the fovea of the other. If there is anomalous retinal correspondence, the two lines appear to have

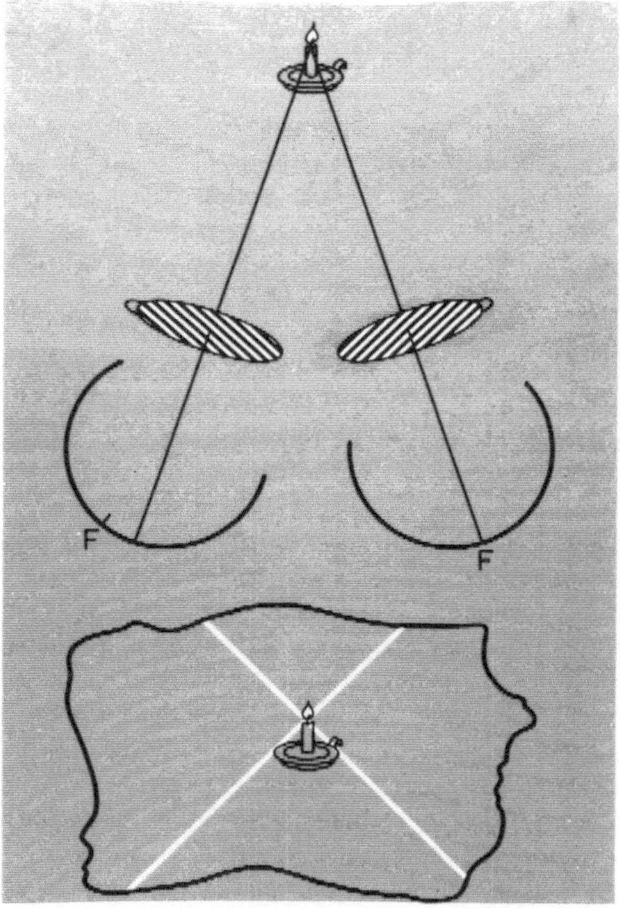

Fig. 3. — Bagolini test for anomalous correspondence.

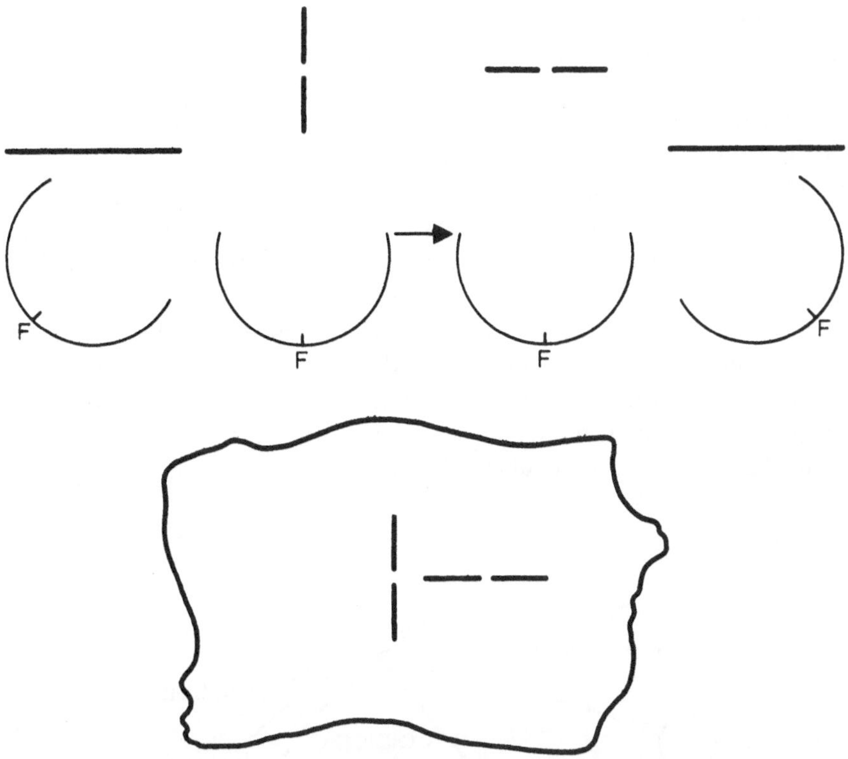

Fig. 4. — After-image test in convergent squint and anomalous correspondence.

shifted sideways instead of being seen as a cross. In this test, especially if it is carried out in a darkened room, binocular stimuli are completely absent, and because the monocular stimuli are not presented at the angle of squint, the dissociation is maximal.

The stability of anomalous retinal correspondence (and, presumably, anomalous binocular vision also) can vary. Anomalous vision is highly consolidated if all tests, including those of a highly dissociating nature, point to anomalous retinal correspondence. It is weak if a minimally dissociating test alone points to harmonious correspondence.

B. *Psychophysics of anomalous binocular vision*

The unstable nature of anomalous binocular vision renders it impossible to analyse anomalous vision in the strict manner employed for normal binocular vision in chapter I.

The *horopter* must be determined by means of dissociated stimuli—as was the case with normal binocular vision—but, as set out above, the evidence for the localization of monocular stimuli in anomalous binocular vision is questionable, and therefore the curious horopter patterns which have been found by a number of investigators demand careful interpretation (47). It is unnecessary, within the scope of this book, to deal with these in detail.

The range of anomalous binocular vision, i.e. the amplitude of sensory fusion, is also difficult to establish. Whereas the zone of normal binocular vision is bounded by diplopia at the front and rear (fig. 5), anomalous binocular vision is often bounded in one direction, or both, by suppression. The aid of monocular stimuli must again be enlisted to draw conclusions—as always, uncertain—concerning the presence of anomalous binocular vision. In the opinion of various researchers, the range of anomalous binocular vision is very great (4)—much greater than that of normal binocular vision (fig. 5). In that large area of sen-

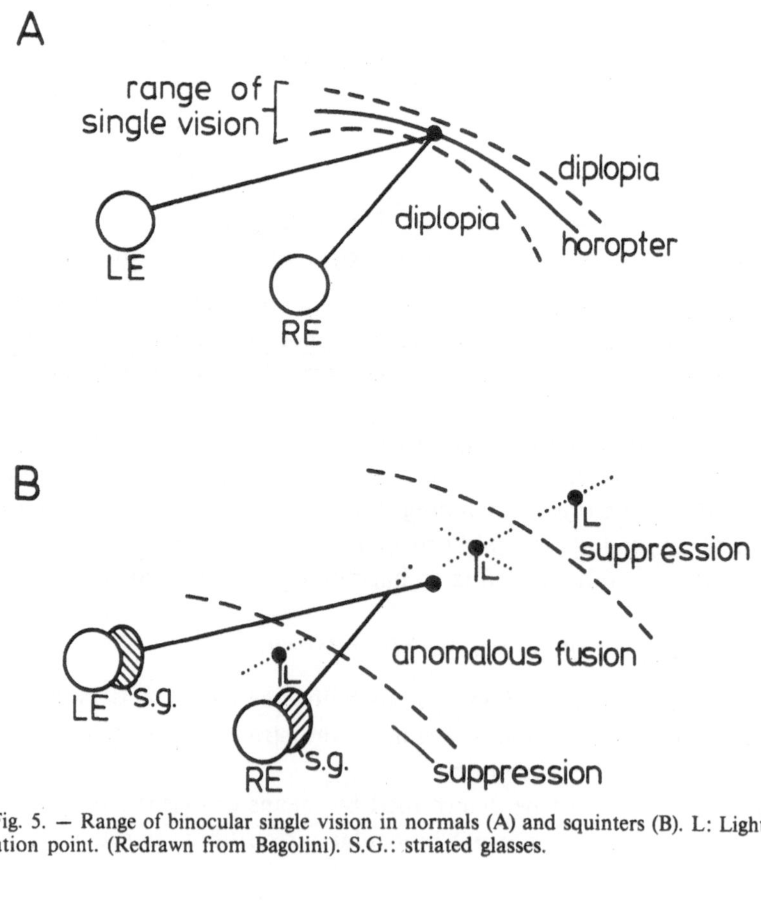

Fig. 5. — Range of binocular single vision in normals (A) and squinters (B). L: Light. P: fixation point. (Redrawn from Bagolini). S.G.: striated glasses.

sory fusion, however, stereoscopic depth perception is often completely absent, or it is markedly subnormal.

Cyclopean localization is absent in all cases of strabismus. Localization is based on the perspective of the fixating eye.

Rivalry cannot as a rule be demonstrated in strabismus by reason of the marked dominance of the fixating eye. Nevertheless, the mechanism must operate in anomalous binocular vision, since in this situation, too, erroneous fusion of disparate image elements must be rejected. The same is true of *globality*, the priority accorded to the fusion of image elements with an identical disparity.

C. *Neuroanatomy and neurophysiology*

Nothing is known about the mechanism of anomalous binocular vision. It is almost universally accepted that anomalous binocular vision is an acquired adaptation in which the basic structure of the visual paths has remained unimpaired. It must therefore be assumed that the afferents reach the visual cortex in the same manner as in normal binocular vision and that neuronal connections by which anomalous binocular vision is possible are made at a higher level. Obviously, the smaller the bridge between disparate elements, the more easily are these connections made. It is therefore not surprising that anomalous binocular vision is particularly well developed where the angle of squint is small. Nothing whatsoever is known about the *neurophysiology of anomalous binocular vision.* Shlaer (1971) fitted kittens with prism spectacles which produced a vertical disparity (72). He later examined the receptive fields of binocular cells in the area striata of the animals. He found cells whose receptive fields had a disparity corresponding to the strength of the prisms, and he concluded from this that new and anomalous connections had arisen between the cortical representations of disparate retinal elements. Further research of this type is needed, and is probably feasible.

D. *Motor aspects of anomalous binocular vision*

Anomalous vision is in most cases highly flexible. Not all cases of convergent squint display strict comitance: for example, the angle of squint may be smaller when gazing upwards than when gazing downwards. Yet in investigations using Bagolini glasses, harmonious anomalous retinal correspondence is observed during both upward and downward gaze (11). The angle of anomaly is then evidently variable to the

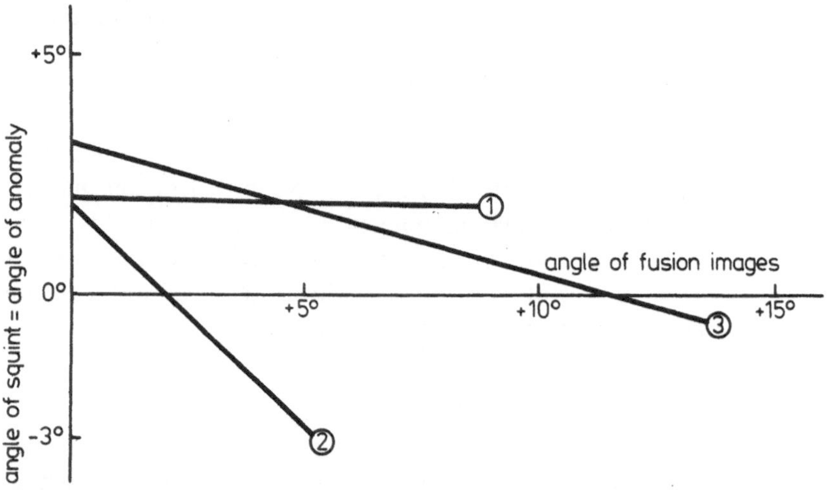

Fig. 6. — Motor behaviour in anomalous fusion. Curve 1: Almost pure anomalous motor fusion. Curve 2: No motor fusion; the angle of anomaly changes with the angle of the fusion slides. Curve 3: Anomalous fusion partially sensory and partially motor.

same extent as the angle of squint. Moreover, harmonious anomalous retinal correspondence can persist at different fixation distances, even though the binocular eye position remains unchanged.

Anomalous fusion of the binocular images upon variation of the fixation distance results not only from changes in the angle of anomaly, but also from true (anomalous) fusional movements. *Anomalous motor fusion* is chiefly observed in strabismus with a very small angle (57, 58, 61). In this respect, the various cases of microstrabismus differ greatly. If in microstrabismus one presents haploscopic images at various angles, some patients follow the angles quite closely by means of motor fusion. They keep their angle of squint—the angle of anomaly—almost constant (fig. 6, curve 1).

In these cases, the motor fusion evidently reaches zero in the binocular pseudofovea (fig. 7). The presentation of fusion images at a more convergent angle (between P and F) then leads to convergence instead of divergence.

Other patients with microstrabismus make no fusional movements, but maintain the abnormal binocular vision by continuously varying the angle of anomaly (fig. 6, curve 2). In others still, the motor fusion lags behind the fusional stimulus presented (fig. 6, curve 3). As explained in chapter I, this lag also occurs in normal motor fusion, when it is known as "fixation disparity". We must assume that in strabismus

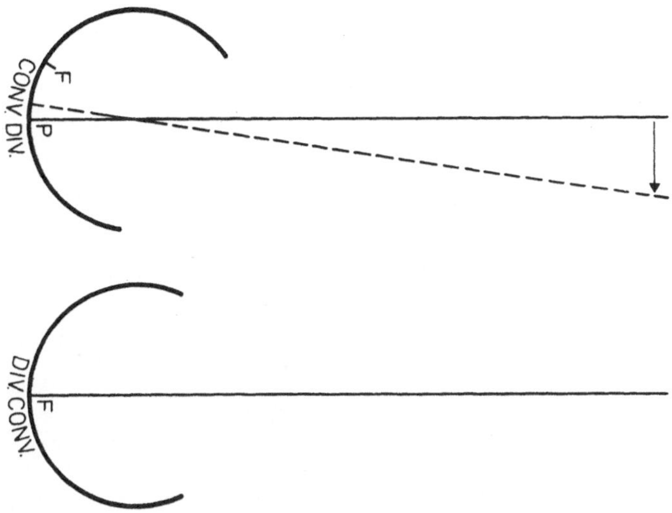

Fig. 7. — The zero point of anomalous motor fusion lies in the pseudofovea.

patients the motor fusion system in principle operates in the same way as in normal subjects, albeit in quantitative terms the eyes lag much farther behind the fusional stimulus than do normal eyes. The study of motor fusion in heterophorias provides still more arguments in favour of the existence of smooth transitions between normal and anomalous binocular vision (25).

E. *Diagrammatic representation of anomalous binocular vision*

Proceeding from what has already been said, we can now draw a diagram representing anomalous binocular vision (fig. 8). It is assumed that the monocular afferents have not been displaced, but that "slanting connections" have arisen which form the basis of the anomalous binocular vision. The direct connections (which represent normal correspondence) have been interrupted.

In anomalous binocular vision there is no cyclopean localization, but absolute dominance of the fixating eye. In the diagram this is clear from the fact that the "arrows of localization" coincide with the central representation of the retina of the fixating eye.

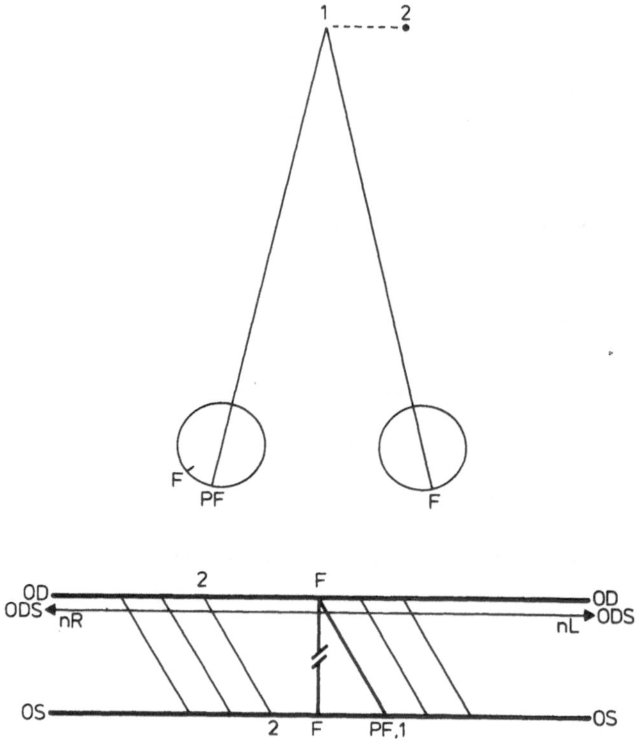

Fig. 8. — Diagram of anomalous binocular vision. PF: Binocular pseudofovea.

Objects which lie in front of, or behind, the point of fixation are seen with the aid of connections which are more, or less, oblique than those which bridge the angle of anomaly (= squint angle). It is conceivable that this is also the manner in which depth perception occurs in strabismus. Where depth perception is present, it is poorly developed, which is not surprising since in anomalous vision the slanting connections which in normal individuals assist depth perception are already employed for vision without depth.

IV. *Sensory anomalies III: Diplopia*

A. *Transient diplopia*

The absence of diplopia is among the characteristic features of concomitant squint. The young child possesses great powers of adaptation to the squint, which it achieves by way of suppression, anomalous retinal correspondence and amblyopia. Transient diplopia, however, not infrequently accompanies squint. At the onset of squint, a child will often be seen to close the deviating eye, indicating the presence of double vision. The symptom is observed particularly in squint of late onset which is easily understandable since the longer the period of development of normal binocular vision, the stronger are the links between the central representations of both retinae. Therefore it will be more difficult to disrupt these links by suppression or to mollify them by abnormal retinal correspondence.

Transient diplopia can occur also during the orthoptic treatment of squint. The elimination of suppression is an important facet of all orthoptic techniques. The prognosis for the recovery of binocular vision following surgery is never more favorable than when pre-operative spontaneous diplopia (and fusion at the objective angle) has been achieved by the orthoptist.

Post-operative diplopia may be considered under two headings:

1) diplopia with normal retinal correspondence. The modified eye position which has not led to bifoveal fixation demands a change in the pattern of regional suppression. This change requires some time to complete, and during this period the patient sees double. Breaking through the suppression can be of benefit in as much as it may pave the way to binocular vision, but if this does not occur, suppression will usually recur as a result of shifting or enlargement of the suppression area.

2) Diplopia with anomalous retinal correspondence. After an operation for squint, the angle of anomaly must adapt itself to the new objective angle, or suppression must recur. Both processes take time, which may be measured in days or months, with the result that diplopia is often observed for some time following such an operation. This is known as "incongruous diplopia" because the mutual positions of the double images do not correspond to the angle of squint. When the eyes are straight the distance between the images is identical to the angle of anomaly; if the image in the squinting eye falls between fovea and pseudofovea, crossed diplopia occurs in cases of esotropia and uncrossed diplopia in cases of exotropia. This is known as paradoxical diplopia.

B. *Persistent diplopia*

Persistent diplopia is in principle of the same type as transient diplopia, differing only in that the double vision is of longer duration or even may be permanent. Because of this, persistent diplopia is characterized as a failure of the adaptive mechanism. Persistent diplopia may in rare cases be present from the onset of squint but much more often, the adaptation is lost at a considerably later date. The process of suppression develops to the full extent shortly after the onset of strabismus and is thereafter gradually dismantled by the development of anomalous retinal correspondence. Suppression is thus a process which, by reason of its own nature, is doomed to retreat. The possibility that suppression will recur is not precluded and indeed this is usually the case following an operation for squint where diplopia exists temporarily. Such recurrence, however, can only occur at an early age. In older patients recurrence is less common and it is impossible to say when the power to suppress finally fails; individuals differ widely in this respect.

The development of anomalous retinal correspondence is more closely allied to age than suppression. The basis for anomalous retinal correspondence is in most cases laid in the first few years of the patient's life, but the power to vary the angle of anomaly subsists. Whether a given anomalous retinal correspondence remains static or changes is presumably not determined solely by factors related to the individual adaptive mechanism, but also to a marked degree by the magnitude of the angle of anomaly. The smaller the angle of anomaly, the more constant it is; where the angle is greater, the flexibility is also greater. Where anomalous retinal correspondence fails to adapt itself to the angle of squint and suppression is absent, "incongruous" or even paradoxical diplopia will persist.

Persistent diplopia, whether congruous or incongruous, is not frequent. The disruption of suppression and anomalous retinal correspondence can have several causes:

- Operative therapy. The higher the age of the patient at the time of surgery, the greater is the risk of diplopia ensueing.
- Overcorrection. The incidence of persistent diplopia following overcorrection is remarkably high.
- Postoperative incomitance. Adaptation is impeded not only as far as the suppression is concerned, but also the anomalous retinal correspondence.
- Treatment for amblyopia. Persistent diplopia occurs sometimes during treatment of the amblyopia.
- Orthoptic therapy. The resulting diminished suppression may cause persistent diplopia where binocular vision is not achieved.

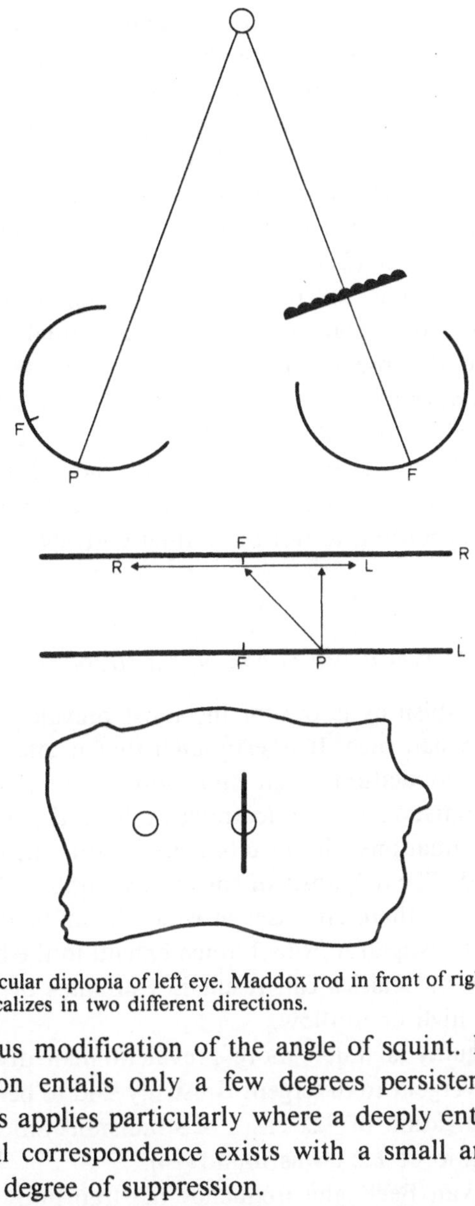

Fig. 9. — Monocular diplopia of left eye. Maddox rod in front of right eye. The binocular pseudofovea P localizes in two different directions.

— Spontaneous modification of the angle of squint. Even when such modification entails only a few degrees persistent diplopia may result. This applies particularly where a deeply entrenched anomalous retinal correspondence exists with a small angle of anomaly and a low degree of suppression.

Horror fusionis is an exceptional form of persistent diplopia. A priori, one might anticipate that, with diplopia, superimposition would be feasible if images were presented haploscopically at a certain angle. However, this is not always so. Where superimposition is not achieved, the images dance round each other and stand, alternately uncrossed and crossed, next to each other. "Horror fusionis" then exists. The term "horror of fusion" adequately describes the situation, for the patient appears to attempt actively to avoid fusion. The stability of the objective eye position is lost, and the patient experiences unpleasant sensations as a result of his inability to unite the images. The cause of horror fusionis is not clear. The customary tests for correspondence reveal normal retinal correspondence. An extremely small angle of anomaly may however be present (21).

Monocular diplopia is the result of the simultaneous existence of anomalous retinal correspondence and normal retinal correspondence. It is more frequently observed in the course of orthoptic training than within the framework of persistent diplopia. In the situation of figure 9 monocular diplopia is provoked by a Maddox rod in front of the right eye. The fixating light is seen to coincide with the red line of the Maddox rod (anomalous correspondence) and a double image of the light is seen at the left (according to normal retinal correspondence).

V. *Prevalence of convergent strabismus*

Convergent strabismus is one of the most prevalent ocular defects among the Caucasian race. It is estimated that it affects between 2% and 4% of the population. Men and women are affected in equal degree. Precise statistical data concerning strabismus are relatively scarce. In mass examinations, the results depend to a large extent on the criteria employed. The diagnosis of convergent strabismus is frequently a simple matter, but there are cases in which it can be discovered only by very precise investigation, which must extend to the binocular functions. Diagnostic difficulties can result in estimates of the percentage being either too high or too low.

Convergent squint is much more prevalent than divergent squint. The ratio of convergent to divergent is usually said to be of the order of 5:1. In an investigation of 922 cases of strabismus among children in Amsterdam, a ratio of 13:1 was found (14).

According to van Beek, the frequency of strabismus in Holland is 4% (7). Frandsen's figures for Denmark are also worthy of mention: she observed a prevalence of 4½% among schoolchildren (32).

Among the non-Caucasian races, the percentage of convergent strabismus is considerably lower. In a population of 12,000 in the U.S.A., researchers found strabismus in 2% of whites and 0.6% of negroes (35).

In Gabon, a country with a negroid population, only 0.52% were found to have the condition (42).

Strabismus is also less prevalent among the mongoloid race. Among the Japanese and other eastern peoples, the divergent form is more prevalent than the convergent (44). In Indonesia, convergent strabismus is rarely observed, the divergent form being the more prevalent (70).

The figures given above apply only to the normal population. Strabismus is found more frequently among individuals with other pathological characteristics. Of these we would mention:

- Cerebral palsy. According to some authors, convergent strabismus is ten times more prevalent among this group than among normal subjects. Many in this group were born prematurely.
- Albinism. In the tyrosinase-negative form, squint is almost obligate. It is also frequently found in achromatopsia, another defect involving foveal hypoplasia.
- Various eye diseases. "Secondary" squint is said to exist if one of the eyes sees poorly as a result of an ocular defect. A unilateral condition which is congenital, or which occurs at an early age, is frequently accompanied by squint, which is nearly always of the convergent type. The occurrence of convergent squint often serves to draw the attention of parents and doctors to a more serious eye condition, such as congenital toxoplasmosis or retinoblastoma.

VI. *Age of onset of convergent strabismus*

Convergent strabismus commences at an early age. Approximately fifty per cent of all children develop a squint during the first year of life. The frequency declines sharply with the rise in age, and after five is only one or two per cent. The graph reproduced (fig. 10) here embodies data from Lang (52) and Keiner (48). There is a remarkable discrepancy between the two curves. Formerly, the age of onset was said to be higher, but now the predominant view is that half of all children develop a squint before their first birthday (64).

It is difficult to arrive at a correct picture regarding the age of onset. The risk of error is greatest if one relies entirely on anamnestic data. Some parents have been late in recognizing a squint because, although it had existed for some time, it was not obvious. Others, having confused a pseudo-strabismus caused by wide nose bridge and epicanthus with convergent squint, pre-dated the onset.

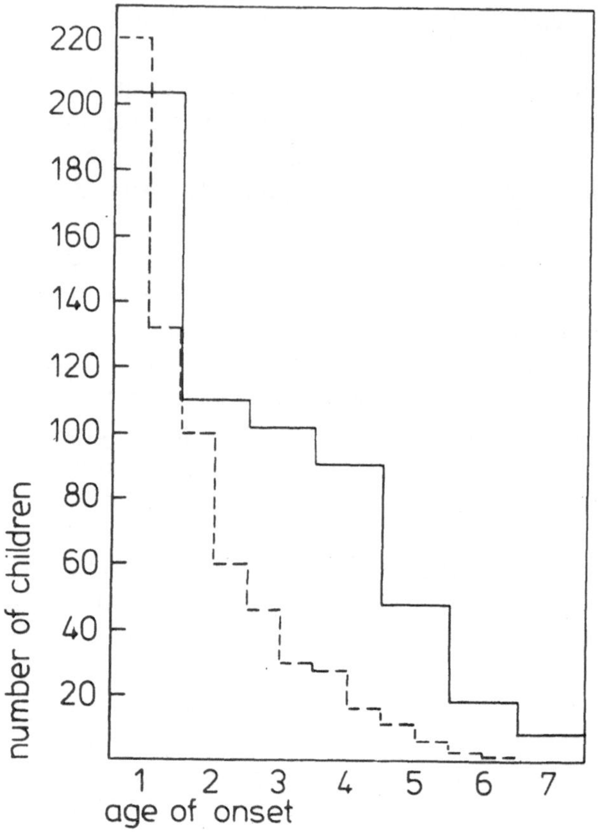

Fig. 10. — Age of onset of squint according to Keiner (-----) and Lang (———).

Even when one personally examines a group of children, and does not proceed from the anamnesis, there is a risk of error. The eye position and eye movements of newborn babies are difficult to judge. During the first few weeks of life, the eye movements are often dissociated and the eye position unstable. A convergent eye position, as an incidental finding, need not be of great significance. As a result, it is not known with certainty how many children suffer from squint from birth. Some authors attempt to circumvent this problem by classifying all strabismus which occurs during the first few months of life as congenital. Thus, for example, Taylor (76) estimates that at least 50% of squints are congenital. This is an imprecise definition and one which can lead to false conclusions. Keiner examined many newborn babies. He took the view that strabismus was never congenital, but in all cases occurred after a period of dissociated eye movements. While accepting that there was a predisposition to strabismus at birth, he believed that "congenital squint" was an acquired defect.

VII. *Strabismus and convergence*

A. *Types of convergence*

In dealing with convergent strabismus, we must obviously examine the phenomenon of convergence. This we can best do on the basis of its physiological function, which is to bring about bifoveal fixation at short distance. Normal eyes converge with an accuracy of a few minutes of arc. Only in heterophoria can the deviation (fixation disparity) be somewhat greater, but even then it seldom exceeds 10 minutes of arc. Convergence is accompanied by accommodation and pupillary contraction. These three actions are summed up in the terms "near reflex" and "convergence synergy".

Convergence can be more closely examined in experimental situations which differ from the normal. In this manner one arrives at an (artificial) classification of the various types of convergence, which largely goes back to the work of Maddox (56):

1. Accommodative convergence ("blur-induced convergence") is produced by stimulating accommodation and simultaneously eliminating fusion.
2. Fusional convergence ("disparity-induced convergence") can be studied by stimulating fusion in the convergent direction with the aid of prisms while the subject fixates at a constant distance.
3. Voluntary convergence is revealed most clearly by convergence without optical stimuli.
4. Proximal convergence is convergence caused by the awareness of proximity. This element of convergence is found by comparing the eye position during distant vision with that during near vision, fusion and accommodation being eliminated in both situations. Proximal convergence is very well known in the field of orthoptics, and usually results in the convergent angle of squint being greater when measured in the synoptophore than when measured by the reflex image method at a distance.
5. Tonic convergence. Anaesthesia usually brings about a change of eye position in the divergent direction. This element of convergence is not only influenced by anaesthesia, since sleep and variation in the condition of the vegetative nervous system and emotions also produce changes in the basic position of rest of the eyes.

Although convergence in all its aspects is of importance in relation to convergent strabismus, two forms, accommodative and tonic, merit particular attention in this context. These will be dealt with separately.

B. *Accommodative aspects of convergent strabismus*

In normal individuals, convergence (the bifoveal fixation of a near point) and accommodation (the correct focusing on the retina) are precisely matched. In emmetropic subjects with sound binocular vision, this implies that the accommodation, measured in diopters, is of the same magnitude as the convergence, measured in metre angles (ma). The latter unit requires some explanation. The convergence angle—the angle at which the lines of gaze intersect—is equal to n metre angles when the bifoveal fixation occurs at a distance of 1/n metres. The metre angle can be converted into prism diopters by multiplying it by the pupil distance in centimetres. A person with a PD of 7 centimetres who fixates at a distance of 0.5 metres has a convergence of 2 metre angles, or 14 prism diopters.

One may wonder why, in normal near vision, accommodation and convergence are precisely matched. In principle, the two reflexes could come about independently—correct focus as a result of elimination of the unsharpness of the image, and bifoveal fixation as a result of eliminating the disparity. In fact, it transpires that a synergy exists, in which the convergence plays a dominant role. If, in a near vision experiment, the stimulus to accommodate is lacking, it is found that the accommodation (measured objectively) keeps precisely in step with the convergence; that is to say, the accommodation/convergence ratio is 1 (D/ma).

This suggests that there is a very strong link between convergence and accommodation. Yet in other respects this link is less rigid. If, conversely, the stimulus to converge is removed (for example, by occluding one eye), the convergence during near vision does not keep in step with the accommodation. The ("accommodative") convergence/accommodation ratio, or AC/A ratio, is usually less than 1 ma/D (0.5 being a typical figure) and seldom more than 1.

The AC/A ratio is easy to measure provided one does not attempt to measure the accommodation objectively, but deduces this from the accommodation stimulus. To this end, the heterophoria is measured at, say, 2.5 metres, before and after interposing a spherical lens of −1 D (accommodation stimulus of 1 diopter). If the PD is 6 cm, and the difference between the two heterophoria measurements 3 prism diopters, the AC/A ratio is 3/6 = 0.5 ma/D.

Alternatively, one can interrupt the fusion and measure the eye position during fixation at 2.5 metres and 30 cm. The subject will then accommodate 3D and, at an AC/A ratio of 1, converge 3 ma; at a PD of 6 cm, that is 18 prism diopters. If the heterophoria during near vision is 9 prism diopters greater (in the eso direction), the AC/A ratio is $1/3 \times (18+9)$ pr. D/D = 1.5 ma/D.

There are two situations in which the abovementioned link between convergence and accommodation can lead to difficulty: refraction anomalies and disturbed binocular vision.

1. Refraction anomalies. To bring a distant object into sharp focus, a child with hypermetropia of 4D, a fixed congenital link between accommodation and convergence and an AC/A ratio of 0.5 would have to converge 2 ma, or approximately 10 prism diopters, or, if the binocular fusion were to resist this, would have to have an esophoria of 10 prism diopters. In reality it is far from being a general rule that hypermetropic children are esophoric. Young children evidently possess a degree of flexibility in matching convergence and accommodation. Only when this flexibility is lacking does hypermetropia lead to esophoria.
2. Squint. If the bifixation mechanism is poorly developed, or absent, the convergent position is determined by the accommodation of the fixating eye and thus by the AC/A ratio. If this ratio exceeds 1, the angle of squint is greater during near vision than distant vision ("convergence excess").

If a child with convergent squint is also hypermetropic, correction of the hypermetropia will reduce the squint angle. This "accommodative component" is governed by the severity of the hypermetropia and the magnitude of the AC/A ratio.

On the basis of the foregoing, the relationships between accommodation and convergent strabismus can be classified as follows:

1. *Purely accommodative squint.* Hypermetropia can lead to esophoria, which can decompensate to convergent strabismus if the power of fusion is less than adequate. The result is then "accommodative squint". The more pronounced the hypermetropia, the more rigid the congenital link between accommodation and convergence, the greater the AC/A ratio and the weaker the power of fusion, the more probable this becomes.

Babies commence to accommodate during the early months of life. Themen (1956) carried out retinoscopic examination on 457 normal babies (77, 13). He distinguished four stages in the development of accommodation and convergence. In stage I, both are absent. In stage II there is convergence, which is always accompanied by "passive" accommodation. In stage III, "active" accommodation may occur in response to a monocular near stimulus; this is initially monocular. The infant appears to discover its accommodation independently of convergence. In stage IV, accommodation occurs bilaterally, even if the stimulus is presented to only one eye (fig. 11). Only in stage III did intermittent strabismus occur, in 72 babies. Ten of these retained the squint. Obviously, the period during which the "active" monocular accommodation is discovered holds dangers for binocular vision.

Various authors have described accommodative squint during the first year of life (6, 63). It is initially intermittent, and is attributed to periodic fusion insufficiency. Accommodative strabismus, particularly in the intermittent phase, can be counteracted by correcting the hyper-

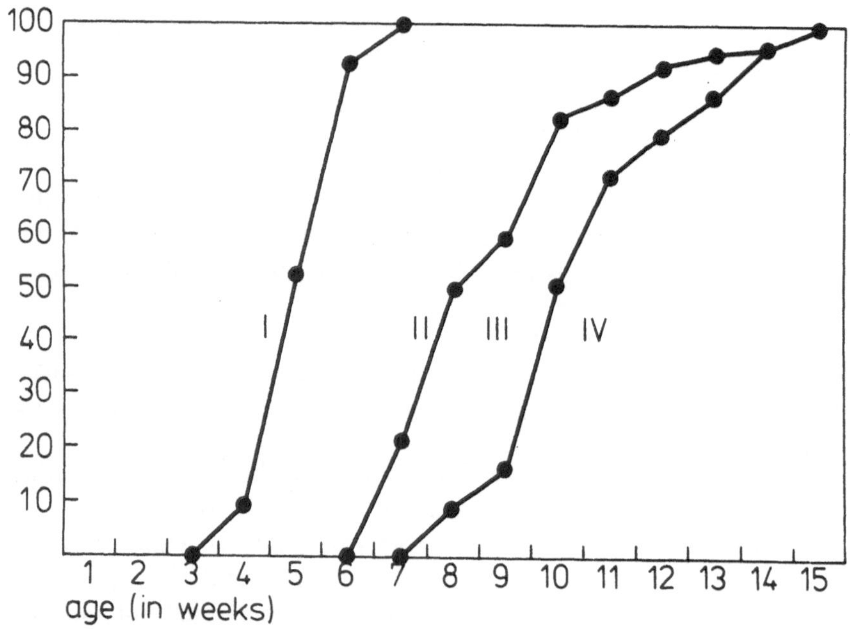

Fig. 11. — Age breakdown of the various stages of the development of convergence and accommodation (as percentage).
I : No accommodation.
II : Passive accommodation, elicited by convergence.
III : Active monocular accommodation.
IV : Active binocular accommodation, even in monocular stimulation.

metropia, or by miotics. Miotics stimulate the ciliary muscle, thereby reducing the accommodative impulse. Moreover, the miosis reduces the blur, thus decreasing the stimulus to accommodation.

If the accommodative squint ceases to be intermittent as a result of progressive weakening of the fusion, miotics and glasses will not immediately result in the restoration of binocular vision. The intermittent phase may be brief, especially in infants. Older children with strabismus of later onset are frequently found to have accommodative squint with a protracted intermittent phase.

2. *Atypical accommodative strabismus.* If the binocular vision (the power of fusion) is weak and the AC/A ratio exceeds 1, the eyes may be straight when fixating in the distance (after the correction of any hypermetropia), but are convergent during near fixation. This "atypical accommodative squint", in which the AC/A ratio is always greater than 1, can be remedied by reading glasses, bifocals, or a miotic.

The etiology of atypical accommodative strabismus is unknown. In some cases there are signs which point to a primary weakness (1, 15) of the accommodation; but one could also conceive of a primary overaction of the accommodative convergence.

This is not to say that every squint in which the angle is greater at near vision than at distant vision is "atypically accommodative". One could think of overaction of the proximal convergence, or variation of the tonic convergence with changes in visual distance.

3. *Partially accommodative squint.* This exists in all cases of convergent strabismus where the angle of squint is reduced by correction of the hypermetropia or with the aid of a miotic, or where the angle is greater at near vision than at distant vision. In such cases, the squint is said to have an "accommodative component". It is not easy to assess the magnitude of this component. The hypermetropia must be known exactly. Some investigators content themselves with retinoscopic determination of the refraction after administering one or two drops of cyclopentolate; others take the view that protracted instillation of atropine, in conjunction with overcorrective glasses, is the only way to completely relax the accommodation. Reference has even been made to a residual atropine-resistant accommodation of several diopters (36).

Whatever the answer may be, the "accommodative component" can manifest itself in two ways—typically by the reduction of the angle of squint during distant vision, following correction of the hypermetropia; and atypically by an increase in the squint angle during near vision when the hypermetropia has been fully corrected.

C. *Tonic and spastic convergence in strabismus*

Where there is no clear evidence of accommodative factors in strabismus, the obvious course is to seek a connection between convergent squint and Maddox's "tonic convergence". This connection does indeed appear to exist, because many patients with a large-angle convergent squint are straight, or even divergent, when anesthetized. If such patients have a widely fluctuating squint angle, there is fluctuating hypertonicity of the convergence: the convergence assumes a spastic character.

It should be realized that this is no more than a description: young patients have a non-accommodative convergent squint with a varying angle, and the squint disappears during anesthesia. Most importantly, it is not stated that the synergistic mechanism of convergence, accommodation and miosis in strabismus is hypertonic or spastic.

Convergence spasms are not among the symptoms of convergent strabismus. The combination of fluctuating esotropia, pupil contraction and accommodation spasm is occasionally observed in older, psychically unstable children who, through persistent diplopia or other causes, have acquired a psychic fixation on the disturbed binocular vision. True convergence spasms are characterized by "pseudo-abducens palsy" (fig. 12). If, during lateral gaze, the adducting eye is allowed to fixate and the abducting eye is occluded, the latter appears unable to abduct. Moreover, the pupils contract. If the adducting eye is occluded, there is no spasm and the abduction is normal.

Although convergence spasms do not form part of the syndrome of convergent strabismus, a pseudo-abducens palsy is sometimes observed in such cases. It may be that there is then a spastic element in the convergent strabismus; but other interpretations are possible.

Thus, a weak gaze innervation and a large convergent angle might bring about full adduction in one eye but little abduction in the other. A strong gaze innervation, however, might bring the abducted eye to the external canthus while check ligaments prevent further adduction of the other eye.

Corcelle described the abduction defect of the occluded eye as the "signe du stop" (14). Others, too, pointed to a spastic element in the esotropia. The disappearance of the squint during anesthetization, referred to above, may be attributable to the elimination of a spastic contraction of the internal muscles. Besides anesthesia, darkness can cause the angle of squint to decrease (48, 84). It is conceivable that

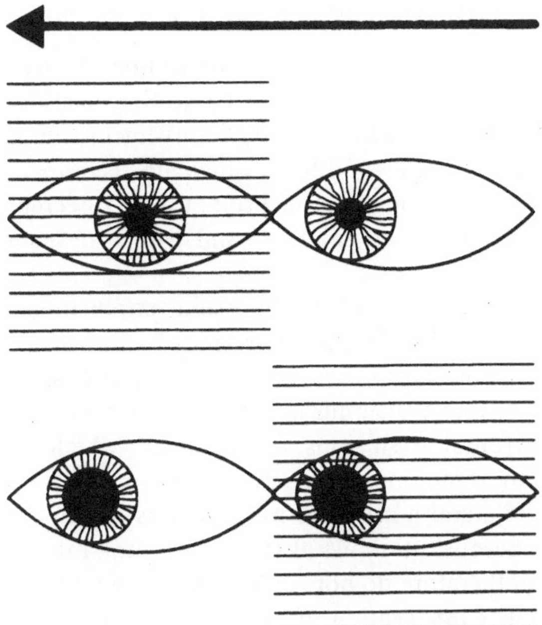

Fig. 12. — Spasm of convergence. Miosis and convergent squint only when the adducting eye fixates.

emotion and neuro-vegetative instability can produce fluctuation of the squint angle by varying the tonus of the "convergence". In none of these cases do true convergence spasms occur, because pupil and accommodation do not participate.

Adelstein and Cüppers (2) provided a completely new view of the hypertonic and spastic elements of convergence. Their explanation is teleological: convergent squint occurs in order to block nystagmus. This concept is chiefly based on the fact that the convergence synergy is capable of arresting certain forms of congenital pendular nystagmus. The extent to which it applies to strabismus convergens is difficult to judge. The term "nystagmus blocking" has come to be widely accepted, but it is not easy to point to cases in which the blocking possesses evident causal significance (85). There is certainly no accompanying miosis or accommodation spasm. As will emerge from the following section, one particular type of congenital nystagmus, occlusion nystagmus, is so closely linked to strabismus that there is little reason for regarding the strabismus as a product of the nystagmus, or vice versa.

VIII. *Nystagmus and related deviations*

Squint in cases of nystagmus. The connections between squint and nystagmus are many and varied. In the section dealing with the frequency of strabismus, it was stated that convergent squint is very often observed in patients with conditions which are accompanied by pendular nystagmus, e.g. albinism and achromatopsy. In cerebral palsy, too, strabismus frequently goes hand in hand with a nystagmus; this is a jerk nystagmus.

Nystagmus in amblyopia (22). In young strabismus patients with severe unilateral amblyopia, the amblyopic eye may display a unilateral pendular nystagmus. This is usually vertical. The conspicuous and pronounced form of this nystagmus is not often observed. Even rarer is the unilateral horizontal nystagmus amblyopicus, which occurs only in infants and can sometimes be made to disappear by the therapy for amblyopia. Unilateral amblyopic nystagmus is of importance in theoretical terms, because it shows that visual-motor mechanisms can be monocular and therefore do not conform to Hering's law relating to the obligate-binocular innervation of eye movements.

A. *Occlusion nystagmus*

In addition to the forms of nystagmus which were mentioned above, and many others which were not, there is one—latent or occlusion nystagmus—which has a much closer relationship with strabismus, in the sense that it seldom if ever occurs in individuals with sound binocular vision, but is often observed in patients with a squint. Latent nystagmus is a jerk nystagmus, which implies that it has a slow and rapid phase. It is also known as "occlusion nystagmus" because the most obvious way to render it manifest is to occlude one of the eyes. Occlusion causes a jerk nystagmus in both eyes, the rapid phase being towards the seeing eye. Nystagmus latens is a frequent phenomenon, and it is estimated that it occurs in at least one of every ten cases of convergent strabismus.

Not only occlusion of one eye, but indeed any disturbance of the visual balance between the two eyes—for example, placing a dark glass, or a strong glass, in front of one eye—can render latent nystagmus manifest. As is to be expected, the latter method has no effect in cases of pronounced amblyopia. If any binocular fusion exists, the disruption of this fusion by, say, the interposition of a prism is sufficient to provoke the nystagmus. As Van Vliet demonstrated, shifting the attention from one eye to the other is in some cases sufficient to reverse the direction of the nystagmus (79).

Occlusion nystagmus can be of large amplitude—so large indeed as to make it very difficult to determine the monocular visual acuity. In other cases, it can only be seen upon very close inspection, particularly if the fixating eye is in abduction (in adduction the amplitude is usually smaller). Many cases of latent nystagmus are recognized only during examination with the ophthalmoscope or the visuscope. Even in very weak cases there is often a manifest disturbance of the optokinetic nystagmus when the stripes are moved towards the fixating eye. Latent nystagmus sometimes has a rotatory component—a rotatory jerk nystagmus with a rapid phase in the direction of the fixating eye.

When the eyes are not occluded, those of a patient with latent nystagmus do not always remain still. Sometimes there is a true *rotatory pendular nystagmus*, but much more frequently there are slight irregular rotatory movements which in many cases become apparent to the investigator only in the slit lamp examination or ophthalmoscopy.

Latent nystagmus occurs in *various forms*, depending upon the visual circumstances:

1. If the inhibition is strong, it plays the role of the occluding hand, rendering the nystagmus manifest without occlusion. In alternating strabismus, and depending upon the fixation, there is then manifest nystagmus which alternates between one side and the other.
2. If one eye is amblyopic, the amplitude of the nystagmus is greater when the good eye is occluded. In very severe amblyopia, the rapid phase is sometimes absent and, upon occlusion of the good eye, the eyes assume only a tonic deviation in the direction of the slow phase.
3. In cases of congenital unilateral blindness, occlusion of the seeing eye is sometimes accompanied by a nystagmus in the direction of the blind eye.

The cause of occlusion nystagmus is unknown. A connection may be sought with the physiological asymmetry of the optokinetic nystagmus in animals with poorly developed binocular vision, and "flash-induced nystagmus", a type which can be evoked by a stroboscopic stimulus and which also beats in the direction of the stimulated eye (16, 27). One could speculate that, with monocular stimulation, the "motor zero point" is nasal with respect to the fovea (22) and that the sharpness of focus must be maintained by refixation (rapid phase). But although some interesting discoveries have been made (45), there is as yet no definitive explanation.

B. *Occlusion hypertropia*

Occlusion hypertropia, which is more widely known as alternating hyperphoria, is a curious motility disturbance which bears a close resemblance to nystagmus latens (18). The two phenomena usually occur in conjunction. The occluded eye slowly elevates behind the hand ("occlusion hypertropia") and falls again as the hand is withdrawn. The alternating hyperphoria, however, is not a true "phoria", because, as is the case in latent nystagmus, binocular vision is nearly always absent, and also because with a phoria, if one eye elevates when occluded, the other depresses in response to occlusion. In alternating hyperphoria, this vertical association of the eyes appears to be interrupted. This explains the use of the term "dissociated hypertropia" to describe the condition.

Dissociated vertical deviations can be provoked in precisely the same manner as described above in connection with latent nystagmus, namely occlusion, interposition of a dark glass and interruption of the fusion. Cases in which fusion exists are rare, and even then the binocular vision is extremely unstable. Bielschowsky described exceptional cases with fusion in his classic publication on this subject. It is a remarkable fact that patients with alternating hyperphoria and binocular vision, even if the latter is poorly developed, may have a very large amplitude of vertical fusion.

Alternating hyperphoria has a rotatory component. The elevating eye undergoes an excycloduction. The unoccluded eye simultaneously performs an incycloduction. In some cases the rotatory component is weak; in others it is more pronounced than the vertical component.

The dissociated vertical deviations vary according to the circumstances:

1. With strong inhibition, "alternating hypertropia" occurs. In alternating strabismus, the non-fixating eye is hypertropic, but the hypertropia does not increase with occlusion. The non-fixating eye may elevate spontaneously and intermittently. This phenomenon chiefly occurs in the squinting eye in uniocular strabismus; the dissociated vertical deviation is sometimes completely unilateral.
2. In severe amblyopia, occlusion of the good eye results in depression of the amblyopic eye. But this phenomenon can also be observed

other than in amblyopia if one places a dark glass in front of the fixating eye, which undergoes an intorsion (Bielschowsky test).

The cause of alternating hyperphoria is unknown. Bielschowsky attributed it to the activity of the centres which control vertical vergence, and therefore took the view that it did not contravene Hering's law. Others ascribed it to monocular mechanisms. In any explanation, due account must be taken of the close clinical relationship between alternating hyperphoria and latent nystagmus.

IX. *Incomitance in convergent strabismus*

Strabismus convergens concomitans is not always concomitant in the strict sense of the term. Just how frequently it is, or is not, depends upon the criteria imposed. For example, it is still held to be physiological if there is a tendency towards slight esophoria during downward gaze, and towards exophoria during upward gaze. On the basis of the (vague) criterion of "appreciable visible incomitance", an estimated 25% of cases reveal incomitance. There are four main types of incomitance, two vertical and two horizontal:

1. Vertical incomitances in lateral directions of gaze: oblique strabismus.
   (a) *Hypertropia in adduction* is the most common. This is sometimes unilateral (and then usually in the non-fixating eye), but usually bilateral. It is also referred to as "strabismus sursoadductorius" or "hyperfunction of the inferior oblique muscles".
   (b) *Hypotropia in adduction*, the opposite picture, is far less frequent. Other names for it are strabismus deorsoadductorius and hyperfunction of the superior oblique muscles.

   In oblique strabismus, vertical incomitance occurs only in horizontal directions of gaze. In the vertical directions, the vertical angle of squint does not change. Nor is this usually the case when the head is tilted towards the shoulders. The result of the Bielschowsky head tilting test is negative or inconclusively positive.
2. Horizontal incomitances in vertical directions of gaze: A and V patterns.
   (a) The *V pattern* is often observed. The eyes are more divergent, or less convergent, during upward gaze than downward.
   (b) The *A pattern* is the opposite: the eyes are more divergent, or less convergent, during downward gaze than upward.

Vertical and horizontal incomitances may occur in isolation, but usually hypertropia in adduction is accompanied by a V pattern, and hypotropia in adduction by an A pattern. Incomitances in other combinations, such as strabismus sursoadductorius with A phenomenon, are highly exceptional.

There is still a great deal of uncertainty concerning the nature of the incomitances (24). It was realized at an early stage that they were not paralytic. Admittedly, the combination of strabismus sursoadductorius and V syndrome closely resembles a bilateral superior oblique muscle palsy, but the essential symptom of palsies of the superior oblique muscle—the influence of head tilting on the vertical deviation—is absent. In many cases, the head tilting test produces a paradoxical result, and this more or less justifies the use of the term "hyperfunction of the inferior oblique muscle".

American authors have opined that the "upshoot" in adduction was linked to a palsy of the superior recti. This is also improbable, since palsies of the superior recti are seldom if ever concomitant in vertical directions of gaze. Nor is there ptosis in case of "upshoot".

An important anatomical view was provided by Urrets-Zavalía (78). He carried out a comparative test on two population groups, whites and Indians. Of the cases of convergent squint among the whites, the majority proved to be strabismus sursoadductorius with a V pattern. Among the Indians, hypotropia in adduction with an A pattern was more prevalent. He drew a connection between these findings and the differences in the skull configuration: the poorly developed cheekbones of the whites, in comparison with those of the Indians. The shape of the palpebral fissure also differed, being mongoloid in subjects with the A pattern, anti-mongoloid in those with the V pattern. Urrets-Zavalía expressed the view that the build of the facial bones determined the type of incomitance. Although he was still thinking in terms of muscle hyper- and hypofunctions, his findings suggest that in strabismus sursoadductorius with V pattern an extorsion of the orbit has taken place, and in strabismus deorsoadductorius with A pattern an intorsion. Weiss (83) demonstrated these torsional deviations by means of photographs of the fundus; others (55) have done so with the aid of campimetry. Unfortunately, these are comparatively coarse methods of investigation; the more sensitive subjective methods of determining torsional deviations fail us, however: besides the fact that there is usually suppression, a subjective readaptation—a sort of torsional abnormal retinal correspondence—may have taken place, with the result that subjective data do not afford an accurate impression of the respective positions of the vertical retinal meridians (38).

Another anatomical theory is supported by Gobin (33, 34). He bases his opinion on the anatomical researches of Fink (31). In the 1960s this author demonstrated on cadavers that the superior and inferior oblique muscles were capable of making widely differing angles with respect to the vertico-sagittal plane. If the inferior oblique muscle was more "sagittalized" than the superior oblique, Gobin stated, the primary consequence was an incyclotropia and the secondary, caused by an impulse to excyclovergence, a hyperfunction of the inferior oblique muscles. In the reverse situation—sagittalization of the superior oblique muscles—the result was hyperfunction of the superior oblique muscles (fig. 13).

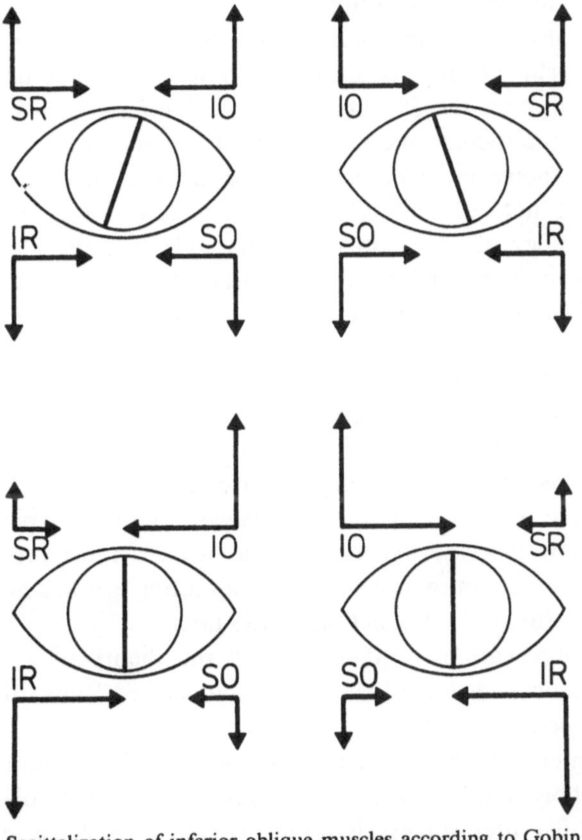

Fig. 13. — Sagittalization of inferior oblique muscles according to Gobin (1969).
A. Vertically acting muscles are in balance. Sagittalization of inferior obliques causes incyclotropia.
B. Excyclovergence compensates intorsion but causes elevation in adduction and V phenomenon.

The distinction between this theory, on the one hand, and the paretic theory and those of Urrets-Zavalía and Weiss on the other, lies in the special, inverse, ratio between vertical and torsional deviations. In bilateral palsy of the superior oblique muscles, and in the cases described by Urrets-Zavalía and Weiss, there will be extorsion of the eyes. In the theory expounded by Gobin, the situation is reversed: sagittalization of the inferior oblique muscles implies a strengthening of the vertical action at the expense of the torsional. Sagittalization of the inferior oblique muscles should result primarily in an intorsion.

Unfortunately, it is not easy to provide exact proof of anatomical mechanisms. From time to time, abnormally situated insertions of the rectus muscles in cases of strabismus sursoadductorius have been described, but this is the exception rather than the rule. It is even more difficult to investigate the path of the oblique muscles in a patient. Even the trochlea cannot be localized on an X-ray plate or a CT scan. This does not alter the fact that anatomical anomalies will play a certain part in the incomitances which exist in concomitant squint.

Anatomy, however, cannot fully explain these incomitances. Their behaviour is not sufficiently static and is too closely linked to the symptomatology of strabismus. It is possible that the hypertropia in adduction—to mention but one incomitance—is not merely one of a number of factors which predispose to squint, e.g. hypermetropia, but rather a symptom of the "squint disease" itself.

Piper (1949) was the first to analyse the incomitances from a non-anatomical point of view (62). He saw a connection between these and alternating hyperphoria, by reason of the fact that in unilateral incomitances it is usually the squinting eye which is too high. He saw this hypertropia as a consolidated, or congealed, occlusion hyperphoria. He took the view that the hypertropia was usually most pronounced in adduction because, in that position, the squinting eye was most strongly inhibited by the occluding action of the nose.

Clinical observations tend to support the theory of a relationship between dissociated deviations and "cyclovertical" incomitances. We would mention two of these:

1. One sometimes observes children who, prior to a squint operation on the horizontal recti, have a pronounced hypertropia in adduction, which after surgery is found to have completely disappeared but to have been replaced by an alternating hyperphoria. This suggests that "upshoot" and alternating hyperphoria are related and that the one can take the place of the other.

2. In some instances, hyperfunction of the inferior oblique muscles of the squinting eye occurs only during fixation with the habitually fixating eye. During fixation with the habitually squinting eye, there is no trace of incomitance. The hypertropia in such cases is dissociated and thus again allied to alternating hyperphoria.

Just how precise is the influence of the sensory system on the motor system, we do not know. As will emerge when we come to deal with the cause of strabismus, we know so little about the fundamental mechanism of this condition that it is as yet impossible to make a definitive statement concerning the incomitances which accompany it. In dealing with oblique strabismus and the A and V patterns, therefore, it would be wise to keep an open mind as to whether the causes are anatomical or innervational.

X. *Clinical pictures*

Strabismus convergens is a multiform disease. There are numerous criteria upon which individual types could be distinguished on the basis of the squint angle, the presence of incomitance, abnormal correspondence, refraction anomalies, nystagmus, amblyopia, nervous factors or heredity. Some investigators draw a distinction between a "pure" or "essential" convergent squint and one in which demonstrable factors such as incomitances or refraction anomalies appear to play an important part. We shall not follow this tradition. Too much uncertainty still surrounds the etiology of squint, and thus there is little point in making sharp divisions. Let us rather place the emphasis on clinical descriptions of the syndrome, and as far as possible refrain from dividing this into individual types. This is not completely feasible, for some characteristics automatically lend themselves to grouping, either on the basis of the age of onset or the angle of the squint. Thus do we arrive at a description of strabismus convergens in three manifestations: strabismus, early onset; strabismus, late onset; and microstrabismus. These are *not* three different types of convergent strabismus, or differing, independent conditions, but rather constructed "ideal types". In the vast majority of squints, the symptomatology is intermediate. No good purpose would be served by describing that intermediate type as such, since it reveals, in varying combinations, the characteristics of the three "ideal types".

A. *Strabismus, early onset*

Congenital or early acquired strabismus has a number of characteristics which are found less frequently, if at all, in cases of later onset. The picture of early onset strabismus is not stationary, but evolves. A characteristic feature of the initial phase of "congenital squint" (which, presumably, is seldom congenital) is *strabismus bilateralis* (48). Both eyes are in the nasal corner. The angle is often large and variable. In typical cases there is no significant refraction anomaly. The right eye fixates in the left half of the field of gaze, and the left eye in the right half. There is sometimes an alternating torticollis caused by the fact that when the child desires to look straight ahead, the fixating eye continues to deviate nasally. It is difficult, if not impossible, to make the eyes abduct by employing optical stimuli, and this applies particularly if the adducting eye is allowed to fixate. Yet there is no true abducens palsy. If the child's head is moved to and fro about a vertical axis, thus activating the vestibulo-ocular reflexes, the eyes are seen to move to the outer corner. If the child is anesthetized, the eyes become straight. The abducens palsy is therefore illusory. If one of the eyes is occluded for a time, the power of abduction of the other will often be stimulated, albeit the movement is of a nystagmoid nature. It is important in therapeutic terms that this occlusion should be started early, as otherwise contracture of the internal muscles will occur, limiting passive mobility.

This syndrome of bilateral strabismus has been described by Keiner and Ciancia. Keiner expressed the view that it was related to a disturbance in the visual abduction reflexes in each of the eyes. Adelstein and Cüppers (2) gave another interpretation. They attributed the syndrome to a nystagmus which was suppressed with the aid of convergence, with the result that the eyes were "blocked" in the adduction position. Whatever one may think of this interpretation, it is a fact that an occlusion nystagmus, or latent nystagmus, soon develops, especially if the unoccluded eye has moved into the primary position or the position of abduction. This is a jerk nystagmus which occurs when one of the eyes is occluded. The rapid phase beats towards the seeing eye.

Step by step, a characteristic type of strabismus (fig. 14) is developing which has the following symptoms (18, 50):

— occlusion nystagmus;
— alternating hyperphoria;
— torsional movements following occlusion;
— vertical deviations in lateral directions of gaze;
— torticollis.

Although the motility of the eyes, and in particular the power to abduct in response to visual stimuli, becomes unrestricted after a time,

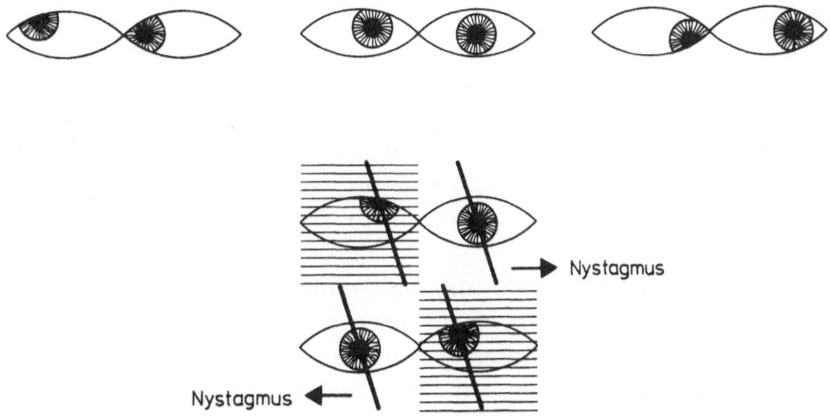

Fig. 14. — Early strabismus with elevation in abduction. Occlusion causes hypertropia, nystagmus and torsion (Crone 1952).

a torticollis remains in many cases. If the head is turned about a vertical axis and in the direction of the fixating eye, the purpose of the torticollis may be to suppress the nystagmus. After all, latent nystagmus is often less than completely latent, and is of smaller amplitude when the eye is in adduction than when it is in abduction. Moreover, there is frequently torticollis about the sagittal axis, the head being tilted towards the shoulder on the side of the fixating eye. The cause of this torticollis is hard to explain.

Owing to the restricted nature of the eye movements and the difficulty of accurately investigating young children, it is not easy to determine whether vertical incomitances, torsions and alternating hyperphoria have existed from the outset. The clinical impression is that alternating hyperphoria occurs only at a later stage. Keiner observed vertical deviations in only 9 out of 568 cases of early onset strabismus.

The so-called congenital squint is by no means alternating in all cases. Yet early onset squint is much more frequently alternating than late onset squint.

In early onset squint, the accommodative factor is usually weak, and anisometropia is a rare phenomenon. The angle of squint fluctuates to a remarkable extent and continues to do so after atropinization and correction. There are some grounds for comparing the fluctuating angle of squint to spasms. Nevertheless, there are also cases of pure accommodative squint in the first six months of life. This squint disappears after adequate (or over-) correction with glasses.

B. *Strabismus, late onset*

Late onset strabismus is of a completely different nature (52). After being straight for, say, two years, the eyes commence to squint. The strabismus is in many cases intermittent in the initial phase and coincides with situations such as fatigue and excitement. There is often a demonstrable source of the squint: a feverish sickness, concussion or emotional stress.

An accommodative factor may be completely absent in late onset strabismus, but as a rule this factor plays a significant role. The squint is often purely accommodative. Incomitances, such as hyperfunction of the inferior oblique muscles and V pattern, do occur in late onset strabismus, but appear to be less common as the age of onset increases. This applies even more to nystagmus, torticollis and dissociated vertical deviation, which are far more characteristic of early onset strabismus.

It is difficult, especially in non-accommodative cases, to determine why the eyes are sometimes straight and at other times markedly convergent. A latent squint cannot usually be found during the straight phase, and certainly not an esophoria with a latent angle of the same magnitude as the manifest angle. One is then almost obliged to conclude that it is an instability, i.e. spastic variations, in the "tonic convergence". This is certainly true of the remarkable cyclic, or "alternate day", squint (40), in which the eyes are straight one day, with insignificant esophoria and hypermetropia, while on the next there is a large angle with suppression. Emotional problems seem to be of importance in this type of squint.

If, prior to the onset of the squint, a substantial period has elapsed, during which the binocular vision has become consolidated, the squint may commence with diplopia. The term "strabismus convergens acutus" is used to describe acute onset squint accompanied by diplopia. In some cases accommodative factors are involved and there is a hypermetropia, or a myopia which has recently been corrected by new glasses, stimulating the accommodation to greater activity than before. In acute convergent squint there is often a pre-existent heterophoria, and the syndrome must be seen as that of an acute decompensated esophoria (21). The following section will show that microstrabismus, too, can decompensate with diplopia. This picture must not be confused with the typical acute strabismus.

In late strabismus, the visual system has had time to build up nor-

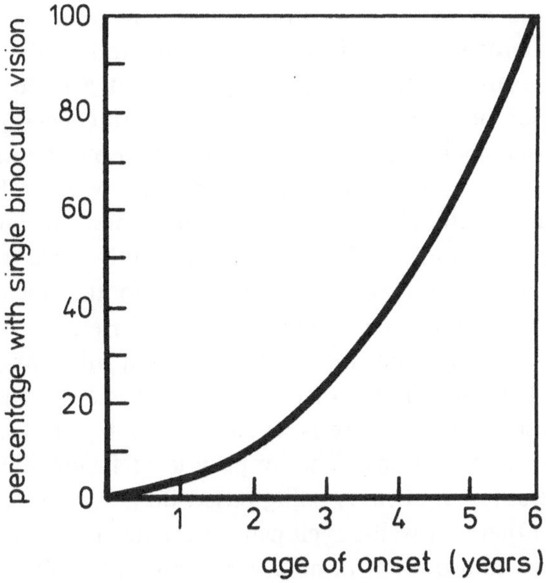

Fig. 15. — Relation between age of onset and postoperative vision (after Douglas, 1952).

mal—though obviously unstable—sensory relations. This explains why the disturbing factors, of accommodative, spastic or anatomical nature, at first only temporarily disrupt binocular vision. Only later can permanent strabismus occur. Even then, it is much more difficult for anomalous binocular vision to develop in late onset squints than in those of early onset.

The prognosis of late onset squint is much more favorable than that of early onset squint, because there is already a basis for normal binocular vision. Glasses may suffice to cure the squint, and operations in many instances lead to the restoration of binocular vision. This is especially true of acute convergent strabismus, where, with adequate therapy, there is almost 100% chance of success. There is without doubt a great deal of truth in the graph produced by Douglas (29), which correlates the prognosis with the date of onset (fig. 15).

C. *Microstrabismus*

In convergent squint, the angle may be as much as 60° yet in other cases be scarcely discernible. The smallest angle of squint which can be demonstrated with clinical aids is of the order of 1°. Squints with an angle of between 1° and 5° are termed "microstrabismus" (53).

In many respects, microstrabismus convergens occupies a place of its own. The microstrabismus is inconspicuous and is discovered only upon closer examination. It often happens that a child or an adult, during a school medical examination or a medical check-up, is found to have subnormal acuity in one eye, and that the ophthalmologist subsequently discovers convergent microstrabismus with amblyopia. The diagnosis can be difficult, particularly if the monocular and binocular pseudo-foveae coincide; in other words, if the angle at which the amblyopic eye fixates eccentrically is equal to the angle of anomaly (39). The occlusion test is negative in such cases.

Binocular vision is more highly developed in microstrabismus than in any other type of squint. Correspondence tests always point to anomalous correspondence. There is usually—though not always—a small foveal suppression scotoma. The amplitude of fusion may be tens of prism diopters, in some cases being based on a variable angle of anomaly and in others on well-developed motor fusion. Even stereoscopic vision is sometimes present in microstrabismus (41), albeit the disparity with which depth is perceived is usually much greater than in normal subjects (in excess of 60 seconds of arc).

Although microstrabismus, as a variant of squint, merits a separate description, it is by no means a separate entity. On the one hand, there are smooth transitions to large-angle convergent squint, and the limit of 5°, below which the term "microstrabismus" is employed, was chosen arbitrarily; on the other hand, there are transitions to heterophoria. In heterophoria there is often a small manifest deviation, the "fixation disparity", which is less than 1° and cannot be demonstrated with the occlusion test. The angle which occurs upon dissociation is a characteristic feature of heterophoria. In many cases of microstrabismus, the manifest angle lies at the boundary of discernibility and increases significantly upon dissociation. Heterophoria and microstrabismus can closely resemble each other and do not belie their mutual affinity (20, 25).

People have asked themselves whether the pathogenesis of microstrabismus differs from those of other forms of convergent squint. Attention has been drawn to the primary importance of anisometropia; as a result of amblyopia and a central scotoma, one of the eyes may have abandoned foveal fixation. This explanation cannot be universally applicable, because microsquinters are often but by no means always amblyopic. Furthermore, the anisometropia may be secondary to the squint by reason of disturbed emmetropization.

Some have considered the anomalous binocular vision to be the primary pathogenic factor (53). All microsquinters undoubtedly have harmonious anomalous correspondence. However, it cannot be proved that the anomalous vision is the cause of the abnormal eye position. The reverse would seem to be more plausible.

As a rule, microstrabismus is divided into primary and secondary types:

Primary microstrabismus is an accidental discovery which is usually made during examination for reduced visual acuity of one eye. The angle in primary microstrabismus can remain constant throughout the subject's life. It is impossible to determine the age at which primary microstrabismus commences. The development of anomalous vision suggests that microstrabismus is a variant of early onset strabismus. Microstrabismus can sometimes decompensate to large-angle squint— for example, under the influence of accommodative factors. It is important to bear this possibility in mind. In a strabismus which is of relatively late onset, and seems therefore responsive to therapy, closer examination will reveal a small angle of anomaly which is a sign of pre-existent microstrabismus. This discovery, of course, adversely affects the prognosis. With suitable therapy (operation, glasses), the original microstrabismus can be restored, but not normal binocular vision.

Secondary microstrabismus is often the terminal point in the treatment of squint with glasses, operation or orthoptic exercise. In early onset strabismus, in particular, surgery or correction of hypermetropia leads much more frequently to microstrabismus than to a perfectly straight eye position with normal binocular vision (43). While this is without doubt a positive therapeutic result, it does not absolve ophthalmologists of the duty to protect the non-fixating eye against amblyopia for a long time.

Clinically, secondary microstrabismus after early operation closely resembles primary microstrabismus. Secondary microstrabismus of later onset has a somewhat different character, because the anomalous sensory relations are less deeply rooted and thus more variable.

XI. *Pathogenesis of convergent strabismus*

A. *Symptom or disease?*

We can point to numerous causal factors in convergent strabismus:

1. Birth trauma is quite often referred to in the anamnesis. Serious perinatal complications which lead to cerebral palsy have, in a very high percentage of cases, led to strabismus. A cerebral lesion is evidently an important pathogenetic factor.
2. Quite a few children develop a squint after a feverish illness such as measles, or after an accident or a psychic trauma. It is not easy to point to the pathogenetic mechanism which leads to strabismus in such cases. Thoughts are turning to a sudden increase in the "tonic" convergence.
3. The incidence of hypermetropia among cases of convergent squint is relatively greater than in a non-squinting population. This applies especially to the higher degrees of hypermetropia. The mechanism is clear: the coupling between accommodation and convergence. Where this coupling is not only strong, but also abnormal, one observes the atypical accommodative squint.
4. Unilateral refraction anomalies, such as monocular hypermetropia, severe myopia and astigmatism, can lead to squint. The same is true of other unilateral eye diseases such as congenital cataract, retinoblastoma, toxoplasmosis, etc. The common pathogenetic mechanism is disturbance of binocular vision. This explains why the straight eye position is not maintained. Why, at a young age at least, strabismus convergens always occurs, and not another deviation, is as yet unexplained.
5. Orbital structural anomalies can in principle disturb binocular vision and thus lead to convergent squint. This applies to the "incomitances" which were discussed in a previous section. There, we also touched on the problem of whether the incomitances preceded the squint, or whether they were rather a consequence of it.
6. Strabismus is exceptionally frequent in albinism and other congenital defects with a fixation nystagmus. In the case of albinism, there is a demonstrable cause of the disturbed binocular vision, namely faulty decussation of the optic fibres from the temporal half of the retina (fig. 16). In achromatism and hereditary nystagmus, the pathogenetic mechanism of the squint is unknown.

From what has been said, one could obtain the impression that strabismus is no more than a symptom, sometimes caused by an error of refraction, sometimes by an anatomical or nervous disturbance. It could then be compared to anaemia, being more a symptom than an illness, in one case caused by a deficit of iron or vitamin B12, in another by a bone marrow defect.

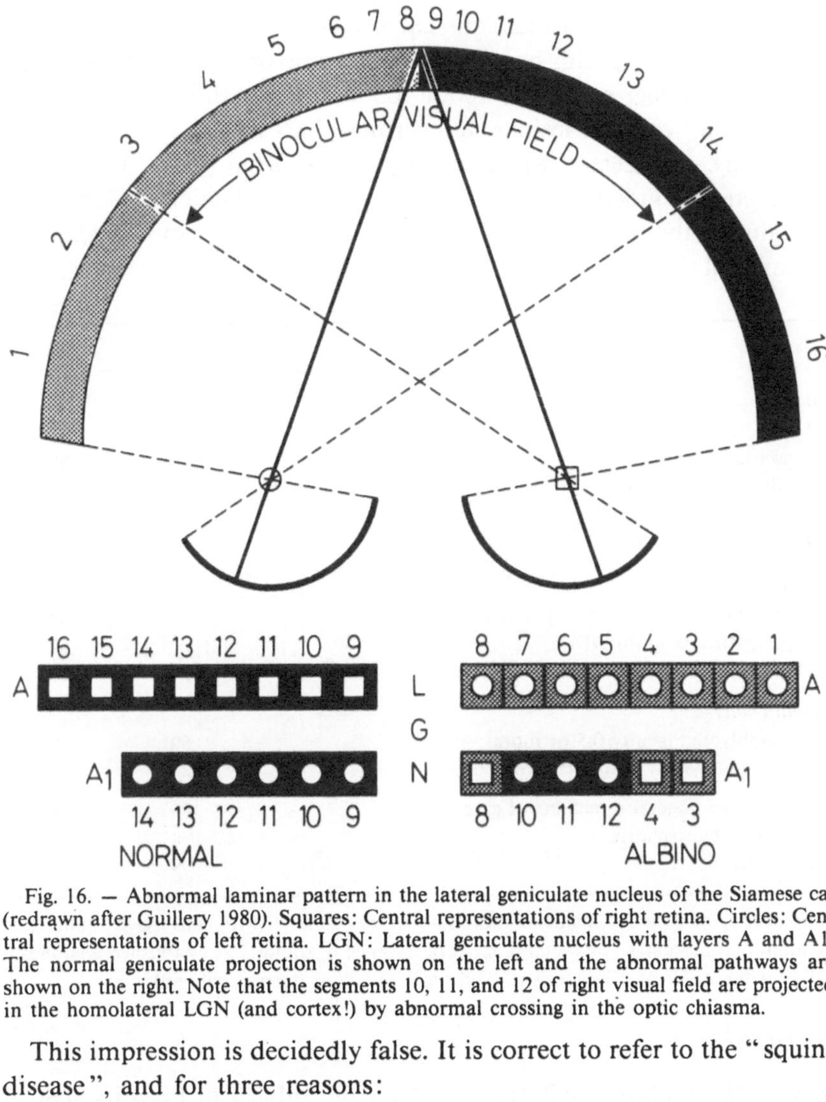

Fig. 16. — Abnormal laminar pattern in the lateral geniculate nucleus of the Siamese cat (redrawn after Guillery 1980). Squares: Central representations of right retina. Circles: Central representations of left retina. LGN: Lateral geniculate nucleus with layers A and A1. The normal geniculate projection is shown on the left and the abnormal pathways are shown on the right. Note that the segments 10, 11, and 12 of right visual field are projected in the homolateral LGN (and cortex!) by abnormal crossing in the optic chiasma.

This impression is decidedly false. It is correct to refer to the "squint disease", and for three reasons:

1. It is impossible to draw a clear distinction between the various types of convergent squint. Young patients with severe hypermetropia can commence to squint during a brief illness and simultaneously display a V syndrome.
2. There are cases of squint in which no specific cause can be identified; yet this type (which is sometimes known as "essential" squint) does not differ fundamentally from those for which a demonstrable "cause" exists.

3. All types of strabismus are equally hereditary, with or without hypermetropia, with or without nystagmus or incomitances. Crone and Velzeboer examined about 900 children with squint, but without other cerebral lesions, for various characteristics (19). The percentage of cases in which strabismus occurred in the family was practically independent of the type of squint. Dufier et al. recently came to the same conclusion; they found that 65% of the cases was familial (30).

	%	%
Anamnesis		
Onset before 18th month	42	64
Onset after 4th year	19	59
Squint in family	63	
Birth trauma	10	57
Precipitating diseases	13	60
Refraction		
Emmetropia	72	63
Hypermetropia up to 3½D	21	67
Hypermetropia of 4D or more	21	67
Visual acuity		
No amblyopia (acuity 0.5 or more)	60	60
Severe amblyopia (acuity less than 0.1)	23	66
Hypertropia in lateral directions of gaze	26	58
Dissociated hyperphoria	9	63
Nystagmus	9	68

Frequency of different characteristics in about 900 children with convergent squint (first column) and percentage in which familial occurrence of squint was established anamnestically for the different characteristics and types of squint (second column).

B. *Heredity*

Something more needs to be said on the subject of heredity. Let us start with some facts. On average, a child's chances of developing strabismus lie between 1 in 33 and 1 in 25; if either of the parents has a squint, the risk is four times as great. Approximately 60% of children with squint have a close relative with strabismus (19, 30). If one of a pair of identical twins has a squint, there is a 2 to 1 chance that the other has also (28, 54, 80).

There is as yet no certainty regarding the method by which strabismus is transmitted. Among the possibilities considered are a recessive autosomal heredity (71) and a monohybrid dominance with incomplete penetrance (81). On the basis of investigations on twins, it was even argued that strabismus is not hereditary, but only the ametropia which causes it (82). Richter (68) concluded that the answer lies in a multifactorial transmission, one in which various genes can lead additively to strabismus: genes for weakness of binocular vision, ametropia and motor anomalies. This explanation is at present held to be the most probable (37).

One can imagine that strabismus becomes manifest through a combination of various factors:

1. Non-hereditary factors (skull trauma, toxoplasmosis, measles, asphyxia at birth, etc.)
2. Hereditary factors:
   - structural anomalies;
   - refraction anomalies;
   - disturbances in the accommodation-convergence relation;
   - defects in the optical path system.

The many possible hereditary factors must include one which is responsible for "essential" convergent squint. This is the "essential" gene, the significance of which is difficult to estimate.

C. Theories concerning squint

There is an urge among scientists to group numerous clinical phenomena under a single heading. In the area of strabismus, some have already succumbed to this urge. To them, accommodative, anatomical, spastic or sensory factors were the true cause—or at least the principal cause—of convergent squint. Others, such as Chavasse, adopted a more eclectic attitude (10).

The obstacle theory

Chavasse argued that everyone was by nature born with sound binocular vision which must be strengthened by exercise in the early years of life. Strabismus arose in the form of obstacles of many types, such as refraction anomalies, disturbances in convergence and accommodation, or structural anomalies, which impeded that development. Chavasse's ideas lead to therapeutic optimism: provided that the obstacles are removed early enough, normal binocular vision must be able to develop. Supporters of Chavasse, such as Taylor (76), claim good results from squint operations performed at a very early age, and maintain that these results support the obstacle theory.

The accommodative theory

One of Donders's greatest achievements lay in pointing to the connection between convergent squint and hypermetropia. Themen's investigation, which is referred to on page 148, clearly reveals that the co-operation between convergence and accommodation can be disturbed even in the first year, and can give rise to convergent squint. It is, however, fairly generally accepted that only a limited number of cases of strabismus are accommodative. Yet to this day ophthalmologists of the Hungarian school, in particular, continue to argue that strabismus convergens is nearly always accommodative. Kettesy, for example, states that even minimal degrees of hypermetropia—commencing with half of one diopter—can cause squint (49). "If glasses do not help in squint, they were wrongly prescribed: too late, too weak, insufficiently permanent". Réthy (67) has gone farthest with the consistent application of Donders's theory. He takes the view that in retinoscopy the accommodation is insufficiently relaxed by atropine. He therefore prescribes overcorrective glasses and protracted atropinization. Further retinoscopy reveals increasing hypermetropia with the passing of the months. Réthy claims a very high percentage of cures and argues that this vindicates Donders's theory.

The anatomical theory

The notion that anatomical changes in the horizontal recti are the cause of squint is not new. The leading modern advocate of the anatomical theory is Gobin. His views on the genesis of cyclovertical incomitances were explained earlier in this chapter. Gobin believes that cyclovertical incomitances are the principal obstacle to the development of binocular vision. He considers accommodative factors to be of such low importance that as a rule glasses are unnecessary. An operation on the oblique muscles to correct the cyclovertical incomitances is the essential component of squint therapy. Gobin claims that this treatment has produced very favorable results and that these prove that he is right.

The spastic theory

On many occasions in the past, hypertonicity of the convergence mechanism has been named as the true cause of strabismus (3). During the past decade, numerous investigators have again assumed that hypertonicity and spasms of the convergence are responsible for the majority of squints. The impulse towards the spastic theory emanated from Cüppers and Adelstein (2), who opined that the syndrome of infantile strabismus with pseudo-abducens palsy and cross fixation described by Keiner and Ciancia was based on "blocking" of nystagmus by spastic convergence. As time passed, many recognized an element of spasm and blocking in up to 80% of the types of convergent strabismus: cases with a fluctuating angle of squint, accommodative squint and even cases of esophoria and strabismus convergens acutus (26). Quéré lent support to Cüppers's view with his electro-oculographically determined "dyssynergy" (64, 65). In many instances the supporters of the "blocking" performed a "Fadenoperation" in order to eliminate the "dynamic" component of the squint angle (60). They claim significantly better therapeutic results in retroequatorial myopexia than were previously obtained with conventional recession and resection of the horizontal muscles, and they regard these as evidence of the validity of the spastic theory (8, 73).

The theory of defective binocular vision

According to Worth (87), the defect in squint lay in the binocular vision itself. He described the defect as "congenital fusion insufficiency" and expressed the view that hypermetropia and incomitances were merely precipitating factors. Keiner, more explicitly, described the fundamental disturbance of binocular vision as a dominance of optomotor reflexes to adduction (48). The babies with "strabismus bilateralis" and pseudo-abducens palsy were the Crown witnesses in support of his theory. Crone attempted to follow this line of thought and to explain convergent squint, alternating hyperphoria, latent nystagmus and the A and V syndromes by a single mechanism (18).

Those who support the theory that strabismus involves a primary defect in binocular vision are pessimists in therapeutic terms. Their belief is that the earlier the onset of a squint, the greater is the primary disturbance of the binocular vision. They therefore maintain that late onset, rather than early therapy, is decisive for the prognosis (29, 51). They interpret the disappointing results of early operation as a strong argument in favor of the theory of a primary defect of binocular vision.

D. *Inadequacy of the theories*

1. The obstacle theory has the merit of doing justice to various pathogenetic factors, but it conflicts with the genetic facts. These indi-

cate that strabismus convergens is a disease, and not a symptom, secondary to a more or less accidental cause, sometimes hereditary and sometimes acquired.

2. The accommodative theory is convincing when applied to a limited group of moderately severe hypermetropias. It is true that hypermetropia of more than 2-3 D is observed much more frequently among children with convergent squint than among those without strabismus (10). But this does not detract from the fact that countless squinters have a smaller hypermetropia, and that the vast majority of moderately hypermetropic children do not squint. There is also the point that the causal connection between strabismus and hypermetropia can at times be reversed. As long ago as 1909, Straub assumed that disturbed binocular vision could inhibit emmetropization (75). Newborn babies have on average a refraction of 2D hypermetropia with a wide statistic spread and substantial astigmatism; adults are emmetropic with a narrow statistic spread. It has been established that visual activity is vital for this "emmetropization" (86). The large degrees of hypermetropia found by supporters of the accommodative theory after protracted atropinization may represent not the "true" refraction, but a disturbed emmetropization.

3. The anatomical theories can scarcely lay claim to universal validity. Lack of uniformity in the length of the horizontal ocular muscles will certainly impede the restoration of binocular vision, but everything points to the fact that anatomical changes develop secondarily to a process which at the outset is purely dynamic (2). The notion that cyclovertical deviations are the cause of strabismus (33, 34) is attractive in those cases where such structural anomalies are evidently present. In many cases of convergent squint, however, cyclovertical deviations are not present in appreciable degree, so it is unlikely that these are an "obstacle" to binocular vision. Furthermore, since cyclovertical deviations are not usually observed prior to the onset of squint, the causal connection between strabismus and cyclovertical deviations is open to more than one interpretation.

4. As soon as one discounts anatomical factors, tonic and spastic disturbances of the convergence become the cause of convergent squint. This assertion is no more than a tautology if convergence and convergent eye position are employed as identical terms. If, however, one explains strabismus by a hypertonicity or spasm of the convergence mechanism (in which convergence goes with accommodation and miosis), the tonic-spastic theory becomes problematical. The infantile stra-

bismus bilateralis of Keiner is—again—the Crown witness for the "blocking syndrome". A convergence spasm, it is said, serves to suppress a nystagmus. Yet one sees no miosis or hyperaccommodation. It is therefore improbable that hypertonicity of the convergence mechanism is caused by nystagmus. A more obvious explanation is that esotropia and latent nystagmus have a common—and unknown—cause. Nystagmus latens is a loyal companion of strabismus. It is therefore not surprising that disturbed following movements and an abnormal optokinetic nystagmus—in short, all forms of "dyssynergy"— are often observed in strabismus. The hypothesis of a blocking of nystagmus is therefore superfluous (85).

5. The notion that a primary defect of binocular vision exists can neither be proved nor refuted, for the simple reason that a disturbance of binocular vision is always present in strabismus. The probability of this theory is enhanced by the fact that there are many cases of strabismus in which not a single obstacle can be demonstrated, and abnormal vulnerability of the sensory co-ordination is the most logical explanation. Patients with microstrabismus are an example. Inversely, there is the important fact that severe motor "obstacles", e.g. ocular muscle palsies, do not as a rule disturb binocular vision (69). Finally, the immensely high prevalence of convergent squint among children with cerebral palsy and cerebral growth disturbances raises a presumption that an as yet unspecified cerebral dysfunction lies at the root of strabismus.

According to the current genetic theory, in which strabismus is held to be multifactorial, a primary defect of binocular vision need not be the sole cause of strabismus, nor even the principal genetic factor, but is perhaps a frequent, or even obligate, factor in the background; this even applies where the significance of another factor (for example, severe hypermetropia) is abundantly clear.

In the light of modern discoveries, there is little point in speculating on the nature of the primary defect in binocular vision. Until this was observed in albino animals, no one could have envisaged the existence of a fault in the decussation of the optic fibres. This can now even be demonstrated in human albinos (17). The coarse signs of faulty decussation of the optic nerves are not found in non-albinotic squinters (59); however, it is quite conceivable that a similar, but more subtle and as yet undemonstrable, defect of the optokinetic system exists in ordinary convergent squint. New data concerning the afferent optical paths are becoming available all the time. The axons (74) of the X, Y and W

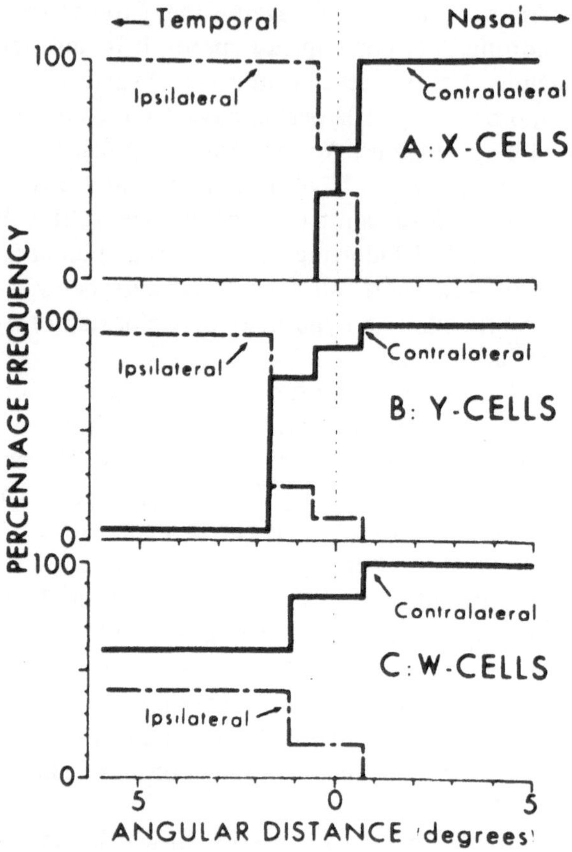

Fig. 17. — The crossing of fibers from X, Y and W cells in cat (from Stone and Fukuda, 1974).
A. Axons from temporal C cells cross, except from part of the parafoveal cells.
B. 5% of the axons of peripheral temporal y cells cross.
C. 60% of the axons of temporally located W cells cross at the chiasma.

ganglion cells of the retina behave very differently among themselves and display different decussation patterns in the chiasma (fig. 17). Even at this first level, a deviation could disturb the binocular vision. At higher neural levels, the conceivable deviations are so numerous that it would be unwise to speculate on them at this juncture. All the theories of strabismus are now obsolete; but we have not yet arrived at the decisive facts.

BIBLIOGRAPHY

(1) ABRAHAM, S.V. — Classification of non-paralytic strabismus. *Amer. J. Ophthal.*, 1949, *32*, 93-98.
(2) ADELSTEIN, F.E., CÜPPERS, C. — Zum Problem der echten und der scheinbaren

Abducenslähmung (Das sogenannte "Blockierungssyndrom"). *Bücherei des Augenarztes*, 1966, *46*, 318-324. F. Enke, Stuttgart.
(3) ADLER, F.H. — Pathologic physiology of convergent strabismus. *Arch. Ophthal.*, 1945, *33*, 362-380.
(4) BAGOLINI, B., CAPOBIANCO, N.M. — Subjective space in comitant squint. *Amer. J. Ophthal.*, 1965, *59*, 430-442.
(5) BAGOLINI, B. — Sensorial anomalies in strabismus. *Docum. Ophthal.*, 1976, *41*[1], 23-43.
(6) BAKER, J.D., PARKS, M.M. — Early onset accommodative esotropia. *Amer. J. Ophthal.*, 1980, *90*, 11-18.
(7) BEEK, C.J. VAN — Over de frequentie van het strabismussyndroom en enkele consequenties daarvan. Thesis Utrecht, 1964.
(8) BEHRENS-BAUMANN, W., WÖLZ, U. — Ergebnisse der "Fadenfixation" nach Cüppers bei Schielern mit schwankendem Winkel. *Klin. Mbl. Augenheilk.*, 1978, *173*, 814-824.
(9) BIELSCHOWSKY, A. — Die einseitigen und gegensinnigen ("dissoziierten") Vertikalbewegungen der Augen. *Albrecht v. Graefes Arch. Ophthal.*, 1930, *125*, 493-553.
(10) CHAVASSE, F.B. — Worth's Squint, 7th ed. Balliere, Tindall & Cox, London 1939.
(11) CIANCIA, A.O. — Sensorial relationship in A and V syndromes. *Trans. Ophthal. Soc. U.K.*, 1962, *82*, 243-251.
(12) CIANCIA, A.O. — La esotropia con limitación bilateral de la abducción en al lactante. *Arch. Oftal. B. Aires*, 1962, *37*, 207.
(13) COLENBRANDER, M.C. — Ontdekking van de accommodatie als oorzaak van scheelzien. *Maandschr. Kindergeneesk.*, 1955, *23*, 2.
(14) CORCELLE, M.L. — Séméiologie du signe du stop. *Bull. Soc. Ophtal. France*, 1962, *62*, 303-305.
(15) COSTENBADER, F.D. — Clinical course and management of esotropia. Strabismus ophthalmic symposium II, ed. J.H. Allen, C.V. Mosby, St. Louis, 1958.
(16) COSTIN, A., CHAIMOVITZ, M., BERGMANN, F. — Nystagmus evoked by intermittent photic stimulation of the rabbit's eye. *Experientia*, 1965, *21*, 167-168.
(17) CREEL, D.J., WITKOP, C.J., KING, R.A. — Asymmetric visual evoked potentials in human albinos: evidence for visual system anomalies. *Invest. Ophthal.*, 1974, *13*, 430.
(18) CRONE, R.A. — Alternating hyperphoria. *Brit. J. Ophthal.*, 1954, *38*, 591-604.
(19) CRONE, R.A., VELZEBOER, C.M.J. — Statistics on strabismus in the Amsterdam youth. *Arch. Ophthal.*, 1956, *55*, 455-470.
(20) CRONE, R.A. — From orthophoria to microtropia. *Brit. Orthopt. J.*, 1969, *26*, 45-51.
(21) CRONE, R.A. — Diplopia (1973). Excerpta Medica, Amsterdam; American Elsevier, New York.
(22) CRONE, R.A. — Amblyopia, the pathology of motor disorders in amblyopic eyes. *Documenta Ophthal. Proc. Series*, 1977, *11*, 9-18.
(23) CRONE, R.A. — Anomale Korrespondenz und anomales Binokularsehen. Bücherei des Augenarztes 72, 1978, 49-62. Ferdinand Enke Verlag, Stuttgart.
(24) CRONE, R.A. — Les composantes torsionelles et verticales dans les troubles oculomoteurs. *J. Fr. Orthop.*, 1981, *13*, 79-89.
(25) CRONE, R.A. — Anomalous and normal motor fusion in esophoria and microesotropia. *Trans. Ophthal. Soc. U.K.*, 1980, *100*, 464-466.
(26) CÜPPERS, C. — Ergänzungen zur Indikation der Fadenoperation. Arbeitskreis Schielbehandlung 9, 1977.
(27) DALEN, J.T.W. VAN — Flash induced nystagmus. Thesis Amsterdam 1978.
(28) DECKER, W. DE, FEUERHAKE, C. — Schielen bei eineiigen Zwillingen. Deutsche Ophthal. Ges., Band 75, Kongress 1977. Bergmann, München 1978, p. 490-493.
(29) DOUGLAS, A.A. — Value of orthoptics in the treatment of squint. *Brit. J. Ophthal.*, 1952, *36*, 169-201.
(30) DUFIER, J.L., BRIARD, M.L., BONAITI, C., FREZAL, J. — Inheritance in the etiology of convergent squint. *Ophthalmologica*, 1979, *179*, 225-234.

(31) FINK, W.H. — Surgery of the vertical muscles of the eye. Thomas, Springfield, 1951.
(32) FRANDSEN, A.D. — Occurrence of squint. Thesis Copenhagen 1960.
(33) GOBIN, M.H. — Cyclotropia and squint. Thesis Leiden 1969.
(34) GOBIN, M.H. — La sagittalisation des obliques. *J. Fr. Orthopt.*, 1979, *11*, 153-165.
(35) GOVER, YANKEY (1944). cit. Duke-Elder, System of Ophthalmology vol. IV, 1973, p. 584. Henry Kimpton, London.
(36) GREGERSEN, E., PONTOPPIDAN, J., RINDZIUNSKI, E. — Intra- and interindividual variation in atropine-resistent residual accommodation. Strabismus Proc. third Meeting I.S.A. Ed. R.D. Reinecke, p. 117-121. Grune and Stratton, New York, San Francisco, London, 1978.
(37) GRÜTZNER, P., YAZAWA, K., SPIVEY, B.E. — Heredity and strabismus. *Survey Ophthal.*, 1970, *14*, 441-455.
(38) GUYTON, D.L., VON NOORDEN, G.K. — Sensory adaptations to cyclodeviations. Strabismus, Proc. third Meeting I.S.A. Ed. R.D. Reinecke, p. 399-403. Grune and Stratton, New York, San Francisco, London, 1978.
(39) HELVESTON, E.M., VON NOORDEN, G.K. — Microtropia: a newly defined entity. *Arch. Ophthal.*, 1967, *78*, 272-281.
(40) HELVESTON, E.M. — Cyclic strabismus. *Amer. Orthopt. J.*, 1973, *23*, 48-51.
(41) HENSON, D.B., WILLIAMS, D.E. — Depth perception in strabismus. *Brit. J. Ophthal.*, 1980, *64*, 349-353.
(42) HOLM, S. — Le strabisme concomitant chez les palénégrides au Gabon, Afrique équatoriale française. *Acta Ophthal.*, 1939, *17*, 367-387.
(43) ING, M., COSTENBADER, F.D., PARKS, M.M., ALBERT, D.G. — Early surgery for congenital esotropia. *Amer. J. Ophthal.*, 1966, *61*, 1419-1427.
(44) ING, M.R., PANG, S.W.L. — The racial distribution of strabismus. Strabismus, Proc. third Meeting I.S.A., Ed. R.D. Reinecke, p. 107-109. Grune and Stratton, New York, San Francisco, London 1978.
(45) ISHIKAWA, S. — Latent nystagmus and its etiology. Strabismus, Proc. third Meeting I.S.A. Ed. R.D. Reinecke, p. 203-214. Grune and Stratton, New York, San Francisco, London, 1978.
(46) JAMPOLSKY, A. — Characteristics of suppression in strabismus. *Arch. Ophthal.*, 1955, *54*, 683-696.
(47) JOHNSTON, A.W. — Clinical horopter determination and the mechanism of binocular vision in anomalous correspondence. *Ophthalmologica*, 1971, *163*, 102-119.
(48) KEINER, G.B.J. — New viewpoints on the origin of squint. Tjeenk Willink, Zwolle, 1951.
(49) KETTESY, A. — Die Brille als Heilmittel des Schielens. *Klin. Mbl. Augenheilk.*, 1972, *161*, 160-164.
(50) LANG, J. — Der kongenitale oder frühkindliche Strabismus. *Ophthalmologica*, 1967, *154*, 201-208.
(51) LANG, J. — Welche Schielfälle können geheilt werden? *Ophthalmologica*, 1968, *156*, 190-196.
(52) LANG, J. — Strabismus. Huber; Bern, Stuttgart, Wien, 1971.
(53) LANG, J. — Mikrostrabismus. Bücherei des Augenarztes 62, Ferdinand Enke, Stuttgart 1973.
(54) LANTHONY, Ph., ITHIER, N., PICARD, M.P. — Les jumeaux strabiques. *J. Franc. Orthopt.*, 1977, *9*, 93-100.
(55) LOCKE, J.C. — Heterotopia of the blind spot in ocular vertical muscle imbalance. *Tr. Amer. Ophthal. Soc.*, 1967, *65*, 306.
(56) MADDOX, E.E. — Discussion on heterophoria. *Trans. Ophthal. Soc. U.K.*, 1929, *49*, 31-44.
(57) MAILLETTE DE BUY WENNIGER-PRICK, L.J.J.M. — Binoculair zien bij microstrabismus. Thesis, Amsterdam 1981.
(58) MARAINI, G., PASINO, L. — Variations in the angle of anomaly and fusional movements in cases of small-angle convergent strabismus with harmonious anomalous retinal correspondence. *Brit. J. Ophthal.*, 1964, *48*, 439-443.
(59) McCORMACK, G.L. — Electrophysiologic evidence for normal optic nerve fiber projections in normally pigmented squinters. *Invest. Ophthal.*, 1975, *14*, 931-935.

(60) MÜHLENDYCK, H., LINNEN, H.J. — Die operative Behandlung nystagmusbedingter schwankender Schielwinkel mit der Fadenoperation nach Cüppers. *Klin. Mbl. Augenheilk.*, 1975, *167*, 273-290.
(61) NOORDENBOS, A.M., CRONE, R.A. — Motor fusion in small-angle esotropia. Orthoptics: Past, presence, future. 3rd Int. Orthoptic Congress, Boston 1975, Eds. S. Moore et al. Stratton, New York 1976.
(62) PIPER, H.F. — Die Schielkrankheit. *Albrecht v. Graefes Arch. Ophthal.*, 1948, *148*, 555-616.
(63) POLLARD, Z.F. — Accommodative esotropia during the first year of life. *Arch. Ophthal.*, 1976, *94*, 1912-1913.
(64) QUERÉ, M.A., DELPLAGE, M.P. — Les troubles opto-moteurs dans les strabismes et les paralysies oculomotrices. *Ann. Oculist.*, 1973, *206*, 449-475.
(65) QUERÉ, M.A., CLERGEAU, G., FONTENAILLE, N. — Die Lähmungsdyssynergien. Die Schieldyssynergien und das Cüppersche Syndrom. *Klin. Mbl. Augenheilk.*, 1965, *167*, 162-178.
(66) QUERÉ, M.A., PECHEREAU, A., CLERGEAU, G. — La nouvelle chirurgie des esotropies fonctionnelles. Opération du fil et techniques classiques. *J. franç. Ophtal.*, 1978, *1*, 51-60, 151-161, 221-228.
(67) RÉTHY, S., GAL, S. — Ergebnisse der konservativen Schielbehandlung durch Überkorrektur der manifesten Hypermetropie. *Klin. Mbl. Augenheilk.*, 1967, *150*, 170-180.
(68) RICHTER, S. — Untersuchungen über die Heredität des Strabismus concomitans. Abhandlungen aus dem Gebiete der Augenheilkunde 23. Thieme, Leipzig 1967.
(69) RICHTER, S. — Untersuchungen über binokulare Funktionen bei Lähmungsschielen. *Ophthalmologica*, 1969, *159*, 328-332.
(70) SANJOTO HARDJOWIJOTO: personal communication.
(71) SCHLOSSMAN, A., PRIESTLEY, B.S. — Role of heredity in etiology and treatment of strabismus. *Arch. Ophthal.*, 1952, *47*, 1-20.
(72) SHLAER, R. — Shift in binocular disparity causes compensatory change in the cortical structure of kittens. *Science*, 1971, *173*, 638-641.
(73) SPIELMANN, A., LAUDAN, J. — Action of recessions and resections when associated with Cüppers' Fadenoperation in esotropia. Statistical results. Strabismus. Proc. third Meeting I.S.A. Ed. R.D. Reinecke, p. 355-369. Grune and Stratton, New York, San Francisco, London 1978.
(74) STONE, J., FUKUDA, Y. — The naso-temporal division of the cat's retina re-examined in terms of Y-, X- and W-cells. *J. Comp. Neurol.*, 1974, *155*, 377-394.
(75) STRAUB, M. — Über die Aetiologie der Brechungsanomalien des Auges und den Ursprung der Emmetropie. Albrecht v. *Graefes Arch. Ophthal.*, 1909, *70*, 130-199.
(76) TAYLOR, D.M. — Congenital strabismus. The common sense approach. *Arch. Ophthal.*, 1967, *77*, 478-484.
(77) THEMEN, C.G.W. — De ontwikkeling van het accommodatie-vermogen in de eerste levensmaanden. Thesis Leiden, 1956.
(78) URRETS-ZAVALíA, A., SOLARES-ZAMORA, J., OLMOS, H.R. — Anthropological studies on the nature of cyclovertical squint. *Brit. J. Ophthal.*, 1961, *45*, 578-596.
(79) VLIET, A.G.M. VAN — Nystagmus latens. Van Gorcum, Assen, 1966.
(80) VRIES, B. DE, HOUTMAN, W.A. — Squint in monozygotic twins. *Documenta Ophthal.*, 1979, *46*, 305-308.
(81) WAARDENBURG, P.J. — Squint and heredity. *Docum. Ophthal.*, 1954, VII-VIII, 422-494.
(82) WEEKERS, R., MONREAU, P., HACOURT, J., ANDRÉ, A. — Contribution à l'étiologie du strabisme concomitant et de l'amblyopie par l'étude de jumeaux unis et bivitellins. *Bull. Soc. Belge Ophtal.*, 1956, *112*, 146-172.
(83) WEISS, J.B. — Syndrome d'extorsion. *Bull. Soc. Ophtal. Fr.*, 1966, *66*, 585-586.
(84) WEISS, J.B., MENAGER, P. — Spasme et contracture spasmodique chez le strabisme convergent. *Bull. et Mem. Soc. Fr. Ophtal.*, 1967, *80*, 548.
(85) WEISS, J.B. — Le «blocage» existe-t-il? *J. Franç. Ophtal.*, 1979, *2*, 715-722.
(86) WIBAUT, F. — Über die Emmetropisation und den Ursprung der sphärischen Refractionsanomalien. *Albrecht v. Graefes Arch. Ophthal.*, 1926, *116*, 596-612.
(87) WORTH, C. — Squint. Its causes, pathology and treatment. 6th ed. Bailliere, Tindall & Cox, London 1929.

Bull. Soc. belge Ophtal., **195**, 179-244, 1981.

CHAPTER VI

METHODS OF EXAMINATION

E. VEREECKEN (*)

Introduction

The delay between the onset of strabismus and the first consultation has been considerably shortened these last 20 years. This most important fact had a great influence on the methods of examination. The objective examination methods, in which the cooperation of the patient is reduced to a minimum, steady fixation, became preponderant. The sequence of our examination methods is as follows:

I. History taking.
II. Inspection.
III. Corneal reflection
IV. Cover test type I and type II.
V. Prisms examination.
VI. Ocular motility:
   - versions,
   - ductions,
   - Bielschowsky test,
   - convergence
VII. Cycloplegia.
VIII. Fundus examination.
IX. Visual acuity.
X. Measurement of angle of deviation.
XI. Tests of binocular vision.
XII. Preoperative examinations:
   - prism compensation test,
   - post-operative diplopia.

(*) Park Ryvissche 66, 9710 Zwijnaarde, Belgium.

The first subjective method of examination, where the examiner relies on the answer of the patient, is only number nine in our survey.

The sequence of examinations, after history taking and inspection, which are the common base of every strabismus examination, depends upon two factors:

— Is for us, eye doctors or orthoptists, the squint obvious or not (presumptive squint)?
— The age of the child.

In this study we started from the case of a child, less than two years old with a presumptive squint. The sequence of examinations is:

I. Presumptive-squint in the young child (less than 2 years).
   Prerequisites: Experience and patience.
   1. Corneal reflection.
   2. Cover test type I.
   3. Prisms examination.
   4. Ocular motility.
   5. Cover test type II.
   6. Refraction and ophthalmoscopy.

The other possibilities in daily practice are:

II. Presumptive squint in the older child.
   Examinations no. I and as early as possible:
   1. Visual acuity.
   2. Prisms examination + subjective answers.
   3. Less-dissociating tests for binocular vision.

III. Obvious squint in the young child (less than 2 years).
   Predominance: detection of amblyopia.
   1. Uniocular or alternating fixation.
   2. Corneal reflection.
   3. Cover test type I.
   4. Ocular motility.
   5. Measurement of angle of deviation.
   6. Refraction and ophthalmoscopy.
   7. Fixation.

IV. Obvious squint in the older child.
   Examination nr. 3 and as early as possible:
   1. Visual acuity.
   2. Tests for binocular vision:
      — less dissociating methods,
      — dissociating methods.

These objective tests offer plenty of advantages:

1. They are simple to perform, require a minimal time commitment and the use of few instruments or apparatus.
2. They can be performed at any age and at any stage in the treatment.
3. They can be performed in "free space", under conditions of casual seeing, in our normal consultation room under the usual everyday real life conditions. By this, we do not reject subjective methods of examination, we use these wherever possible. (This is mostly dependent on age). In many objective methods, we describe the complementary subjective execution of these tests, as the latter may deliver important and sometimes indispensable information to arrive at the correct diagnosis. The exact definition of the sensorial status—so important for prognosis and treatment—is not possible without these subjective tests. We consider objective and subjective examination methods complementary methods.

I. *History*

The history taking is an essential part of a strabismus examination especially with regard to prognosis; it should always be carried out at the first examination. During the history taking, the doctor observes the patient, the position of the eyes and looks for any abnormal posture of the head.

a. *The onset*

When was the deviation first noticed? The date of onset, important for diagnosis and prognosis, is likely to be more accurate when the deviation is first observed by a parent and when the first examination is relatively soon after the onset. In cases of very early onset, in the first months of life, one should carefully inquire about pregnancy and delivery and ask if the parents noticed nystagmoid movements of the eyes.

How did the squint appear? As a sudden and definite, gradual or intermittent squint? Are there still moments that the eyes are parallel? Was there any precipitating cause, febrile illness, or were there any psychological factors?

What is the nature of the deviation? Did the affected eye turn in, out, up or down? Which eye is affected, the right or the left one? Is it always the same eye or each eye alternately?

b. *The subsequent history*

Is the squint still intermittent or does it become constant? Has the deviation become more or less (pseudostrabismus) pronounced since first observed? Has any treatment already been carried out? Have glasses been prescribed (after atropine examination or another cycloplegic drug?) Have they been worn? What was the effect of the glasses upon the squint? Has occlusion been carried out? Which eye, how long? Has an operation been carried out? If so, when, upon which eye, and what was the result?

c. *The present nature of the deviation*

Is the squint intermittent? If so, when: in the morning, when the patient is tired or excited (accommodation)? When looking in a particular direction or only when fixing a near object? Is the squint constant? Is the deviation variable in degree and, if so, under what circumstances?

d. *Family history*

Heredity is an important factor in strabismus. Statistical examinations (26, 42) show that if one child of a family squints, there is one chance on four that another child of this family will squint too. If both parents are normal, there are 2.6% chances that one of their children will squint. If one parent squints, the risk for any of their children is 16%.

In any new case of strabismus, an eye-examination of the parents, brothers and sisters is desirable and useful; this permits us also the realization of a family tree. If a brother, sister or parent of a child squints, we consider this child a "high risk-child". A careful and an early examination of this child is mandatory, for the prevention or treatment of amblyopia and/or strabismus.

II. *Inspection*

During the history taking we observe the young child all the time from behind our desk and try to come into contact with the child laughing at it or showing a toy, etc.

Basic examination position

Then we ask a parent to take a seat in the normally illuminated room with the child on his lap, unless the child is old enough to sit on a chair

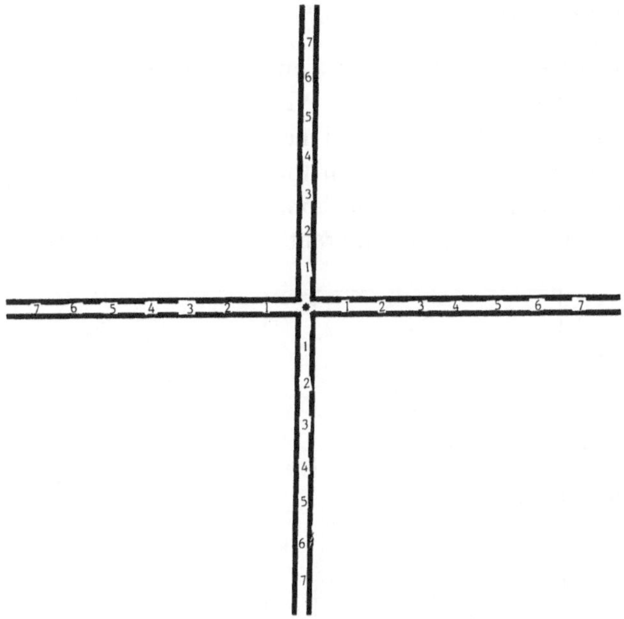

Fig. 1. — The Maddox-cross.

by himself. We adjust the height of the chair so that the eyes of the patient are in line with the central spotlight on the Maddox tangent scale, situated exactly 5 m. directly before the examination chair. The head is kept straight. This is the primary position (fig. 1).

We sit on a chair in front of and a little to the side of the patient, which permits him to fix the central spotlight on the Maddox tangent scale, with his head straight. It is practically impossible to make a young child (less than 2 years old) gaze steadily at the spotlight at 5 m. Therefore many ingenious systems were proposed, i.e. Lang (23) uses an illuminated coloured turning disc, coupled to a music box. We examine these young children with a little non dazzling spotlight held at 60 cm., which can be flashed on and off to attract and retain the child's attention. Such fixation object presents the advantage of rarely eliciting accommodation and permits us to observe the position of the corneal reflections. Otherwise we use keys or a toy with a squeaker to attract the child's attention (auditive stimulus). For the relatively rare cases where it is imperative to examine these young children at 5 m. fixation, we might ask a parent to move a coloured glass before the central spotlight at the Maddox tangent scale and we ask the child "to blow out the light".

A. *Abnormal head posture (torticollis)*

In every case of strabismus we must look for it, as it may have important diagnostic significance. We look for it already in the history taking, but usually the abnormal head position is easier to observe when we ask a visual effort from the child, i.e. examining his visual acuity. Once the presence of an abnormal head posture is noted, we first try to describe it in its different components (fig.. 2):

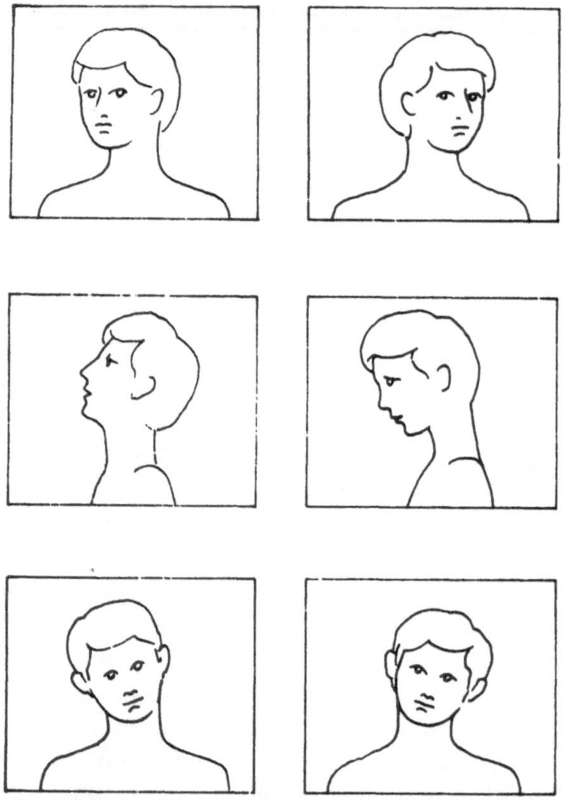

a)

b)

c)

Fig. 2. — Torticollis.
a) turn of the face around the vertical axis: to the right or left;
b) an elevation or depression of the chin around the frontal axis;
c) a tilt of the head around the sagittal axis: to the right or left shoulder.

Then we try to determine the origin. This abnormal head posture can be due to:

a) a primary contraction of the sternocleidomastoïd or exceptionally to congenital anomalies in the cervical vertebrae. In these cases we feel the abnormal sternocleidomastoïd, the mobility of the head is limited and the eye movements are normal whatever the direction of gaze.

b) Ocular reasons:
   1) eye muscle paresis (mostly the superior oblique). In babies, the most common cause is limitation of abduction in the dominant eye; occasionally such children show inversion of the torticollis when the dominant eye is occluded.
   2) Duane's syndrome, sometimes typical squint incomitances (A and V pattern).
   3) Nystagmus.
   4) Optical reasons: uncorrected or poorly corrected astigmatism or overcorrected spherical errors; in these cases the refractive correction is less in the periphery of the glasses.

The diagnosis is chiefly made by putting the head straight or even more by placing the head in the opposite position of the abnormal head posture. The parallelism of the visual axes is lost or nystagmus appears. In long existing cases the diagnosis is sometimes difficult, secondary muscle changes hampering diagnosis. Photographs of different ages may be useful.

Covering separately each eye can be helpful to detect which eye is responsible for the abnormal head posture.

The cover test type I carried out in this posture and not with the head straight and less dissociating examinations of the binocular status (cfr. XI B) tell us if in the abnormal head posture there is binocular single vision or not. In these cases where binocular single vision exists, we carefully explain to the parents that this abnormal head posture is a compensatory protective mecanism that must be conserved. We ask them to return every three months until an exact motor diagnosis is possible in these young children. If the child by this time looses his abnormal head posture and/or if strabismus appears, the patient should return at once.

B. *The eyelid and palpebral fissures*

Does ptosis exist? Or pseudoptosis? Since Urrets-Zavalia (39) and Urist (38) we know that anomalies of the palpebral and facial bones may be associated with A and V patterns. Malar hyperplasia and upward or mongoloïd slant of the palpebral fissure is common to an A pattern esotropia (and underaction of inferior obliques). Malar hypoa)

b)

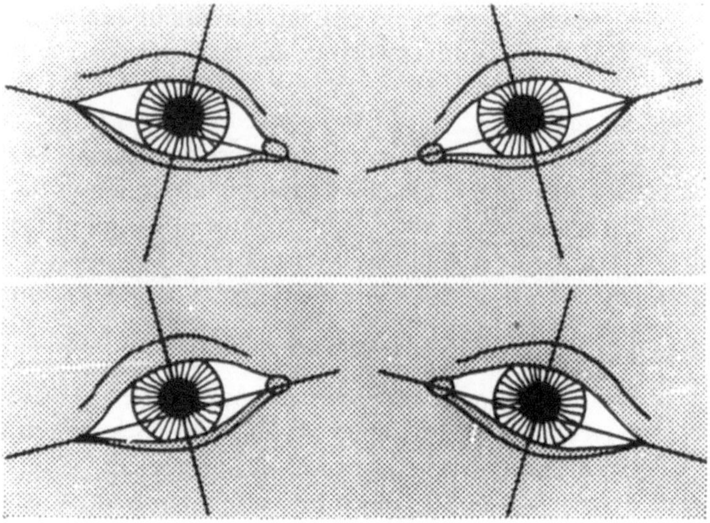

Fig. 3.
a) Mongoloid palpebral fissures : A-pattern.
b) Antimongoloid palpebral fissures : V-pattern.

plasia and downward slanting lids (anti-mongoloïd palpebral fissures) is common with V-pattern esotropia (and overaction of the inferior obliques) (fig. 3).

C. *The pupils*

Are the pupils equal in size or does an anisocoria exist? If the anisocoria in darkness is equal to the anisocoria existing in light, we can consider it not clinically important. An anisocoria greater in darkness than in light is pathological and necessitates further examination. There is evidence that the reflex to darkness is more vulnerable in pathological conditions than that to light (11).

We examine the pupillary reflexes to light, darkness and near; they are normally equal in both eyes.

The Marcus Gunn pupillary sign:

When the pupillary activity to light of one eye is diminished (as in amblyopic pupillary paresis) the consensual darkness reflex derived from the other eye may dominate the pupillary reaction. The test is most readily made by using a swinging flash light (37). Rapidly moving a light from one eye to another instantly substitutes a direct light response for a consensual response. If there is unilateral optic nerve damage, the direct light response in this pupil is less than the consensual response to darkness obtained from the normal one, so that when the flashlight is being moved from a normal eye to one with optic nerve damage, the pupil *dilates.* On returning the light to the normal eye, the pupil constricts.

The Gunn's pupillary sign gives us an easy and valuable opportunity to separate functional unilateral amblyopia (the pupil constricts) from organic unilateral amblyopia with normal fundus, and this even in young children (the pupil dilates).

The pupillary contraction, together with accommodation and convergence on attempting to regard a near object, are three synkinetic reactions which occur normally together, but the pupillary contraction can occur with either accommodation or convergence excluded (12). This pupillary contraction in the near reflex occurs even when one eye is amblyopic or covered.

D. *Nystagmus*

D.1. Nystagmus can be seen directly, or only by putting the head straight in cases of ocular torticollis due to nystagmus, or only when examining versions. If we note the existence of nystagmus, we have to specify, if this is a pendular or jerk nystagmus (in the latter we have to note if the quick phase is to the right or to the left), if the nystagmus is horizontal, vertical or rotatory or a combination of these forms. If the amplitude of the nystagmus is low, we sometimes need careful observation at the slitlamp, or will have to examine the eye fundus with the star of an ophthalmoscope (enlarging 16 × the movement of the eye fundus) or will have to use the nystagmus spectacles of Frenzel to detect the presence of nystagmus.

Does nystagmus exist in the primary position or not? Does a "zero-point" of nystagmus exist anywhere? Nystagmus is often an important neurological symptom; in cases where the apparition of nystagmus is recent or in cases of vertical nystagmus, a complete neurological examination is certainly necessary.

D.2. Latent nystagmus (occlusion nystagmus).

This nystagmus is not ordinarily present but is elicited by occlusion of one or other eye or by certain other forms of uniocular embarrassment. It is a jerk nystagmus with rapid phase to the non-covered eye. This nystagmus is usually associated with some form of squint; it frequently occurs in association with dissociated vertical divergence (alternating hypertropia).

III. *Corneal reflections*

The study of corneal reflection is performed with the aid of a moderately intense light, ca. 60 cm in front of the child's eyes. As an exception to our basic examination position, the observer sits here directly opposite the patient. The patient is being instructed to look at te light, if the young child does not do so, the room light is turned off.

1. When the corneal reflections are symmetrical but not central in both eyes, there is no strabismus but an equal angle Kappa exists in both eyes (fig. 4).

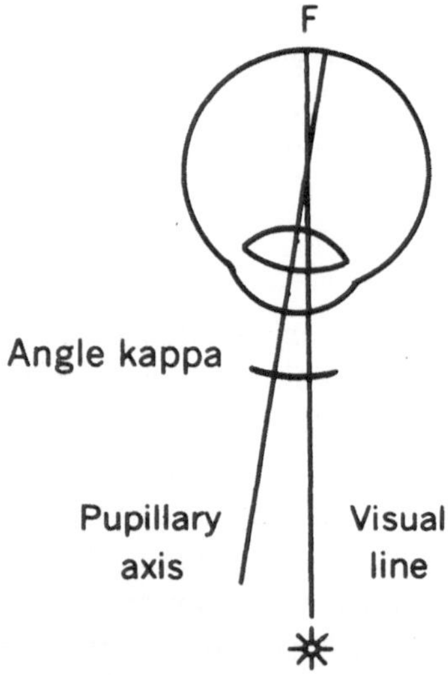

Fig. 4. — The angle Kappa is the angle formed between the central pupillary line and the visual axis.

Normally these axes do not coincide, in the normal eye the visual axis cuts the cornea to the nasal side of the central pupillary line. The angle Kappa is then said to be positive, this is frequently so in hypermetropia. If the visual axis cuts the cornea to the temporal side of the central pupillary line the angle Kappa is said to be negative (sometimes in myopia). In most cases the angle Kappa is of such a small degree that its existence can be neglected.

The presence of a large negative (or temporal) angle Kappa may produce an apparent convergent strabismus (fig. 5, fig. 6).

The angle Kappa can be measured in degrees monocularly on the Maddox tangent scale at a distance of 1 m. The observer sits directly under the central spotlight, and asks the child to look at te observer's

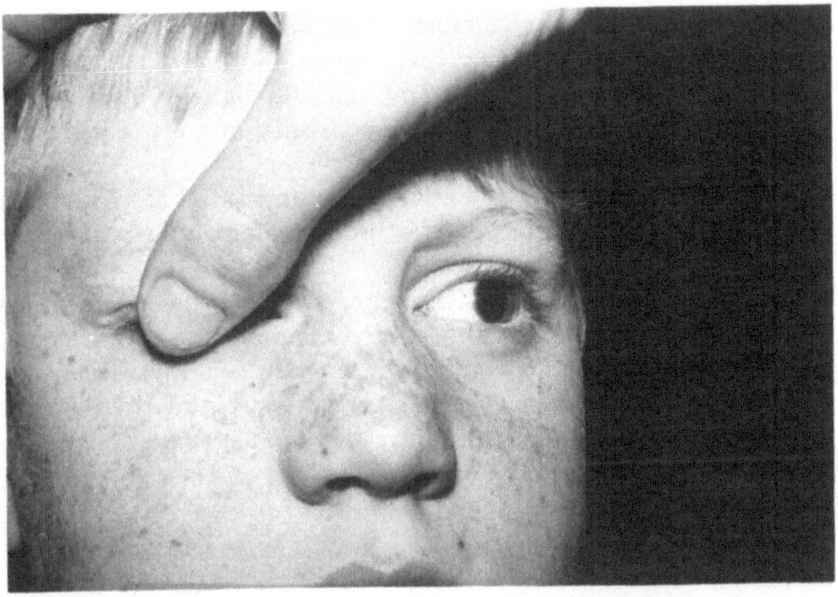

Fig. 5. — A large positive angle Kappa. The patient looks straight ahead.

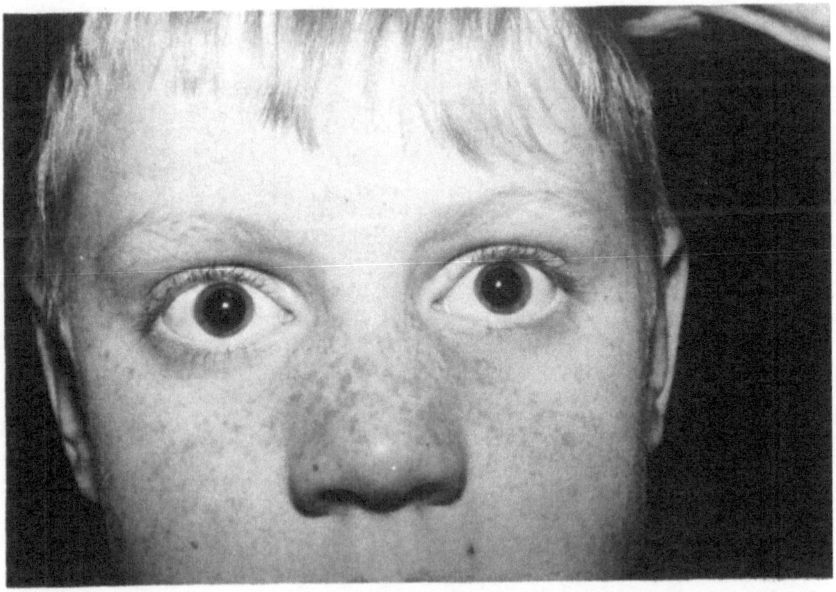

Fig. 6. — Same patient with both eyes open. Pseudo-orthophoria due to the large positive angle Kappa. In reality it is a moderate left esotropia.

finger, pointing to different numbers on the scale, until the reflection of the fixation spotlight on the cornea is central.

The monocular measurement of the angle Kappa can be done at the synoptophore by using a special slide consisting of a row of numbers and letters at intervals of one degree.

2. When the corneal reflections are symmetrical and central in both eyes, there is no strabismus. So we already eliminate the strabismus due to:

a) uni- or bilateral epicanthus. Broad epicanthal folds of skin which partly cover the medial canthus are common in young children, they disappear with the normal growth of face and root of the nose. This appearance of apparent convergent strabismus is especially marked in the position of lateroversion because the adducted eye disappears in the corner (fig. 7).

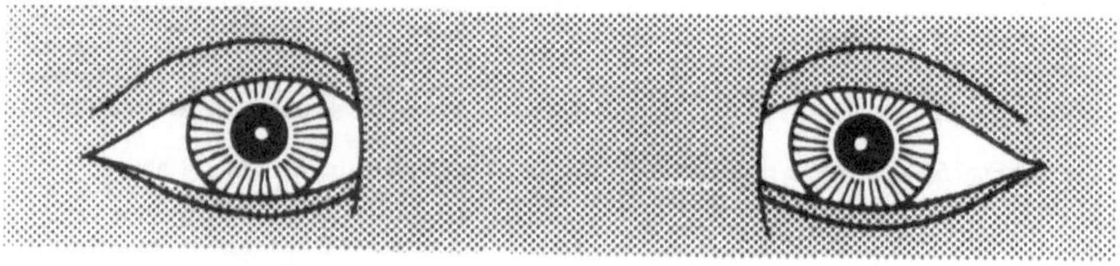

Fig. 7. — Pseudo-esotropia due to bilateral epichanthus.

b) Abnormalities in the orbita configuration (fig. 8).

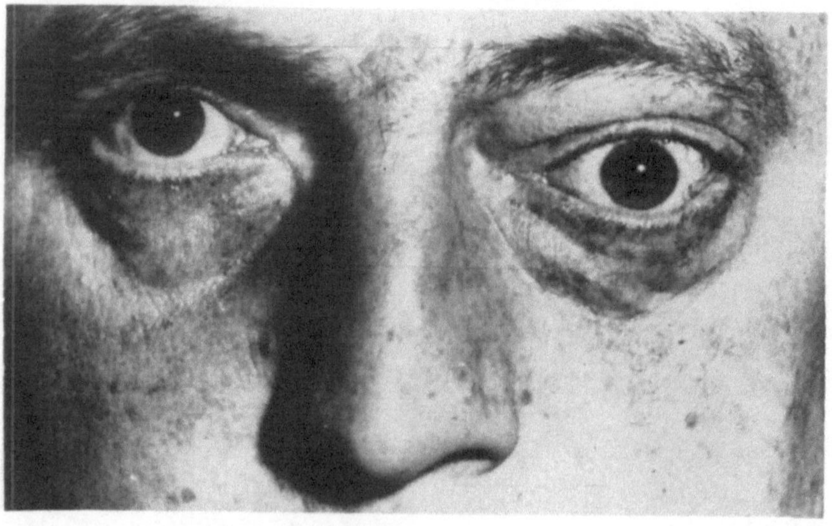

Fig. 8. — Abnormalities in the orbita configuration. Gross displacement of the left eyeball downwards. The visual axes are parallel in the primary position, orthophoria on cover test.

If the orbits are closer together than normal, the interpupillary distance is less than normal and a pseudo-esotropia may be produced. The cover test easily demonstrates the absence of a true squint in both these pseudo-esotropias.

3. When the corneal reflections are asymmetrical, this means strabismus. If the corneal reflection in the squinting eye is displaced temporaly, we have to do with an esotropia. Observation of the position of the corneal reflections will usually enable an approximate estimate of the degree of deviation (Hirschberg method). 1 mm. decentration of corneal reflection corresponds to 7° strabismus at 33 cm. Exceptionally there is no strabismus but an unequal angle Kappa in both eyes; again in this case the negative cover test type I proves the absence of a true squint.

IV. *The cover test*

This objective method, introduced by Donders, is the basic strabismus examination. It is always the first test to be performed. In orthophoria each eye is aligned with the fixation object, covering one eye will not provoke a fixation movement of the fellow eye. In heterotropia one eye is not aligned with the fixation object. Covering the fixating eye provokes a fixation movement of the deviating eye.

Strict fixation control is necessary, especially in young children. Therefore a flashing muscle light, with its corneal reflection control is appropriate. We always attract again the child's attention to the light ("look at the light, blow it out"!) sometimes associating an auditive stimulus, as making noises. If we still doubt, we move the light in different directions and we control by means of the corneal reflection, if the child really fixes.

A. *Cover test type I: The monolateral cover test*

For didactic reasons only we describe this test in three steps.

Step I.: Does the non-covered eye make a movement?

In every case of presumptive strabismus it is mandatory to start with this test, to distinguish between manifest and latent squint (heterophoria). It is essential to disrupt the possibly existing fusion as little as possible. The aim of this step is to determine, if there is a manifest strabismus or not; this step is therefore particularly indicated for pseudo-strabismus and microstrabismus.

Procedure:

We ask the young child to look at the fixation light and we cover quickly, at about 30 cm. (cover at distance), one eye, e.g. the left, *and observe the right eye.* If the child easily accepts this cover, we gently put our hand on his head to fix it and cover again one eye with our thumb. If the child is old enough, we ask him to look at the central spotlight on the Maddox tangent scale at 5 m (fig. 9).

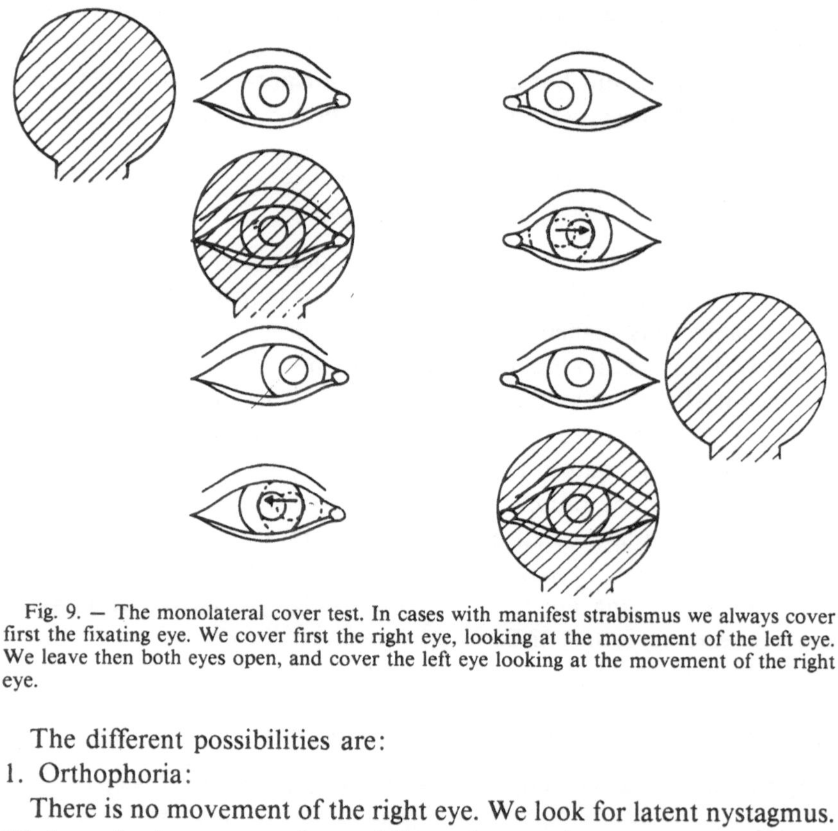

Fig. 9. — The monolateral cover test. In cases with manifest strabismus we always cover first the fixating eye. We cover first the right eye, looking at the movement of the left eye. We leave then both eyes open, and cover the left eye looking at the movement of the right eye.

The different possibilities are:

1. Orthophoria:

There is no movement of the right eye. We look for latent nystagmus. We leave both eyes open for a while, cover the right eye and *observe the left eye.* There is no movement of the left eye.

2. Manifest squint:

On covering e.g. the left eye, the right eye moves horizontally or vertically to take up fixation. The squint is convergent if the right eye moves laterally to fix, divergent if the right eye moves medially. There is right hypertropia, if the right eye moves downwards and right hypotropia, if the right eye moves upwards.

If, on removing the cover, the right eye retains fixation, the squint is alternating. There are different degrees of alternation.

a. Free alternation means that fixation is taken up and retained by the non-covered eye, regardless of which eye is covered. If the child closes and opens his eyes he fixes one time with the right eye, another time with the other eye.

b. In other cases the child can alternate, but there is a predilection for fixing with the same eye. This predilection can exist in different degrees: the child can only, during a few seconds, retain the fixation with one eye, or he can retain the fixation until blinking, or even longer than the blinking reflex. This predilection can depend from the direction of gaze. If change of fixation is only possible in a very lateral gaze, then we must take care that amblyopia does not develop.

If on removing the cover, the right eye reverts to its original position the squint is monolateral. The monolaterality also exists in different degrees: if the left eye is covered in right convergent strabismus, the right eye moves to take fixation but more or less directly on uncovering the left eye, the latter reassumes the fixation. The quicker this refixation by the left eye happens, the stronger the monolaterality and the greater the danger for amblyopia of the right eye. The amblyopia is more pronounced if after covering the fixing eye, the non-covered eye executes searching movements to take the fixation. If after covering the dominating eye the non-covered eye does not move from its squinting position, or if there is a strong reaction of the child on covering the fixing eye, the amblyopia is deep.

The cover test should always be carried out:

a) with right and left eye fixing in turn. Between each covering we always leave both eyes open for about 30 seconds. If the movement is equal in both eyes, whether horizontally or vertically, the squint is said to be concomitant. When the fixation movement is different according to which eye fixates, the squint is said to be incomitant. It is too often neglected that this incomitance can be due to accommodative factors (unequal hypermetropia). The use of an accommodative target for fixation, instead of the spotlight, is mandatory in these cases. The squint is incomitant too if the fixation movements are different in different positions of gaze. This incomitance is not due to accommodative factors.

b) At 5 m. and at 33 cm. When we suspect accommodative factors, we use as accommodative fixation target in the distance, letters, numbers or separate E or picture targets, which demand a good vision to be

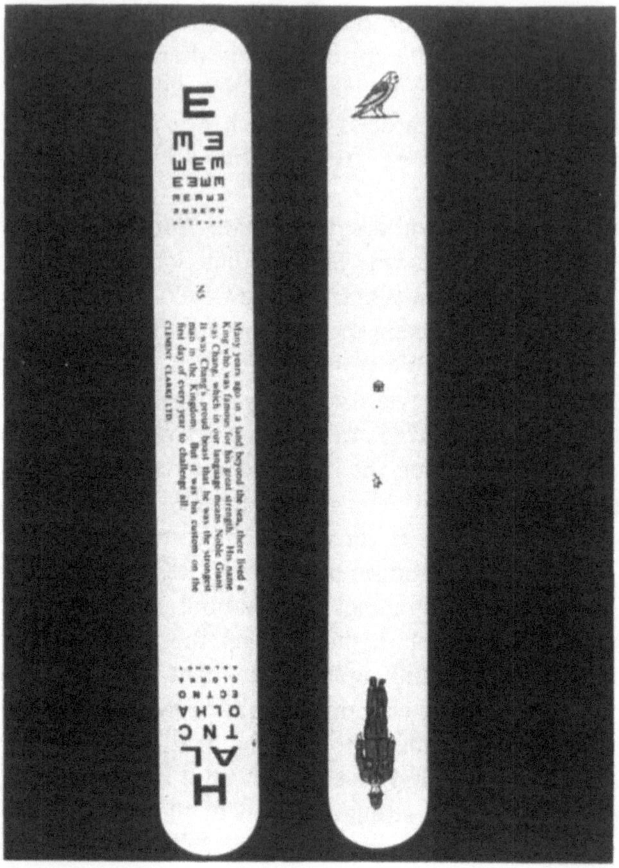

Fig. 10. — This little white plastic bar has four printed pictures of different sizes, two reduced test types and a passage of N 5 script.

seen, and which should be described or read during the test. We always use as fixation target for near the fixation bar (fig. 10).

The fixation bar should be held by the patient in the primary plane at eye level (and not in the reading position). We ask him to describe which picture he sees and to read the test types if possible. So we have our hands free for the cover test.

c) In the different positions of gaze if there is any suspicion of incomitance. In some cases the deviation may only occur in some directions.

An experienced observer estimates quite well the degree of the deviation on the cover test, but we classify only: as small angle (less than 6°), moderate angle (up to 15°) and large angle (more than 15°).

Step 2: WHAT DOES THE EYE DO BEHIND THE COVER?

As a cover we use our thumb or an obliquely held cover paddle which permits us to observe the covered eye. We execute this test again with right and left eye fixing, at 5 m. and 33 cm. Do we see a latent nystagmus? Do we see an horizontal or vertical movement of this eye? This indicates heterophoria (latent squint). If we see that typical slow, upward movement of the covered eye, the diagnosis of alternating hyperphoria is made (8) (fig. 11).

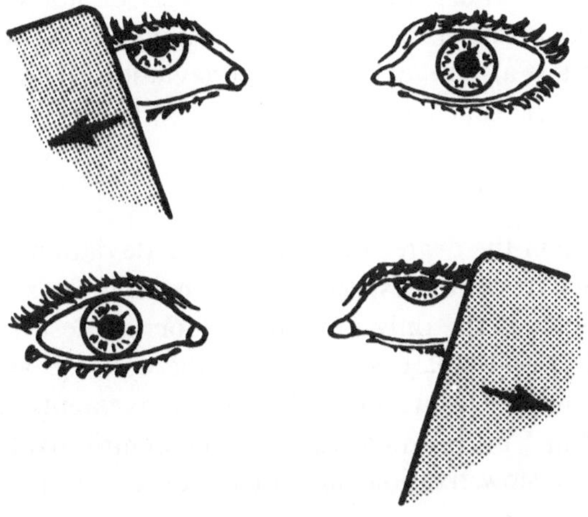

Fig. 11. — Alternating hyperphoria. The eye behind the cover is deviated upwards.

Step 3: WHAT HAPPENS TO THE UNCOVERED EYE?

The uncovered eye does not move: orthophoria.

Only the uncovered eye moves, it recovers its original position: refusion movement (heterophoria). This re-fusion movement can be rapid or does not occur at all; in the latter possibility, the dissociation has caused a latent squint to break down in a manifest one: intermittent strabismus.

We should always carefully control if this re-fusion movement ends up in orthophoria, by covering the good eye. Otherwise we miss the diagnosis of microtropia.

In dissociated vertical divergence (alternating hyperphoria) (8) the under-cover-upwards-deviated eye moves downwards; the recovering from the deviation is sometimes slow. The differential diagnosis with a concomitant or paretic vertical hypertropia is that in the former each eye moves downwards by uncovering, in the latter, one eye on assuming fixation, deviates downwards and the other eye deviates upwards.

Nor must these conditions be confused with bilateral overaction of the inferior obliques, which also shows a deviation downwards of both eyes on uncovering, but this deviation is mainly evident on lateroversion and is not or only slightly provoked by covering the eyes in the primary position. The sluggish downward movement and the often associated latent nystagmus in alternating hyperphoria constitute other elements for the differential diagnosis. The dissociated vertical divergence can be unilateral, and can be associated or not with a vertical deviation. If the former is as great as the associated vertical deviation, then the cover test also reveals a vertical deviation when one eye fixes, and none when the other eye fixes.

Limitations of the cover test

Depending upon the degree of experience, a deviation of less than 1° to 2° may escape detection, especially when nystagmus is associated. As fixation capability is the only prerequisite for this test, it is necessary that the fixation object is easily seen by the eye, e.g. an uncorrected myopic eye cannot execute exact fixation movements on a fixation object situated at 5 m. In microtropia with eccentric fixation, there are often no or very slow fixation movements on covering the good eye.

Conclusion:

Despite these limitations which prove that even the best diagnostic test can fail, the cover test is a simple and quick test, practicable at any age, which produces remarkably accurate information about the motor and sensorial status of the eyes (17). Especially if the visual acuity is normal in both eyes, we are sure, if there is a manifest or latent strabismus, a latent nystagmus or not; we know if the squint is an eso, exo, hypo- or hypertropia; if the strabismus is intermittent or constant, concomitant or incomitant, monolateral or alternating. With some experience we can estimate quite well the degree of the deviation.

The cover test reveals much about the sensorial status too. When orthophoria exists, with normal visual acuity on both sides, we are sure about bifoveal fixation (fusion). Steps 2 and 3 can reveal real fusion movements. The cover test shows us if one eye is amblyopic or not.

We note on the patient's record: e.g. right convergent strabismus of ±10° in the distance, ±15° near. Concomitance. The child can retain fixation with the right eye. It is important, in order to avoid later difficulties in the diagnosis of the motor status, to note which eye is the originally fixating eye, because dominance may—and this is often the aim—be changed by our conservative treatment.

B. *Cover test type II: Alternating cover test*

In cases where there is no manifest or doubtful deviation with cover test type I, we pursue the examination as indicated in the diagnostic plan n° 1 (Introduction). The difference with cover type I is that here the aim is to disrupt any existing fusion (fig. 12).

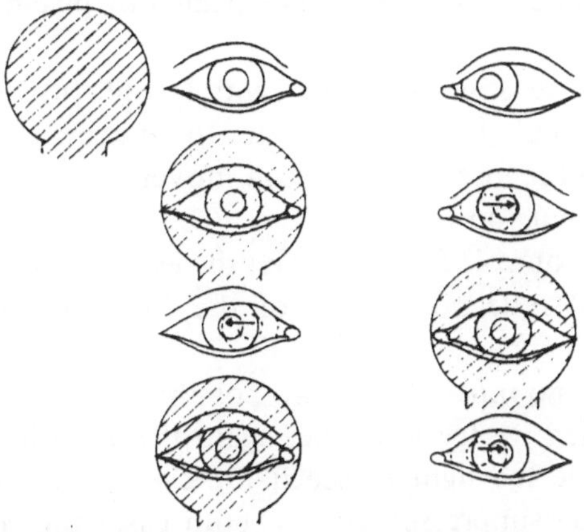

Fig. 12. — Alternating Cover Test. Each eye is covered alternately. Both eyes are never open together. We have to look each time to the uncovered eye.

This test is thus especially appropriate to detect latent strabismus (heterophoria). When there is a fixation movement on type I, step I, there will always be a movement on type II. This movement can be equal; if it is greater it then represents the maximal motor deviation. In cases where surgery is necessary, this maximal motor deviation should be the base for surgery. The smallest manifest angle corresponds to the sensorial deviation.

Adult patients sometimes tell us that on cover test type II they observe a jump of the fixation light, even if we doubt if there is any movement. Sometimes the uncovered eye makes a too big fixation movement, transgresses the midline and returns immediately to the midline to take up fixation. Queré (30) states that this motor phenomenon is an indication for the existence of abnormal retinal correspondence.

V. *Prisms examination*

This further examination to refine our diagnosis of the sensorial status of the eyes should be executed in every case when no or doubtful fixation movement is seen on cover test type I. This examination can be done from the age of 6 months, in so far as we can be sure of the fixation.

A. *Horizontal prism test*

Procedure: an 8 pD base-out prism is placed e.g. over the right eye while the patient fixates a spotlight and the examiner observes the movements of both eyes. The test is repeated by placing the prism over the left eye.

In opposition to Jampolsky (18) and Irvine (16), who use a 4 pD prism we use an 8 pD to better visualize the movements, and we use no more than 8 pD because the refixation movement is more rapid if retinal disparity is not too big.

We have two controls for diagnosis: the eye movements of both eyes and the corneal reflections. Any of the following possibilities may ensue:

a) If there are no movements, two possibilities exist. Either the child does not fix: then we try to attract again the attention to the fixation light or we move the light to see if the eye follows. Or the prism is placed before the suppressed eye. In both cases the corneal reflection will be asymmetrical (fig. 13).

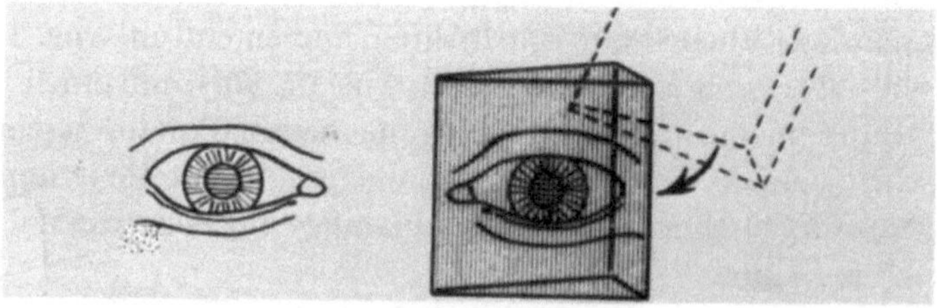

Fig. 13. — Horizontal prism test. Neither eye moves.

b) We observe only a conjugated movement of both eyes in the direction of the top of the prism. There is no fusional movement of the left eye, the left eye is suppressed. The corneal reflection is asymmetrical (fig. 14).

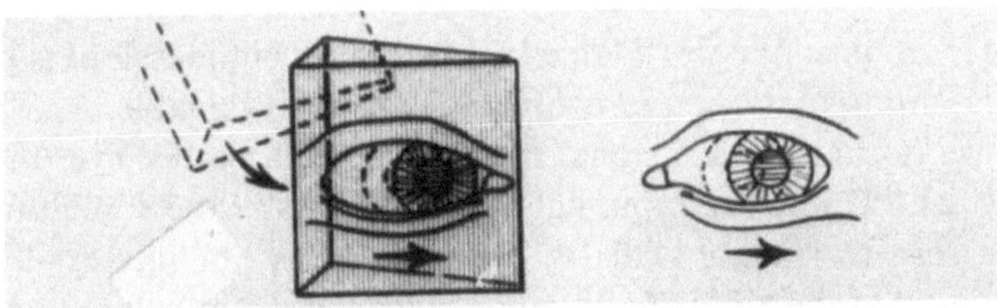

Fig. 14. — Horizontal prism test. O.S. remains turned out after a prism is placed over O.D.

c) Fusional movement. First we see a quick movement to the left of both eyes and after it a slower fusional movement of the left eye to the right to regain fixation. The corneal reflection is symmetrical (fig. 15).

On withdrawal of the prism, the eye behind the prism returns to its original position with symmetrical corneal reflection, or if this eye does not redress (or sometimes only after blinking) the corneal reflection is asymmetrical; this means intermittent strabismus. In some cases we only see a movement of the eye behind the prism, at the end of the movement the corneal reflection is symmetrical (probably in cases of strong dominance of the other eye).

This test should be carried out slowly because fusional movements are slower than fixation movements (cfr. chapter IV).

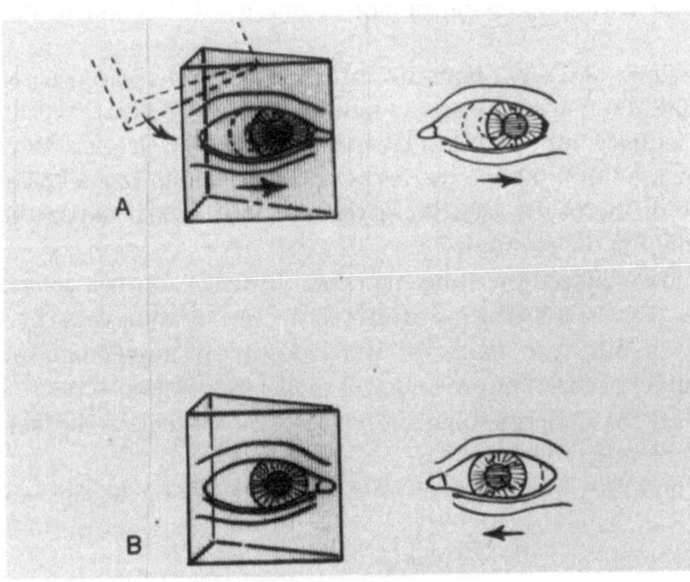

Fig. 15. — Horizontal prism test:
a) Laevoversion on both eyes;
b) a slow fusional movement of O S is observed.

This is an objective test to detect if fusion (or suppression) is present. In older children subjective cooperation can be valuable, e.g. in cases where we do not see a fusional movement of the other eye. If we ask the patient "Do you see one light or two lights?", he sometimes says that he sees two lights. This second light does not interest him. On explaining that the aim is to continue, with the prism before one eye, to see one light, he does this sometimes remarkably well, it is to say that the patient has certainly fusion although the objective procedure of the test seems to exclude it. For these reasons a negative test does not exclude the existence of fusion (except when the subjective complement is possible). It is often difficult to observe exactly the eye movements: the fusional movement is slower and sometimes difficult to evaluate (e.g. a movement in different periods: a movement, a stop, again a movement). A positive test can be found in cases of microtropia and even in cases of slight unilateral amblyopia.

We note e.g.: horizontal prism: fusion +.

B. *Vertical prism test*

This objective test is especially indicated in young children where our previous tests are negative. The aim of the test is to detect if in free space there is suppression or not of one eye (detection of dominant eye).

Procedure: An 8 pD base-up prism is alternately placed before each eye while the patient fixates a spotlight at 5 m (33 cm). We have the same controls: movement of the eye and corneal reflection. We examine here a point 4° above the fovea or above the horizontal joining the middle of the papilla and the fovea, so we are often outside the suppression area in esotropia.

In older children the subjective complement: "do you see one light or two" can be valuable as explained for the previous test. The test is positive if either eye makes that quick downward movement. In a child a negative test does not exclude binocular cooperation because of possible lack of understanding or cooperation, except if the subjective complement is possible.

We note then e.g.: vertical prism: suppression of the right eye.

C. *Prism bar or rotary prism*

This is the objective measurement of fusion-amplitude in cases where the horizontal prism test reveals the existence of fusion (with or without fixation movements), or in cases where the cover test type I is negative.

Controls: corneal reflection and eye movements.

Procedure: We measure the fusional amplitude by alternately placing prisms of increasing strength, first base-in in front of each eye, while the patient fixes a spotlight at 5 m (33 cm), until the corneal reflections are no more symmetrical or until we see a movement of the other eye or no more following movement of the eye behind the prism (divergent fusional amplitude). Then we repeat the same procedure with prisms base-out (convergent fusional amplitude) and finally base-up or down to measure the vertical fusional amplitude. This can be done either by means of a prism bar for horizontal and for vertical fusion or with a rotary prism.

It is important to know that fusion movements are slow and therefore the progression of prisms of increasing strength before the eye should be slow too. The normal limits of fusional amplitude as measured by prisms are as follows:

— divergent fusional amplitude: 4 to 6 pD.
— convergent fusional amplitude: 10 to 25 pD.
— vertical fusional amplitude: 3 to 4 pD.

A further control is the observation of the eye movement to regain fixation on withdrawal of the prisms.

The subjectif complement for older children is extremely valuable here as the observation of corneal reflection behind the prism and observation of the exact eye movement is difficult. We increase the strength of the prisms until the spotlight becomes double, always asking the child to see the light single as long as possible. This subjective control can be refined by placing Bagolini glasses (p. 223) in a clip before the eyes. Normally the patient sees one light crossed by two luminous beams as an X. We increase the strength of the prisms until something is wrong with this image. We note on the record e.g.: Fusion −4 pD to +18 pD.

VI. *Examination of ocular movements*

A. *Versions*

This is the examination of the conjugate ocular movements in the cardinal directions of the gaze (fig. 16).

They are initiated, either in response to a command or peripheral light stimulus (saccades) or by moving a fixation light in the different

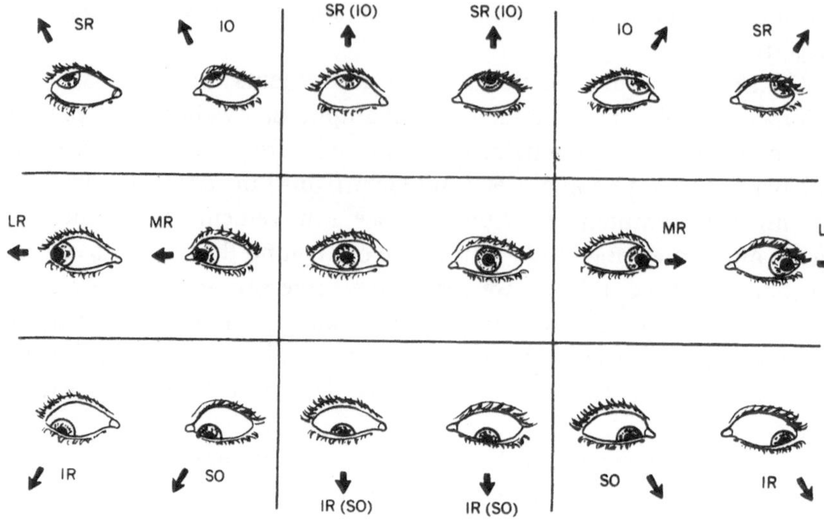

Fig. 16. — The nine cardinal directions of gaze.

positions of gaze. These latter, slower and sliding pursue movements can be elicited in two ways:

a. The head stays immobile, we place the fixation object, e.g. a flashing light, at eye level of the child straight between the two eyes at approximately 60 cm. and then move the fixation object in the different positions of gaze. With very young children the mother gently retains the head of the child and it is the doctor who moves around the child. It is often better to associate the visual stimulus of the fixation light with an auditory one (consisting of sounds articulated by the examiner).

b. The fixation object rests immobile, e.g. the central spotlight on the Maddox tangent scale, we move the head of the patient in the different positions of gaze, always stimulating him to fix the light. This examination of ocular movements is subject to multiple limitations. First of all, an exact motor examination presumes that both synergists could be examined in every direction of gaze up to the extreme end-position alternately with each eye as fixing eye. To discover slight differences, it is essential to reach the extreme end-position in any direction. Because nose and orbital rim prevent this, we can examine the eye movements in the horizontal and diagonal gaze directions only with the abducting eye as fixating eye, the adducted eye is to be examined as non-fixating eye.

Slight differences can by non-extreme versions be covered by fusion, submaximal innervation already suffices to reach these excursions. If a gross horizontal deviation is associated with vertical deviations, it is often very difficult to analyze the vertical deviation e.g. in young children with uni- or bilateral limitation of abduction and with a gross horizontal deviation, it is practically impossible to get a clear picture of the motor status.

Physiological pursue movements presume foveal fixation in both eyes. The excursion of an amblyopic eye is not so smooth and often of lesser extension in comparison with the excursion of the fixating eye.

Serves as control:

1. The corneal reflection. Is there in any direction of gaze a difference in position of the corneal reflection as compared with the primary position? Is there a difference in a certain direction, we always control by means of the cover test. The cover test controls here the eye position in an end-position. We examine the excursion to this endpoint with the following movements.

2. The corneal limbus. If observation of corneal reflection is impossible, e.g. when the adducted eye is covered by the nose, we use the comparison of the level of the corneal limbus as control. In gaze up, we look at the inferior limbus, in gaze down, we look at the superior limbus.

A.1. Horizontal ocular movements

The abducting eye is commonly used as fixating eye; the movement starts from the primary position until maximal abduction and we look if this eye reaches its normal end-position (the temporal limbus touching the external canthus) and if we see nystagmoid movements in either eye. We have to differentiate the normal end position nystagmus (with the quick phase directed to the end position) from abnormal nystagmoid jerks, which signify limitation of movement. These nystagmoid jerks appear before the end position is reached and the nystagmus differs according to whether the right or the left eye is abducted. The movement of the adducted eye is mostly examined as a non-fixating eye. When we examine it as a fixating eye, we look if this eye reaches its normal end point (the nasal pupil border touches the vertical line through the lacrimal points) and if we see nystagmoid jerks.

Failure of the temporal corneal margin of the abducted eye to reach the canthus externus does not indicate limitation of abduction unless this abducting eye is being used for fixation. This is one factor in the frequent pseudo-abducens palsy in small children. Apparent inability to abduct may be due to a lack of effort involved in abducting an habitually adducted eye, or due to habitual inhibition of abduction as seen in the crossed-fixation (the child uses his left eye for viewing objects in the right field of vision and his right eye to view an object in the left field of vision). The differential diagnosis is made by the doll's head phenomenon (a sudden passive turning of the head will frequently reveal good abduction in uncooperative children) or by an occlusion of several hours or days demonstrating in most cases that it is a pseudo-palsy. Abducensparalysis in young children is rare or fugitive (40).

Still more important is to look if both eyes move together; are the movements sliding or with saccades; do the corneal reflections change in executing this movement (large angles of deviation diminish in lateroversion for mechanical reasons already). Special care is taken to detect updrift or downdrift of the non-fixing eye in lateroversion (cfr. A and V pattern). Generally speaking we can say that a limitation of movement is due to a weakness of the agonist or to a mechanical restriction of the antagonist (antagonist contracture) especially in already operated cases. The differential diagnosis is chiefly made by the passive duction test (cfr. operative treatment).

Recording abnormalities of ocular movement should be described in terms of defective movement rather than in terms of defective muscular action. We note also: Abduction right eye: −2 (1 is light, 2 moderate, 3 pronounced, − means hypofunction, + hyperfunction).

A.2. Vertical ocular movements

In young children the head is gently fixed by the mother and we move our fixation object at approximately 60 cm. straight up and down. In older children we depress the child's head while he fixes the central spotlight at 5 m. to examine the maximal straight-up gaze (eventually lifting his spectacles a little), then we lean the head backwards as far as possible, always asking him to fix the light at 5 m. This is very important to avoid confusion between V esotropia and "convergence-excess". A pseudo V esotropia in down gaze and near position is easily diagnosed if the near measurement is taken in depression (role of accommodation and normal increase of convergence in down gaze).

We look carefully if there are differences in height in down and upper gaze between the eyes, differences in the angle of the horizontal devia-

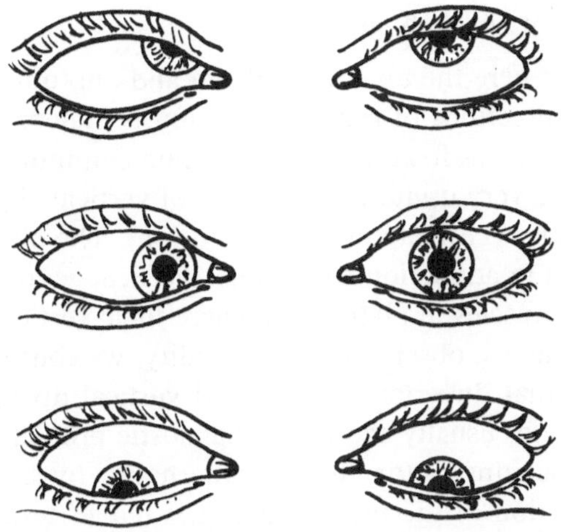

Fig. 17. — A-esotropia with fusion in downward gaze.

tion on looking upwards as compared with looking downwards. These are the alphabetical patterns, first described by Duane in 1897. Costenbader suggested the term A-V pattern (fig. 17).

When there is a more divergent position in elevation than in depression, or more convergent position in depression than in elevation, the configuration ressembles the letter V. When the reverse is present the letter A is simulated.

An X pattern is present when the eyes are more divergent above and below than in the primary position. It is now generally accepted that to diagnose a clinically significant V pattern there must be a difference of at least 15 pD (prismdiopters) between up gaze and down gaze, and 10 pD for the diagnosis of an A pattern. The frequency of occurrence of A and V patterns, if these limits are accepted, range from 10 to maximally 20%.

Establishing the diagnosis of A and V pattern supposes that the angle measurements are determined at 5 m. fixation, with full accommodative control (full refractive error correction being worn and use of accommodative fixation target), with good fixation control, and that these differences are confirmed in repeated control examinations (20). A and V patterns appear relatively late, approximately at one year and a half, there is evidence that early treatment of strabismus (cfr. conservative treatment) largely prevents the apparition of vertical abnormalities. Vertical abnormalities are relatively rare in adulthood strabismus.

A.3. Diagonal ocular movements

We examine here the up and in, down and out, down and in, up and out cardinal directions of gaze. As previously stated, the abducted eye is commonly used as fixating eye. These non commonly used directions in daily life are very useful for diagnosis of vertical abnormalities (nose and orbital rim eventually preventing fusion). The oblique muscles are best examined in adduction where their vertical action is maximal; the vertical recti muscles in abduction, where their vertical action is maximal. Every time we observe an abnormality, we control by executing a cover test in that direction. Dissociated vertical divergencies (alternating hyperphoria) usually causes no diagnostic problem unless the nose acts as a dissociating factor, then the alternating hyperphoria can simulate an overaction of the inferior obliques (cover test step 3).

B. *Ductions*

This monocular examination of eye movements—the other eye is covered—should be carried out when the versions show a limited movement. This often helps to distinguish "inhibition of abduction" from a "defect of abduction". The limitation of movement can be due to a mechanical restriction of movement (contracture of the antagonist) or to a weakness of a muscle (agonist).

C. *The Bielschowsky test*

This is the comparison of the vertical deviation in both eyes when the head is tilted to right and left shoulder. This test should be executed in every case with abnormal head posture and in cases with vertical deviations.

Procedure: The patient looks at the central spotlight on the Maddox scale, the examiner tilts the patient's head 45° first to the right shoulder then to the left one, comparing in these positions the lower corneal margin of both eyes, to see if there is a vertical deviation of one eye. In case of doubt, a control is made with cover test type I in these tilted positions. When there is no vertical difference, the Bielschowsky test is negative. It is homonymous positive, if we see an elevation on tilting the head to the homonymous shoulder, heteronymous positive when the elevation is seen on tilting the head to the heteronymous shoulder (fig. 18, fig. 19).

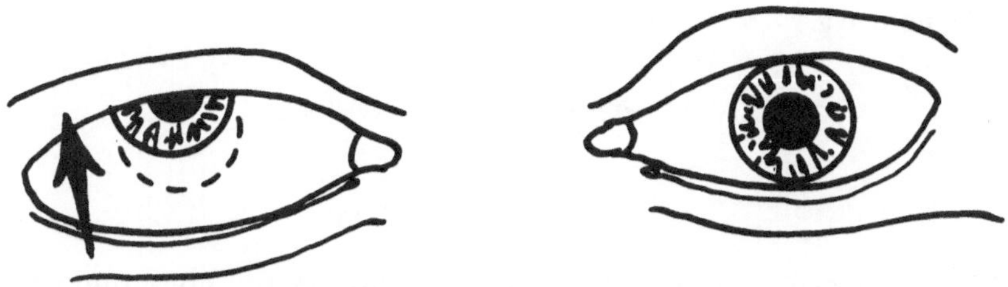

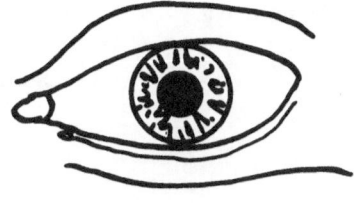

Fig. 18. — The Bielschowsky test is homonymous positive, there is an elevation of the right eye on tilting the head to the right shoulder.

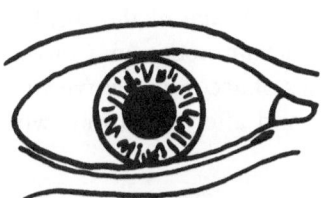

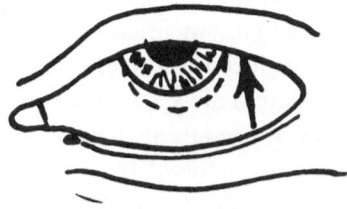

Fig. 19. — The Bielschowsky test is heteronymous positive, there is an elevation of the left eye on tilting the head to the right shoulder.

The Bielschowsky test is the decisive stage in the "3 step procedure" used to diagnose which vertical muscle is affected; it is especially useful to demonstrate superior oblique limitation.

D. *Convergence*

An adequate, at any distance adapted, convergence of both visual axes on the fixation object is only possible with a perfectly normal ocular apparatus.

Procedure:

1. The sliding convergence.

In the examination of symmetrical convergence the fixation object is held on a level with, and about 50 cm. in front of the patient's nose and the patient is asked to keep his gaze fixed upon it. The examiner approaches the fixing object towards the patient's nose until it is at 10 cm., observing the behaviour of the patient's eyes in doing so.

Especially in A and V pattern cases, we also examine convergence on depression and elevation of gaze of about 20°. When the examination of asymmetrical convergence (the fixation light is placed directly before one eye instead of in front of patient's nose) is normal, we are sure that the binocular vision is normal.

We note e.g.:

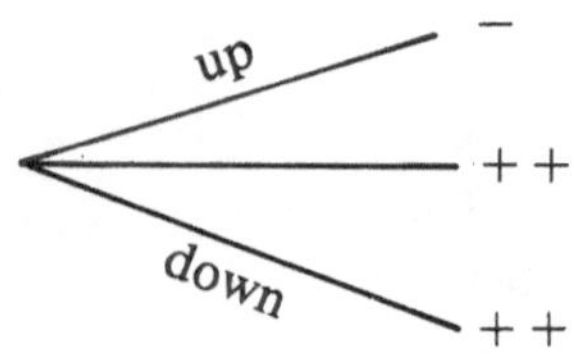

In "convergence insufficiency" one eye (always the non-dominant eye) deviates outward often long before the fixation object is at 10 cm. An adequate correction of the refractive error and the use of the fixation bar is necessary before we may diagnose "convergence insufficiency". The patient must read the text on the bar. Much of the socalled "convergence insufficiency" is due to lack of accommodation. Convergence should always be tested carefully in cases of accommodative strabismus, especially in higher plus corrections and after operations with liberal recessions of the medial recti.

2. The sudden convergence.

We ask the patient to fix the fixation object suddenly presented at different distances between 15 and 50 cm. and in different directions of gaze. Sometimes a marked "convergence excess" of one eye—always the nondominant eye—is seen. The influence of the examination conditions, as the kind of fixation object, the distance of presentation, the method used, is very pronounced in obtaining this excessive convergence response. The presentation of the same fixation object at the same distance at eye level or in the reading position, can change the obtained convergence (the power of convergence increases with depression of the gaze and decreases with its elevation). The same difference can be found in examining convergence in this form or in the sliding form. The same child can show a pronounced "convergence excess" when e.g. a finger is used as fixation object and be completely normal on reading a text presented at the same distance as our finger. In some people the first reaction to this suddenly proposed fixation object is a sometimes enormous over-convergence of one eye; part of them redress their eye completely, part of them only partially, part of them do not redress it at all. Some people show a "convergence excess" with the fixation object presented at 15 cm and not when it is presented at 30 cm. All this explains why there is so much confusion about "convergence excess" still augmented by the discussions of AC/A ratio's.

The study of the AC/A ratio has little or no value in clinical practice, therefore the only thing we do is to measure the angle of deviation at 5 m. and 33 cm. (cfr. X). When the angle of deviation for near, tested with the fixation bar, is greater than the angle of deviation for distance, we are confronted with an "atypical accommodative squint" (cfr. conservative treatment). We do not accept that this difference in angle of deviation between far and near, must be greater than 10 pD, before we can speak of "atypical accommodative squint", as is commonly indicated in the literature.

This "convergence excess" in our experience is strongly related to age. We never see it in congenital squint, it is frequently observed at 3-5 years of age, it can then persist for some months or even years, but it disappears when growing older. In these cases of "convergence excess" it is important to know that a slight amblyopia of the non-dominating eye is frequent. The visual acuity should be carefully tested.

Summary

If we could not in this stage of examination detect a strabismus, we perform a retinoscopy to exclude big errors of refraction (especially anisometropia) and an examination of the ocular media and fundi. In high risk children (p. 182) we perform this retinoscopy under cyclopentolate à 1%; this permits at the same time an easier examination of the fundi. We explain to the parents that their child actually does not squint, but that this is not an absolute guarantee. In our consultation we estimate pseudo-esotropia to be 30% of all young children brought to us for strabismus. We ask the parents to continue to observe the eyes of their young children; if nothing happens, the examination should be repeated every three months, especially for high risk children. Every ophthalmologist discovers strabismus in children previously classified as non-squinters. These are the pseudo-pseudo-esotropias of Ciancia (7). If in the meantime a squint develops, the child should be presented immediately.

VII. *Cycloplegia*

By definition cycloplegia means paralysis of the ciliary muscle and therefore loss of accommodation. Every case of manifest or latent strabismus is an absolute indication for cycloplegia. In present days the choice is practically limited to two drugs, atropine and cyclopentolate hydrochloride. Atropine is the strongest parasympathicolyticum we have. Most people prescribe atropine 0.5% for children up to one year and 1% in children older than one year. The main disadvantage of atropine is that its mydriatic and cycloplegic effects can last up to 8 days.

Cyclopentolate hydrochloride (Cyclogyl, Cyclopentol) is only available in 1% concentration. The 2% concentration has been withdrawn because of its many side-effects. Full cycloplegia starts 45 minutes after two instillations of one drop in each eye with ten-minute interval and should last 30 minutes. The retinoscopy should also be carried out between 45 and 75 minutes after the first instillation. The mydriatic and cycloplegic effect of cyclopentolate disappears completely within less than 24 hours and can be shortened by instillation of one drop of pilocarpin. Resistance to cyclopentolate is especially described in children with dark irides. Somnolence is not rare. This short and presumably full cycloplegia is the main advantage. With cyclopentolate, instillation and measurement of refraction are possible in the same session.

Does cyclopentolate 1% create paralysis of the ciliary muscle? Residual accommodation after the use of cyclopentolate is reported to be between 1.25 and 2.5 D in a general population of older children and adults. In negroes it may be greater (6, 13). We performed a cyclopentolate 1% retinoscopy in 40 orthophoric patients aged 7 to 48, 45 minutes after two instillations. We let them read at 30 cm. a near visual acuity chart, calibrated 1/20 to 1/2 (échelle de Dor) and this with the optical correction found under retinoscopy, giving them 10/10 visual acuity for distance. All 40 read at least 1/12 and at most 1/3 (the main was 1/8).

Conclusion: cyclopentolate 1% does not completely paralyze the ciliary muscle.

Does atropine 1% have a stronger cycloplegic action than cyclopentolate 1%?

The relative accuracy of cycloplegic retinoscopy using cyclopentolate or atropine has remained a subject of debate for pediatric ophthalmologists. Studies on older children and adults indicate comparable cycloplegic activity (6, 13, 35). Ingram and Bar found cyclopentolate 1% to be significantly less effective than atropine in one-year-old children (15). In the group which concerns us especially, esotropic children under the age of six years, atropine is certainly more effective than cyclopentolate in revealing hyperopia, as shown recently by multiple authors (3, 19, 33, 34). Therefore, for the first refraction of a strabismus patient younger than six years, we only use atropine ointment because it is more efficient in this form and never leads to atropine poisoning (dryness of the skin, raised temperature, delirium) as drops might do. We always prescribe atropine 1% ointment 3 times a day, 5 days prior to the examination. We explain to the parents that the pupil will dilate, that the vision for near, and eventually in suspicion of high hypermetropia the vision for distance also, will be worse and that the angle of strabismus may become greater. Especially in the last decade it became more and more evident that atropine, even used as described above, often does not create a full cycloplegia in this group of esotropic children under the age of six years.

1. Some authors (25, 43) found a residual accommodation with atropine in adults. Cüppers and Mühlendyck found more or less residual accommodation in nearly 1/3 of their esotropic children after months of penalisation with atropine in the fixing eye (9).

2. The experiences with penalisation and overcorrection (cfr. conservative treatment) often revealed an increase of the hypermetropia or decrease of myopia, this not only in the dominating eye under long lasting atropine instillation, but also in the over-corrected amblyopic eye (9, 14, 29, 31).

3. Many authors describe an increase in hypermetropia on repeated atropine examinations (21, 28, 32, 44).

We know that in a normal population the hypermetropia increases until the age of 6 to 7 years, but this increase is maximally +1.5 D and the peak of the increase is situated at the age of 3 (4, 22, 36). This can also not be the unique reason to explain the increase; most probably the total hypermetropia releases only progressively under the influence of repeated atropine applications or over-correction. This resistance to atropine is particularly pronounced in young children, in esotropia, and in children with dark irides. The desired total correction of the refraction may also often be known only by repeating regularly the retinoscopy under atropine or and by "overcorrecting" slightly as we describe in the chapter on conservative treatment.

When the child returns the sixth day, we look therefore first of all if cycloplegia is complete: is there still a pupil reaction to light, do we find changing values on repeating our retinoscopy, is there residual accommodation in older children, can they recognize any of the E letters presented at 30 cm wearing their full correction for distance? In any of these cases cycloplegia is certainly not complete.

We also look if the objective angle has changed under atropine. There are three possibilities:

1. The angle of deviation has disappeared. This is an accommodati-

ve strabismus. The strabismus will disappear with the full correction worn.

2. There is an increase in angle deviation, the accommodation is not completely paralyzed. The child reacts against this diminution of vision with the only thing he can change, an increase in accommodation and also an increase in convergence. A prescription of the "total refraction value" found under atropine is then in reality an undercorrection.

3. The angle of deviation did not change.

The retinoscopy can be done by plane mirror and light source behind and above the patient's head, by an electric self-illuminating retinoscope or by a streak-retinoscope. The results of the retinoscopy examination are noted as follows:

e.g.

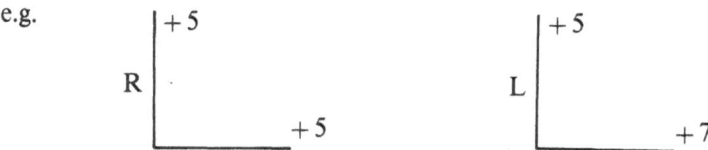

This implies that in the right eye a +5D lens was required to neutralize the reflection in each meridian, whereas in the left eye a +5D lens was required in the vertical meridian and a +7D in the horizontal meridian.

In older children we like to use the coincidence refractometer of Harting, where the total refraction is directly given and where any movement of the two images, one against the other, clearly indicates that accommodation is not fully paralyzed.

VIII. *Examination of ocular media and fundus*

This should be done in every strabismus case to eliminate possible local causes of defective vision such as opacities of the cornea or lens, organic disease of retina or optic nerve head, moderate form of retrolental fibroplasia (where the papil is elongated to the temporal side with many horizontal blood vessels) or even extra-ocular causes, e.g. a brain tumor. These organic lesions may cause a "secondary" squint, which constitutes 4% of Ciancia's esotropes under the age of two (7). The fundus examination has a great importance in the differential diagnosis between functional and organic amblyopia (cfr. amblyopia). In rare cases of an intractable child suspected of fundus pathology, we examine the dilated fundus under anaesthesia.

IX. *Visual acuity test*

Testing visual acuity is dependent on age. The principle nevertheless is to try to determine the visual acuity as soon as possible.

1. Under the age of 3, the responses of visual acuity testing are seldom reliable. In this age group we rely mainly on the cover test for the diagnosis of amblyopia and sometimes on pupillary responses (cfr. pag. 186).

2. Testing visual acuity in children older than 3 years can be done by Landolt's "broken ring"-test constructed on the same principle as Snellen's letter test types. We prefer the separate "E" presented at 5 m. The child, each eye alternately firmly occluded by the palm of the hand of the mother, holding a wooden E in his hand, is instructed to place his E the same way as presented by the examiner. Most of the visual tests for children are inaccurate, but we are not so much interested in the exact vision of each eye as in the fact if a difference does exist in visual acuity between both eyes. The experience of the examiner plays an important role in this age group. In cases of abnormal head posture visual acuity is tested monocularly in the torticollis position, and with the head straight. Testing the visual acuity often presents the best opportunity to diagnose the existence of torticollis. In nystagmus visual acuity is tested monocularly in the three horizontal positions and then with both eyes open in the primary position and in the eventually existing "O zone". In strabismus cases, visual acuity testing starts with the dominant eye. The children often give better answers when the E is vertically presented than when horizontally presented, this can be due to still insufficient lateralisation or to a non-corrected astigmatism.

In the course of amblyopia treatment we have to realize that a vision of 10/10 of separate E is usually not equivalent to 10/10 optotypes or E in rows.

Near vision at 33 cm should always be tested too.

Poor visual acuity for distance may be accompanied with comparatively good visual acuity for near or vice-versa. As soon as glasses are prescribed, visual acuity should be tested with and then without the correcting glasses for each eye separately. In cases of accommodative squint fully corrected by glasses, the binocular visual acuity should be tested also.

3. In children older than six years visual acuity is tested in the distance by means of the Snellen's letter test types and for near with a reading test at 33 cm. Practically all near vision tests are ordinary prin-

ter's types of varying sizes and therefore not very accurate. The ease of the child in reading is very important; we should always compare this between both eyes.

X. *Measurement of the angle of deviation*

The angle of squint is often "variable". The condition of the patient (emotion, fatigue), the conditions of examinations (with or without spectacles), in free space or at the synoptophore, the distance of the object (5 m or 33 cm), the kind of fixation object (accommodative target or not) can all change the angle. Variability of the angle strictu sensu means: in the same condition of examination and especially on direct observation. Different explanations are proposed: mostly insufficient elimination of accommodation, blocked nystagmus (10) or spastic factors (42). These latter are demonstrated by a difference in angle of deviation in darkness or light, or with eyes open and closed.

Therefore we can frequently only state that the angle of deviation as measured by such and such method with right or left eye fixing, at that distance, is so many degrees. As the exact measurement of the deviation is only necessary as a base for the operative indication, it is more important, in the course of our treatment of strabismus, to train ourselves to make a quick but nevertheless careful estimation of the angle of deviation by means of simple inspection, especially by means of the Hirschberg method or by cover test. The cover test type I shows us the manifest deviation, the cover test type II the total deviation.

A. *Estimation of the deviation*

A.1. When fixation is non foveal in the squinting eye

The only possibility is by observation of the corneal reflection. This can be done in three manners:

— Measurement on the Maddox scale. The patient is seated at a distance of 1 m, his eyes at level with the central spotlight. The examiner, sitting under the light and fixing the patient, observes the position of the corneal reflection in the fixing eye as the patient looks at the light (fig. 20).

— Krimsky's prism test. The examiner sits directly in front of the deviating eye, in order to avoid false readings caused by parallax. With these methods, allowance must be made for any underlying angle Kappa and for parallax. These methods give us an estimation of the manifest angle with the usually fixing eye fixating in the primary position.

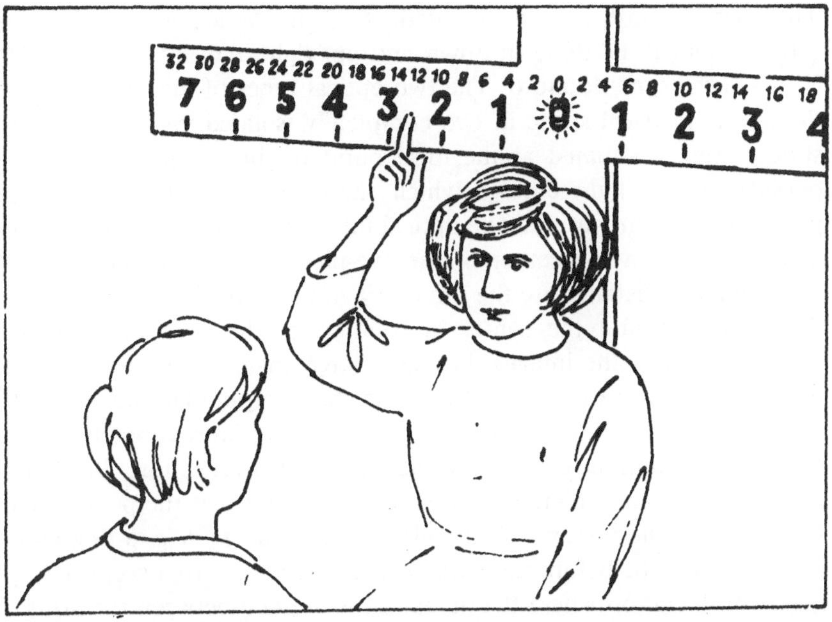

Fig. 20. — Estimation of the angle of deviation at Maddox scale. The patient follows with his good eye the examiner's finger, moved along the scale until the reflex in the deviating eye is central. The small number on the scale, indicated by the finger, represents the angle of squint in degrees.

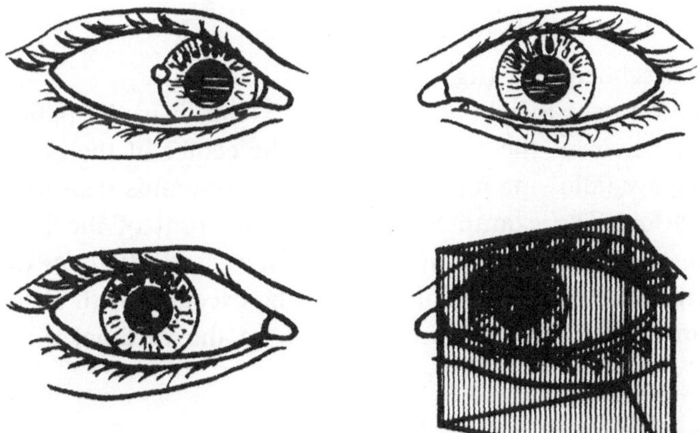

Fig. 21. — The Krimsky test. Prisms, base out of increasing power are placed before the fixating eye until the light reflex is centered on the cornea of the deviating eye. This prism indicates the magnitude of the deviation.

The Krimsky test can be executed at 33 cm. When necessary, these estimations can be done in down and up, right and left gaze (fig. 21).

— On the synoptophore: The two optical tubes of the synoptophore divide the physical space in two completely isolated visual fields. The slide carrier is situated at the focal point of the eye-piece lens, thus parallel rays of light emerge which should ensure relaxation of the patient's accommodation. The optical tubes can be adjusted so that the distance between the center of the eye-piece lenses and the patient's interpupillary distance are the same. When the optical tubes are rotated they move around the center of rotation of the eyes, enabling the patient to follow the images through a large angle. By accurate adjustment of the chin rest, the head rest and the interpupillary distance, the patient's eyes are at level with the eye-pieces, at approximately 1.5 cm so that the examiner easily observes the corneal reflection. Dissimilar and relatively small pictures are chosen to ensure that the patient fixes the center of the picture when called upon to do so (e.g. a dog and a kennel). The tube before the fixing eye is placed at zero, except in large angles of deviation where the deviation is divided between the arms of the instrument. The patient is encouraged to look directly in the center of the picture in front of the fixing eye. The examiner adjusts the tube before the deviating eye so that the corneal reflections are symmetrical in both eyes. The horizontal deviation is compensated for by turning the tubes of the synoptophore, the vertical deviation by adjusting the height of the slides.

A.2. When fixation is foveal in each eye

The Hirschberg test (fig. 22).

A fixation light is held at eye level at 33 cm from the patient; 1 mm of displacement of the reflection from the center of the cornea of the squinting eye (allowing for angle Kappa) corresponds then to 7° of ocular deviation. The examiner sits directly in front of the patient. The precision of this method is not better than 7° as a difference of 1 mm is the limit of discernment. This test can be executed with right and left eye fixing and if incomitance is found, in the cardinal directions of gaze.

B. *Measurement of the deviation*

Strictly speaking, the exact measurement of the angle of deviation is only necessary if the operative decision is taken. This exact measurement must be done:

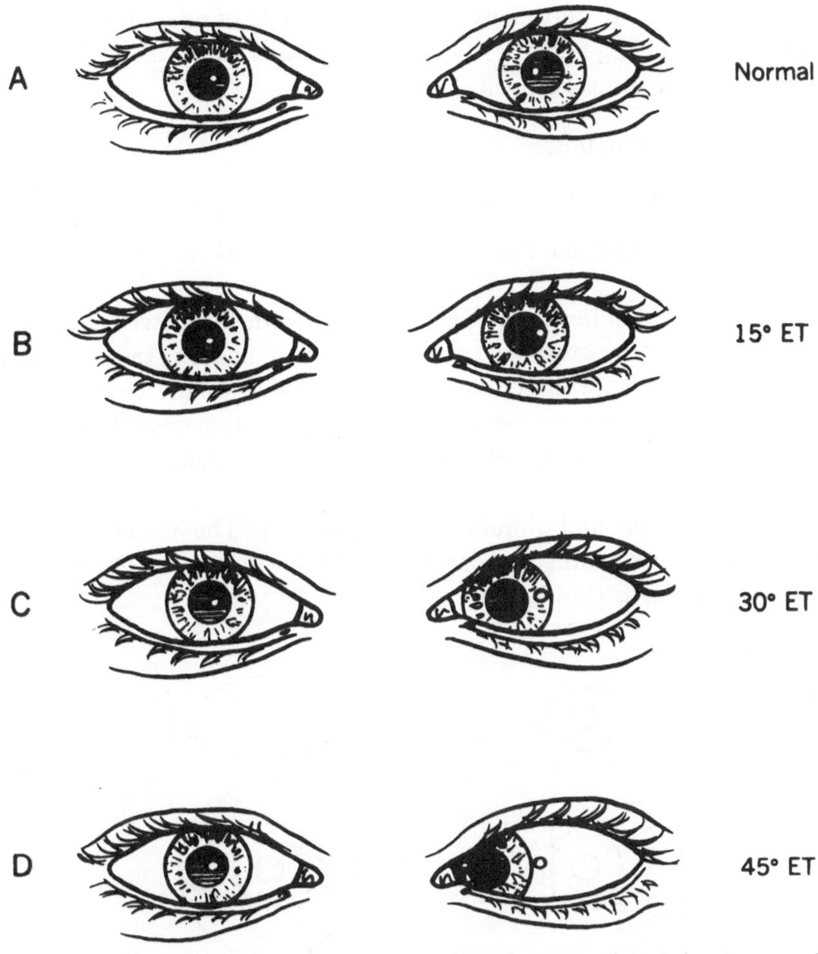

Fig. 22. — The Hirschberg method. Estimation of the angle of deviation by corneal reflection.

1. in primary position with each eye fixing in turn,
2. at 5 m and at 33 cm,
3. with and without spectacles,
4. with accommodative fixation targets,
5. in the cardinal positions of gaze if there is evidence of incomitance.

At 33 cm the examination should be done at eye level, not in the reading position. Classically the angle is measured with and without spectacles. In cases of astigmatism of more than 1D, of anisometropia of more than 1D difference between both eyes and of hypermetropia of more than 3D, we personally measure the angle of deviation only with spectacles, judging that after the operation the patient will still need his spectacles for optical reasons.

B.1. Objective methods of measurement

a. Measurement of the manifest angle

This is the angle detected by cover test type I. It can be measured in three manners:

— on the Maddox scale. The difference with the described method (p. 214) is that the examiner moves a muscle light along the scale in the prolongation of the direction of the visual line of the deviating eye, until, on covering the good eye, there is no fixation movement of the deviating eye. The angle of squint is read off directly on the tangent scale.

— with prism and simultaneous cover test. The patient fixes the central Maddox spotlight. According to H. W. Brown the exactitude of this method is 2° (5) (fig. 23).

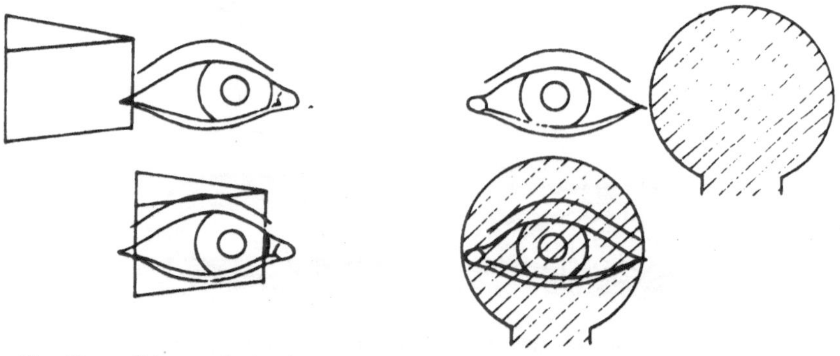

Fig. 23. — Prism and simultaneous cover test. We cover the fixating eye and place simultaneously a prism of increasing strength base out, before the deviating eye, until there is no more fixation movement. That prism measures the angle of deviation.

— on the synoptophore. The conditions of examination are those described earlier (p. 216). In adults the measurement is done with foveolar-sized slides (1° as circle and point). The tube before the fixing eye is on 0° and fixation of the dog is assumed with that eye, the other tube is at the estimated angle. Both tubes are illuminated. The light before the fixing eye is extinguished and the examiner carefully observes the patient's other eye when he is asked to look directly at the center of the kennel. If there are fixation movements the tube with the kennel has to be moved until there are no more fixation movements when the light is extinguished before the fixating eye. Between every repetition of the examination both tubes are illuminated again to allow for binocular vision. The examination is then repeated with the other eye fixing.

This examination corresponds to the cover test type I and to the prism and simultaneous cover test.

Conclusion: It is important to know the exact manifest angle of deviation in order to make the decision: to operate or not.

b. Measurement of the maximum angle

This is the angle as seen by cover test type II. It can be measured in three ways:

— on the Maddox scale. The difference with the described method is that we cover alternately without leaving both eyes open and we ask the

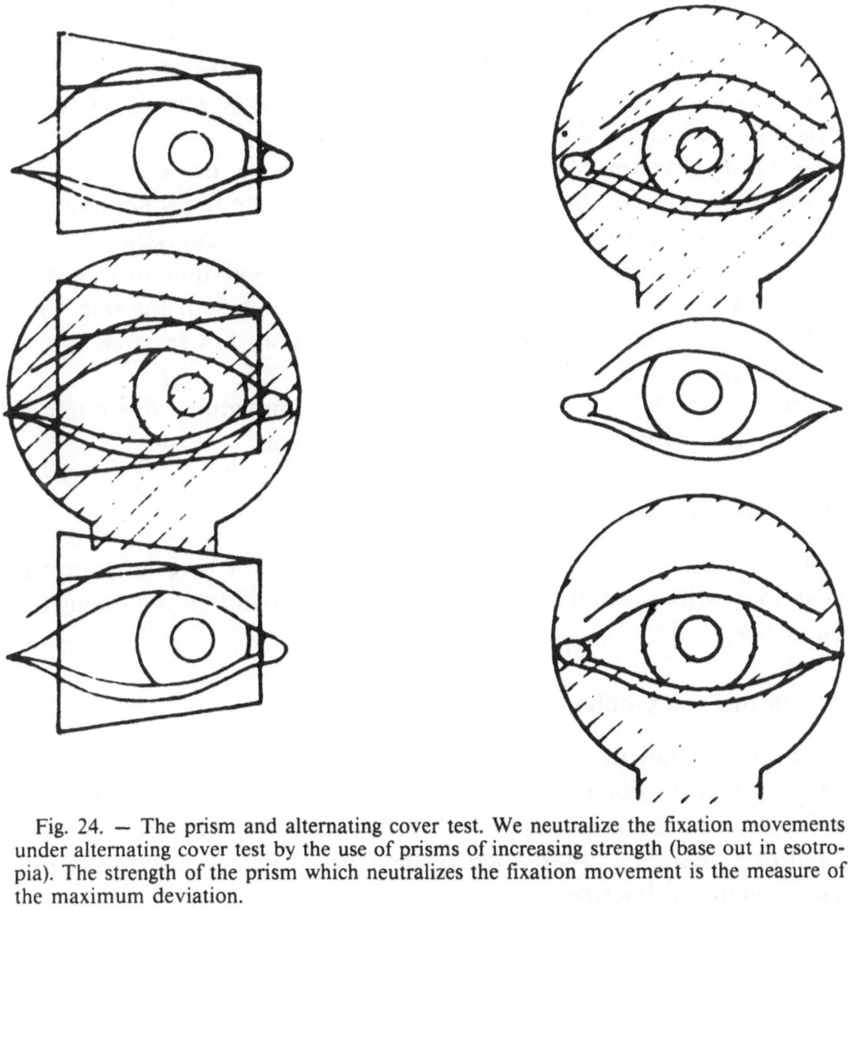

Fig. 24. — The prism and alternating cover test. We neutralize the fixation movements under alternating cover test by the use of prisms of increasing strength (base out in esotropia). The strength of the prism which neutralizes the fixation movement is the measure of the maximum deviation.

patient to look with one eye at the central spot on the scale and with the other eye at our muscle light placed on the estimated angle on the scale. If in executing these demands no fixation movements occur, the maximal angle of squint is read off directly on the tangent scale.

— The prism and alternating cover test (fig. 24).

This method is the generally most employed method, although it demands certain precautions: the prism must be held exactly horizontal and as close to the eye as possible. In measuring the angle of deviation in gaze up and down the prism may not move along with the head. A prismatic effect can occur in looking through the periphery of glasses especially correcting high refractive errors, when measuring angles of deviation in lateral or vertical gaze. Prisms not placed at the center of rotation of the eye can give rise to a considerable error, particularly with large deviations. This error can be minimized by placing the fixation object far away holding the prism as close to the eye as possible. This test can be executed with the prism before the fixating eye and the cover paddle before the deviated eye or, as most people do, with the prism and cover paddle before the deviated eye.

— On the synoptophore. The difference with the described method is that the tubes are illuminated alternately and the tubes are adjusted until no more fixation movements are seen. This examination corresponds to the cover test type II. The angle of deviation in esotropia measured on the synoptophore is generally greater than the one measured in free space (near reflex). Therefore it does not serve as a base for the operative indication.

Conclusion: It is important to know the maximum deviation in order to decide how much surgery must be done.

B.2. Subjective methods of measurement

These methods are only applicable in cases with foveal fixation in both eyes, with normal correspondence, and in children old enough to cooperate.

— On the synoptophore

The measurement is done by the patient himself who adjusts the tubes so that the dog is seen in the kennel. When he reports that he has achieved this, the angle indicated on the scale is the subjective angle. Control is made by observation of the corneal reflections and by previous methods described.

— Dark red glass at the Maddox scale

This measurement is based on the confusion of two objects that are seen foveally. The red glass must be so dark that the patient only sees through this glass the central fixation light on the Maddox scale. The other eye sees, when uncovered, the Maddox scale. As fusion is completely broken, we measure the maximum angle of deviation. The localisation of this dark red point seen by the fixating eye can only be done by the corresponding point of the deviated eye. If the dark red glass is before the right eye and the patient localizes the red light as indicated in the scheme, the deviation is 3° of esotropia and 4° left hypertropia (fig. 25).

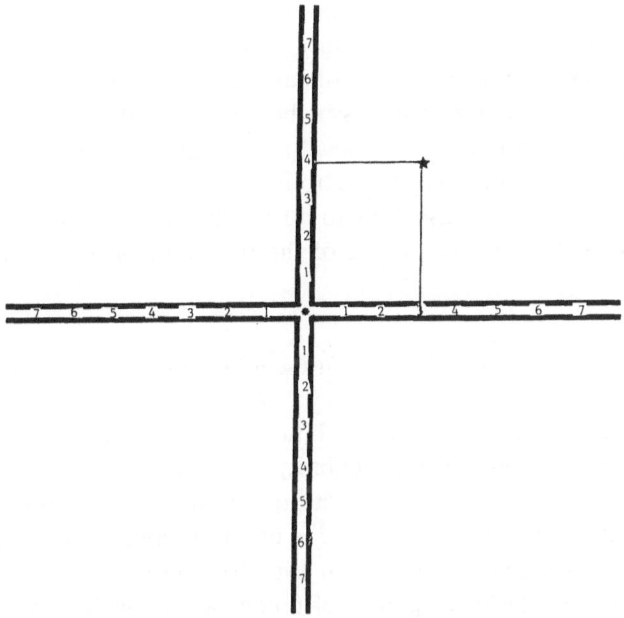

Fig. 25. — Dark red glass at the Maddox scale.

These measurements may be recorded in the form of a chart (fig. 26). We like this method because we can at once measure the maximum horizontal and vertical deviation, in all directions of gaze and in extreme up and down gaze. Alternating hyperphoria is easily recognized (the red point is localized beneath the white light with each eye fixing) and

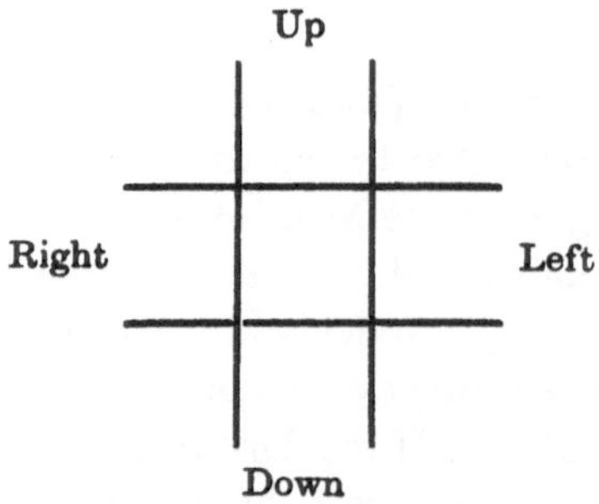

RIGHT EYE FIXING

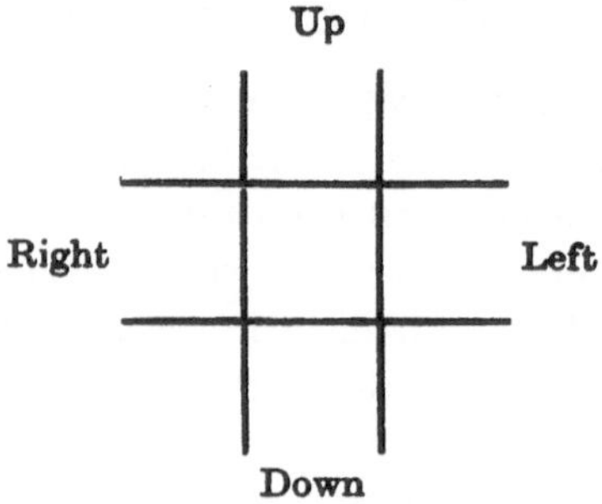

LEFT EYE FIXING

Fig. 26. — Charts for use with the dark red glass + Maddox scale and with the prism and alternate cover test in the primary and eight cardinal positions of gaze.

it is the only method which enables us to follow the course of movement between extreme positions of gaze, e.g. from extreme up to extreme down gaze. The dark red glass is before the right eye. We start from extreme gaze up and move the head of the patient until extreme down gaze, the patient always continues to fix the red light during this movement of his head. We ask him to go to the wall behind the Maddox scale and to show us the course of the red point on the wall (41).

XI. *Examination of binocular vision. The sensorial status*

Suppression and/or anomalous binocular vision characterize the binocular vision in strabismus. Lability is the main feature of both of them. Therefore the answer to the question "How is the binocular vision in this case of strabismus"? is often different, dependent on the examination method or on which eye fixes. For didactic reasons we continue to use the three grades of binocular vision first described by Worth: simultaneous perception, fusion and stereoscopic vision. Most important is to detect that form of binocular vision existing in "casual seeing" as the Anglo-Saxons call it, or in "free space" term preferred on the Continent. Each examination of the sensorial status has therefore to begin with less-dissociating tests. The tendency to disrupt a given sensorial status is called "dissociation".

The possibilities of examination of the sensorial status depends on the age of the patient and on the fact if fixation is foveal in both eyes or not.

Examination of the sensorial status in children less than four years old

The history taking (age of onset, optical treatment and family history) and inspection (manifest strabismus without closing one eye or intermittent strabismus, the pupil reactions in amblyopia) already give us valid information about the sensorial status. As explained, the cover test reveals much about the sensorial status, the possible presence of bifoveal fixation, fusion and fusion amplitude, the existence of a monolateral strabismus with or without amblyopia. The refixation movement on the alternating cover test delivers evidence for the existence of abnormal retinal correspondence. A normal convergence with orthophoria proves good bifoveal cooperation. The examination with prisms can show us suppression of one eye, normal fusion (without fixation movements) or abnormal fusion (with fixation movements). Even in young children, where subjective examinations are not possible, much valid information about the sensorial status is available.

Examination of the sensorial status in children older than four years

A. Foveal fixation in both eyes

1. Less-dissociating examinations

1.1. The striated glasses of Bagolini

These are plenoglasses adaptable to trial frames. If one looks through these glasses, the surroundings remain unaltered, a 20/20 visual acuity is possible. However, when looking at a light, a feeble luminous stripe is due to very fine parallel striations on the glass. The stripe is perpendicular to the striations. A mark is placed on each striated glass so that the orientation of the beam of light seen by the patient can easily be recognized by the examiner. We place the glasses before the eyes with the axis oriented respectively at 45° and 135°; a normal subject sees a light crossed by two luminous beams as an X and the light is situated exactly at the center of the X (2).

The patient may see:

a) one light crossed by two luminous beams (fig. 27a): the patient sees an X. A cover test type I must always be executed (never an alternate cover test which disrupts a weak fusional status). When no movement is noted the binocular vision is normal. When fixation

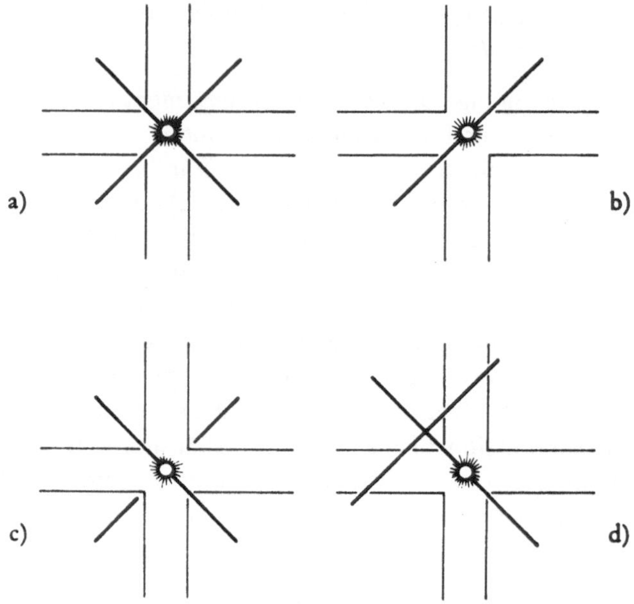

Fig. 27a-d. — Striated glasses of Bagolini. Explanation in text.

movements are seen the binocular vision is abnormal: harmonious anomalous correspondence. This answer is possible in cases of a slight amblyopia with eccentric fixation.

b) The beam of the light corresponding to the deviated eye is not perceived by the patient (fig. 27b). This indicates suppression of the deviated eye, this finding is common in large angle strabismus.

c) One light crossed by two luminous beams, but part of one beam near the light is not perceived (fig. 27c). This indicates central suppression of the corresponding eye with normal binocular vision, if there is no deviation at cover test type I, with anomalous binocular vision if there is a deviation with the cover test (0 point scotoma): harmonious anomalous correspondence.

d) One light is seen with two luminous beams, one beam does not cross through the center of the light, or two lights and each light with its own luminous beam (fig. 27d). When on cover test type I the localisation of the second beam (subjective angle) corresponds to the angle of deviation, we have a manifest esotropia with normal correspondence. If we turn the striated glass corresponding to this second beam so that the beam becomes vertical and after it horizontal, the subjective angle can be read directly from the Maddox cross. When on cover test type I the subjective angle does not correspond to the angle of deviation, we have a squint with dysharmonious anomalous correspondence.

e) In cases where only one luminous beam is seen (suppression of an eye) we turn off the light in the examination room, the suppression often disappears and the same possibilities occur as described. The anomalous correspondence with the striated glasses examination method is practically always harmonious, except after an operation where paradoxical diplopia is frequent. Disadvantage of the method: small angles of anomaly may be overlooked.

1.2. Phasendifferenz haploscope of Aulhorn (fig. 28)

The dissociation of the images of both eyes is attained by rotating sector discs of which the on and off phase are arranged so that the visual field of one eye is free when the visual field of the other eye is covered and vice-versa. The images are presented alternatively but it is impossible to recognize this because the frequency of alternating presentation is much higher than the fusion frequency of the eyes. Each eye sees only the image of the projector destinated for this eye, both eyes see the wall on which the images are presented simultaneously.

Advantages:

1. This is an examination in conditions of casual seeing with only a slight decrease in light intensity.
2. The examination can be executed at any distance, simply by moving the examination screen.

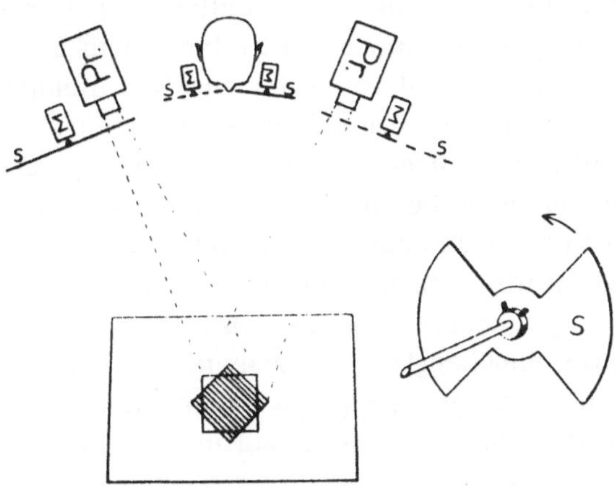

Fig. 28. — Phasendifferenzhaploskop of Aulhorn. M = Motor, S = sector discs, Pr = projector.

3. The only monocular visible images can be presented simultaneously with binocular visible images (third projector). All examinations can also be executed as less or more dissociating.
4. Aniseiconia measurements are possible.

The main disadvantage is the fact that the objective position of the eyes of the patient behind these sector discs is difficult to observe, and it is practically impossible to perform a cover test.

1.3. Diplopia examination

The general principle of this test is to provoke diplopia and to compare the angular distance of the two images (subjective angle) with the angle of deviation. If the objective angle is equal to the subjective angle, the correspondence is normal. These double images may be spontaneous after orthoptic exercices or after an operation, or may be provoked by anti-suppressive devices such as a red glass, a vertical prism or a horizontal prism which compensates for the angle of deviation. In cases where suppression is deep, the red glass is not sufficient to provoke diplopia, the use of the bar of Filters of Bagolini is then indicated.

— with the red glass.

Procedure: The patient fixes the central spotlight on the Maddox scale, the red glass is placed behind the cover before the deviating eye. We uncover that eye, observe carefully if there is no eye movement (to avoid quick alternation). We ask then: "Do you see one light or two?" If the child sees only one light (white) there is suppression of the deviating eye. If the child sees two lights simultaneously (a white and a red one) we ask the child to show us where both lights are seen (fig. 29).

In esotropia with normal correspondence the diplopia is homonymous and the distance between red and white light (subjective angle) is equal to the measured angle of deviation. If the diplopia is heteronymous, or homonymous but the subjective angle is not equal to the angle of deviation, the anomalous correspondence is dysharmonious. If both lights are localized together notwithstanding a manifest squint, the anomalous correspondence is harmonious.

Disadvantages: Small angles of anomaly may be overlooked: the angle of deviation may change during this examination (movement of the eyes) and the localisation of this second image is not always accurate.

— Vertical prism

Procedure: The patient fixes the central spotlight on the Maddox

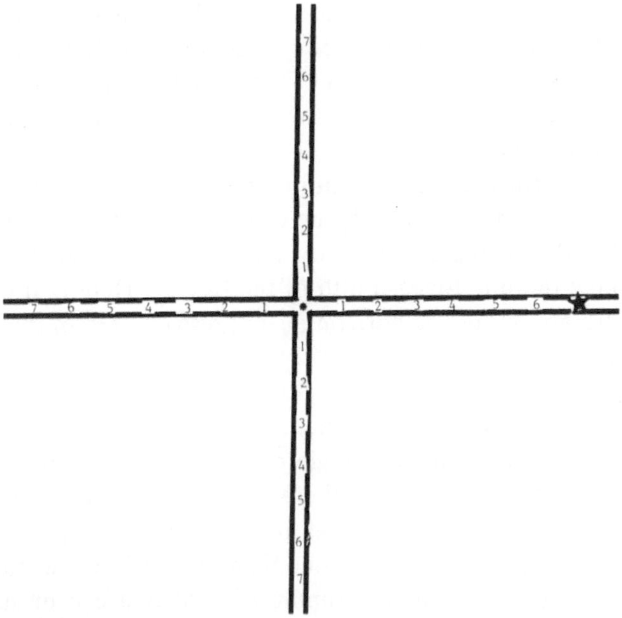

Fig. 29. — The red glass is before the right eye, the angle of deviation is 7°. The red light is localized on the homonymous 7°. The correspondence is normal.

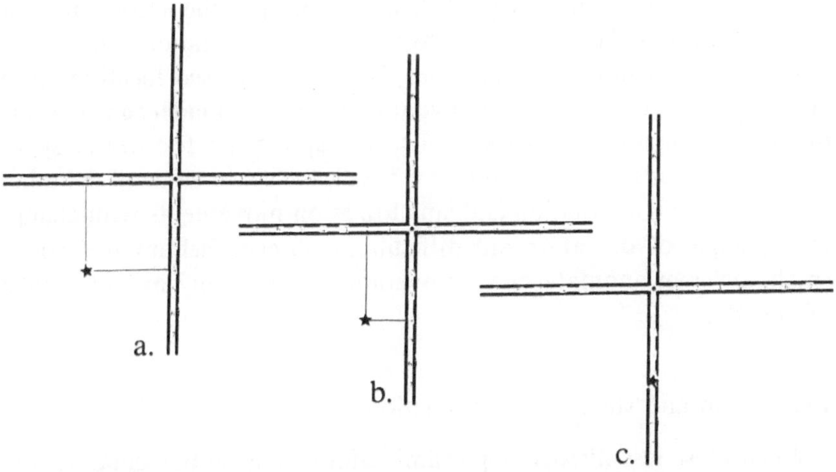

Fig. 30. — Vertical prism procedure in a case of left esotropia of 4°.

a. localisation 4° homonymous and 4° beneath: normal correspondence;
b. localisation 2° homonymous and 4° beneath: dysharmonious anomalous correspondence.
c. localisation 4° beneath: harmonious anomalous correspondence.

scale, a vertical prism of 8 pD base-up is placed before the deviating eye. We ask the child: "Do you see one light or two"? If the child sees only one light there is suppression of the deviating eye. If the child sees two lights simultaneously we ask the child to show where this second light has been seen (fig. 30).

This is a correspondence examination executed in conditions of casual seeing, where the space value of the fovea of the fixating eye is compared with the space value of a peripheral point in the deviating eye, 4° above the line fovea-midth of the papilla. Hereby it often happens that we are out of the horizontal suppression area in the deviating eye.

— Prism compensation examination.

Procedure: We measure the angle of deviation with the prism and alternating cover test (p. 220). If there is no more movement, we leave both eyes open with that prism before the eyes.

We ask the child: "Do you see one light or two"? If the patient sees one light, this can be a foveal suppression of one eye or fusion. To differentiate, we turn the prism some degrees up or downwards, one light indicates suppression, or we combine with the striated glasses: if fusion, the patient sees one light and an X. If the patient sees two lights simultaneously without eye movement, we ask him to show us where he localizes the second image. When in esotropia the second light is cross localized at an angle equal to the angle of deviation, the correspondence is harmonious anomalous. If there is crossed localisation at an angle less than the angle of deviation, the correspondence is dysharmonious anomalous. This very quick correspondence test in free space compares the space value of one fovea with the space value of the other fovea. As quick alternation and small fixation movements with change in the angle of deviation are difficult to observe behind the prism, small angles of anomaly may be overlooked, especially in large angles of deviation.

1.4. Fusion and stereopsis examination

When these less-dissociating examinations indicate binocular vision, we go further and examine:

1. Fusion: in free space (p. 199) and on the synoptophore.
2. Stereopsis: in free space and on the synoptophore.

Stereopsis constitutes the highest degree of binocular vision.

— The coincidence test or test with two pencils (Lang).

This is a quick and easy to perform examination method of the practical perception of depth (fig. 31). It is amazing how even an amblyopic eye contributes to the depth evaluation, what demonstrates the importance of the peripheral retina in the perception of stereopsis.

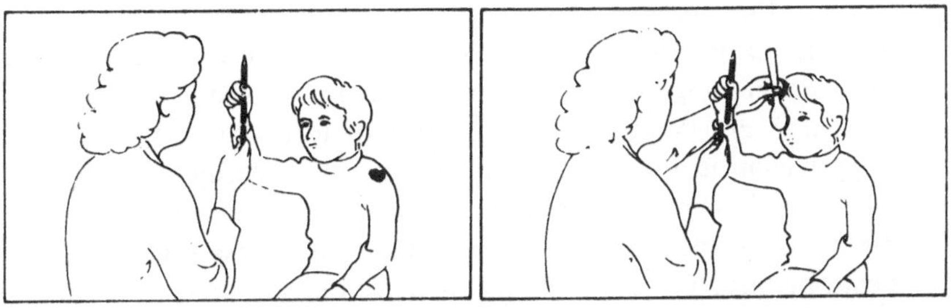

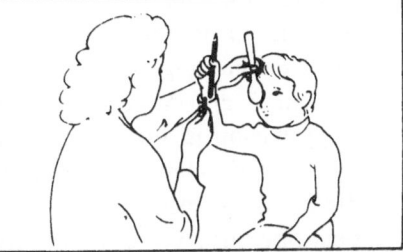

Fig. 31. — The coincidence test. The examiner holds a pencil base-up at eye level. The patient tries to place his pencil base down on the examiner's pencil. Can he perform this, the patient has to do the same thing with one eye closed.

— Examination with stereoscopic images.

Sligthly different images are simultaneously presented to each eye, which by fusion evoke a stereoscopic sensation. This can be done with stereoscopes, with polarized images, on the synoptophore or with the Titmus fly test. In this very popular test, a big enlarged fly is seen "en relief" through polarized spectacles; even by very young children the fear reaction is often present. We ask the child to grasp from the side the wing extremities of the fly. A series of progressively more difficult rings permits the evaluation of stereopsis up to 40 seconds of arc.

In the T.N.O. random dot stereogram the perception of depth is examined by means of red-green goggles. The stereopsis perception on this test demands more time, is more difficult but also more exact (480 to 15 seconds of arc) than with the fly test.

Some children of 5-6 years with normal binocular vision cannot execute this test. On the other hand, lower degrees of stereopsis are often present in microtropia even in cases of anisometropia and in slight forms of amblyopia. It is only when stereopsis on the Titmus test is positive beyond ring 5 or with positive answers on the T.N.O. random dot stereogram, that we can be sure of the existence of really normal binocular vision.

Conclusion of the less-dissociating examinations: it is necessary to start in every strabismus case with these less-dissociating examinations because they are close to the "conditions of casual seeing". They offer the best proof to show:

1. An anomalous type of binocular vision. This binocular vision is usually quite weak in comparison with normal binocular single vision. Therefore the anomalous type is easily "dissociated" by an unusual binocular stimulation. This dissociation will lead to suppression (or diplopia).
2. A weak normal sensorial status as we may find post-operatively in a child developing normal binocular vision, in some directions of gaze in A and V patterns or in cases of torticollis with binocular single vision in the torticollis position, is also easily "dissociated" by more dissociating examination methods, with suppression (or diplopia) as reaction. These less dissociating examinations offer post-operatively the possibility of detecting the first symptoms of the tendency to normalisation of anomalous correspondence, which is of utmost importance.

2. Dissociating examination methods

Monocular stimulations predominate in these examination methods; there are practically no binocular stimulations. These methods (the Worth Four dot test, the synoptophore, the dark red glass and after-image on the Maddox scale and the Hering after-images) deviate progressively more and more from the "conditions of casual seeing" or from "seeing in free space".

2.1. Worth four dot test

Looking through a pair of red and green goggles, the patient views a box with four lights (one red, 2 green and 1 white) situated either at 6 m or at 33 cm (with the four lights mounted on a flashlight). The red glass is always before the right eye.

There are three responses that the patient may give:

- suppression when the patient sees only 2 or 3 of the dots;
- diplopia when he sees 5 dots;
- fusion if he sees 4 dots. In this case correspondence is normal when there is no angle of deviation or anomalous if there is a deviation.

This is a very gross test. To perform a cover test to differentiate between normal or anomalous correspondence is practically impossible with these red-green goggles. In the presence of a dense central suppression scotoma or of small angle deviations or even in large angle deviation, when we approach the test close enough to the patient so that the distance between the lights is greater than the suppression area, the answer may indicate "fusion".

2.2. The synoptophore

This instrument is very useful for investigating the grades of binocular vision; objective and subjective investigations can be done under continuous control of the eye position.

2.2.1. With real objects

— simultaneous perception.

We use macular-sized slides of simultaneous perception (3 to 5°) as e.g. "dog and kennel". The first image is the fixating object (the dog), the second image always constitutes the surroundings of the first (the kennel). The patient is instructed to look steadily at the dog; he must not be allowed to alternate from one picture to the other. He is then asked "to put the dog into the kennel" by moving the tube containing the kennel. The angle at which he superimposes the picture is the subjective angle.

The double objective control: the comparison of the position of the corneal reflection and the notation whether or not the eyes move, when the patient is asked to look alternatively at the center of each picture which remains illuminated, is to be done at every step of the binocular vision examination. The angle of deviation changes frequently on the synoptophore. In the subjective examination (simultaneous presentation of the images) the angle often decreases; therefore this objective control is always necessary. If the subjective angle is equal to the objective angle, the correspondence is normal. Often the child cannot superimpose both images at the angle of deviation.

The different possibilities are:

— When the tubes are moved one picture crosses over the other and this crossing takes place at the angle of deviation. The corneal reflections are symmetrical. The sensorial relationship between the two eyes is normal. If one image disappears at the objective angle of deviation and reappears immediately at the other side of the picture when the tube is carried past the angle of deviation, it indicates that the sensorial relationship between the two eyes is normal but is masked by a central suppression scotoma that can easily be measured. We note e.g. the angle of deviation $+17°$ is practically equal to the subjective angle with a suppression scotoma from 13° to 17°.

— At the angle at which the dog is seen in the kennel, one or other eye has to make a movement in order to take up central fixation and the corneal reflections are asymmetrically disposed on the cornea. The retinal correspondence is abnormal. The abnormal retinal correspondence is dysharmonious with a subjective angle between 0° and the angle of deviation. The difference between objective and subjective angle of deviation is the angle of anomaly. The abnormal retinal correspondence is harmonious if the subjective angle of deviation is at 0°.

— At the objective angle both pictures are seen simultaneously but they appear to be situated in two different directions, they are crossed. The patient may attempt to superimpose the pictures at an angle less than the objective angle, they are close together, until one picture disappears and it appears again at the opposite side of its companion picture after further few degrees of movement. Such cases are diagnosed as attempted abnormal retinal correspondence. The suppression area, corresponding to the fixation point or zero point scotoma, can be measured; this area is greater as in cases with normal correspondence. We note e.g. angle of deviation $+13°$, the subjective angle is approximately at $+4°$, suppression scotoma from $+3$ to $+10°$.

— In some cases the image of the deviating eye is totally excluded.

— fusion

A pair of similar pictures with different controls such as a clown with toys in the hands is used for this purpose.

The tubes are set so that the patient sees two clowns, he is then instructed to move the handles of the synoptophore so that the two clowns blend into one with all the controls. The examiner should always observe the corneal reflections in order to be sure that fusion of the two pictures and not suppression of one of them is taking place. If there is any doubt, control is executed if no fixation movement appears while performing the previously described cover test. These controls are always necessary to distinguish true fusion (fusion at the angle of squint) from fusion in cases of abnormal retinal correspondence (fusion at the subjective angle); in the latter there are fixation movements. It must be remembered that repeated extinguishing of the light may break up the fusion which, in cases of strabismus is usually weak already. If true fusion does exist, the angle of fusion can be different of the previously measured angle of deviation. If the pictures seem satisfactorily fused, we examine the strength of fusion by locking the angle at which the patient joins the picture, the tubes are then moved slowly from side to side while the patient's eyes follow the picture. If the pictures do not remain joined, fusion is said to be weak. Similarly we examine the convergent and divergent range of fusion using the small screw for adjustment of the locked angle to converge or diverge the tubes. In some cases where a vertical deviation is present, we examine the vertical range of fusion by moving one of the pictures slowly up or downwards. The decision as to the presence of true fusion is an important one to be made because the treatment and outcome of treatment depends upon this conclusion. True fusion is likely in three cases: 1) the pictures "jump together" at an angle less than the angle of deviation; 2) diplopia appears when the maximal range of fusion is reached; 3) the pictures can be kept joined when side movements or fusional vergence movements are executed. Lack of fusion should be suspected when one of the following observations can be made:

- inability to maintain superimposition of similar pictures; the patient is unable to keep the pictures joined together because of a slight apparent movement of either picture, or one of the control signs becomes indistinct or is seen at another place, further away or higher.
- the picture joins at an angle greater than the objective angle of deviation. This indicates super-imposition, not a really blending of two images.
- inability to keep the pictures joined when side movements or fusional vergence movements are tested, the pictures break into two as soon as we move the tubes.

— Stereoscopic vision

If fusion is present, we examine the stereoscopic vision with slides for children (as the bucket); this can be used in cases of foveal suppression to determine the presence of peripheral fusion. For adults the slide with the numbers is used; as this test has control details, it cannot be seen stereoscopically in the presence of a foveal suppression in one eye. In cases of abnormal retinal correspondence stereopsis can be positive on the synoptophore, but it is always a little uncertain; near and far away often alternate.

2.2.2. Examination with entoptic phenomena on the synoptophore

The after-image slides. The positive after-images are those seen with the light off, they are seen as a light line against a dark background (e.g. with eyes closed). The negative after-images seen with the light on, are seen as a dark line against a light background. The slide with the vertical after-image is always presented before the deviating eye because the suppression is greatest in the horizontal direction. A patient with

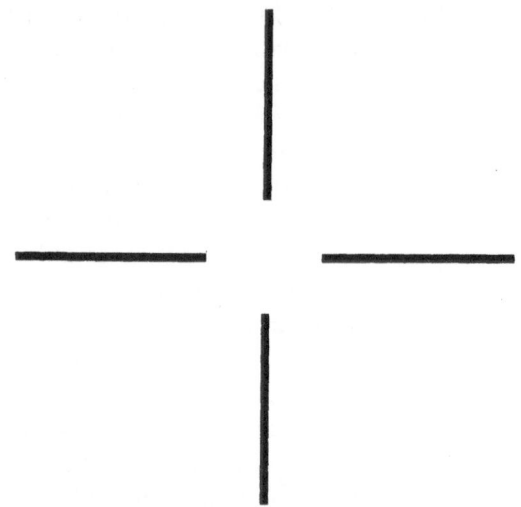

Fig. 32. — After-image in normal correspondence.

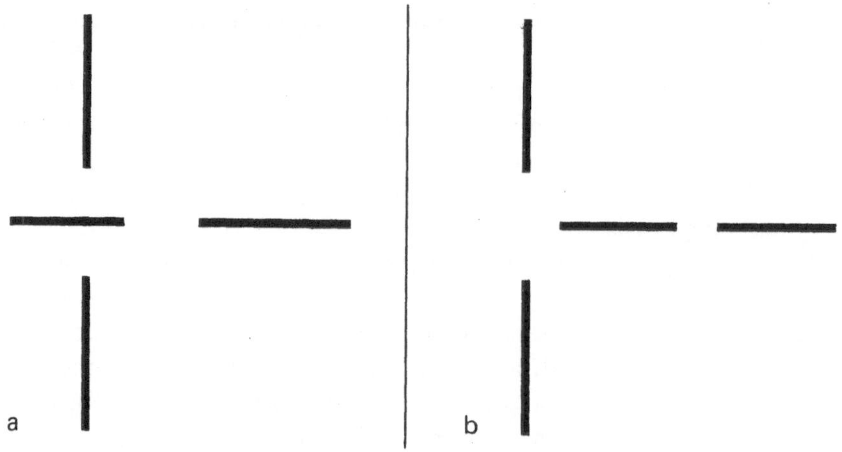

Fig. 33
a. After-image. Small angle of anomaly.
b. After-image. Large angle of anomaly.

normal retinal correspondence will see the after-image as a symmetrical cross. (fig. 32).

In abnormal retinal correspondence the after image is asymmetrical in a great variety of ways. (fig. 33).

Small angles of anomaly may be overlooked with these large post-images. In certain cases the position of the lines may change. During the period of appreciation of the after image, e.g. originally separated lines can momentarily be seen as a cross. This indicates a tendency to normal correspondence. As after-images are the most dissociating stimuli we have, the results of this examination are of prognostic value. If we find an abnormal retinal correspondence with this test, it indicates that it is deeply rooted.

2.3. After-image + Dark red glass examination at Maddox scale

Although this confusion test introduced by Cüppers is the most accurate examination method of the retinal correspondence, we use this method only in these rare cases where doubt still exists about the existence of a little angle of anomaly.

Procedure: e.g. right esotropia of 8°. The vertical after-image is given on the deviating eye by means of an electronic flashing device which has a linear slit in its front surface (fig. 34), thereafter the flashing light is switched on to visualize maximally the after-image. The patient is seated in the darkened room at 2.5 m from the Maddox scale (at 1 m in very large angles). We place the dark red glass before the fixating eye

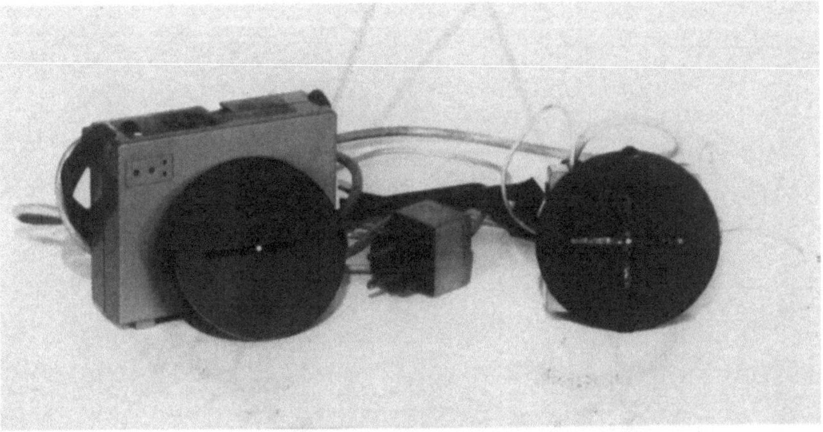

Fig. 34. — Electronic flash device.

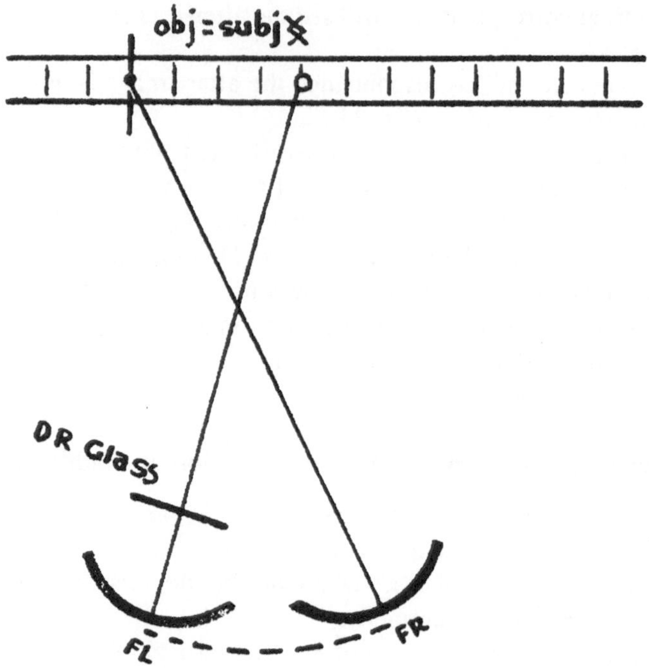

Fig. 35A — Normal correspondence. The red spot is in the center of the after-image.

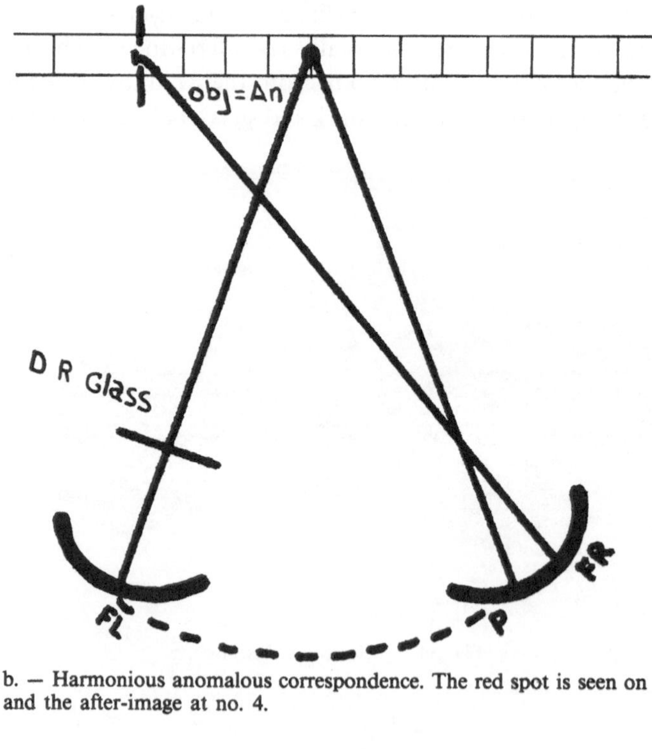

Fig. 35b. — Harmonious anomalous correspondence. The red spot is seen on the central spotlight and the after-image at no. 4.

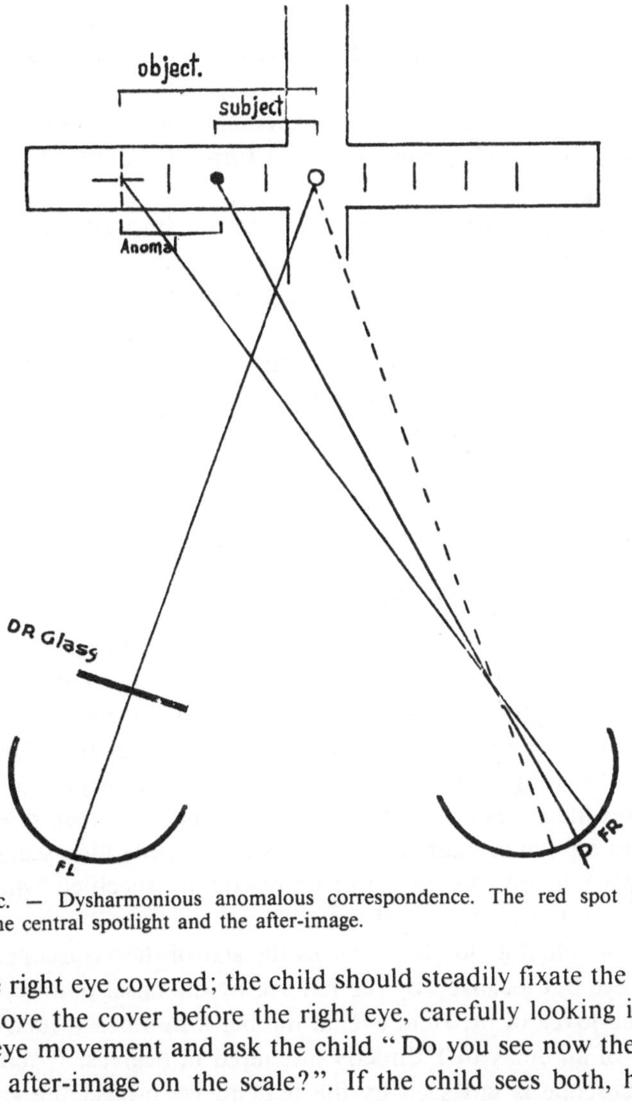

Fig. 35c. — Dysharmonious anomalous correspondence. The red spot is localised between the central spotlight and the after-image.

with the right eye covered; the child should steadily fixate the red light. We remove the cover before the right eye, carefully looking if there is not an eye movement and ask the child "Do you see now the red spot and the after-image on the scale?". If the child sees both, he should indicate on which number on the scale the red spot and after image are seen (fig. 35a, b, c).

Explanation: This is a confusion test. The after image characterizes the fovea of the deviating eye. The red spot seen by the fovea of the left eye is localized on the scale by the corresponding point in the deviated eye. This is the most reliable correspondence test we have.

– the objective and subjective angle of deviation are measured in degrees (with an accuracy of 1°) in the same examination.

- the dark red glass fully dissociates both eyes, the inhibition in the deviating eye is also strongly decreased. Therefore suppression is rare with this test.
- correspondence and angular measurements can be executed with the test with right and left eye fixing in turn and in all possible directions of gaze.

Conclusion of dissociating examinations: the importance of dissociating examination is due to:

1. their diagnostic value. These are the most accurate methods to detect small angles of anomaly.
2. their prognostic value. The more the test is dissociating, the more the abnormal correspondence found is deeply rooted. Abnormal correspondence is the sign of abnormal binocular vision (chapter V).

B. WHEN FIXATION IS NON-FOVEAL IN ONE EYE

1. Foveo-foveolar test of Cüppers

Procedure: The patient is seated at 5 m (or 2.5 m) and parallel to the Maddox scale, the fixating eye is nearest to the scale. The patient fixates the central light of the scale via a plano mirror which for the convenience of the examiner is turned in such a manner that the amblyopic eye looks straight ahead, the visuscope star is projected by the examiner onto the fovea of the amblyopic eye and only then does he ask the patient on which figure (black or red) of the Maddox scale the star is seen. Due to the mirror effect, it has to be specified whether the asterisk is on the black or red figures.

If for example (fig. 36), he localizes the star of the visuscope, seen by the right eye but localized by the left eye by the nasal point corresponding to the fovea of the right eye, at the black number 4, then we have the angle of anomaly (4°), directly measured in degrees. When the star of the visuscope is not seen by the patient, we project the green disc without the star and ask the child to localize this green disc on the Maddox scale. This is a very accurate test for small angles of anomalies which are measured in degrees.

2. Haidinger's brushes and vertical after-image on the synoptophore

Haidinger's brushes are entoptic phenomena seen only by the fovea; therefore they are always presented to the amblyopic eye.

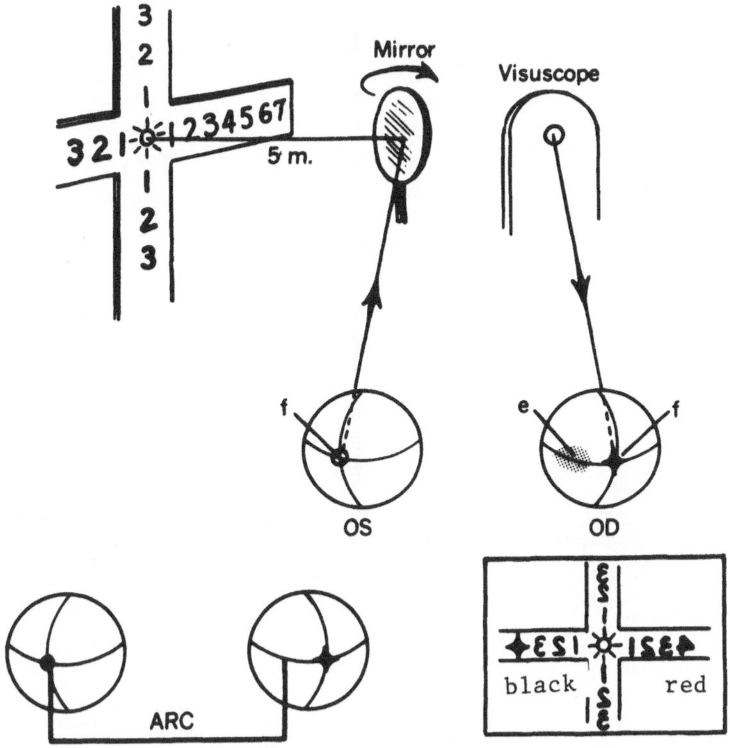

Fig. 36. — Foveo-foveolar test.

Procedure: The fixing eye receives stimulation with the vertical after-image as described in the preceding description. The Haidinger brushes are "switched-on" in front of the deviating eye. The child should always fix the central turning point of the brushes. It is often necessary to diminish the light intensity before the fixating eye or even to place an opal filter before this eye to diminish the suppression of the amblyopic eye until the brushes are seen, as binocular examination often increases the foveal suppression in the deviating eye. If only the vertical after-image is seen, no valid answers can be given. The patient is asked to describe the position of the two images in relation to each other. In practice we draw on a paper the vertical image ourselves and ask the child where he sees the brushes (fig. 37, fig. 38).

If the brushes are displaced, we always ask if the after-image does not move in the direction of the brushes or possibly if the brushes are not seen in the center of the after-image, which should indicate a tendency to normal correspondence.

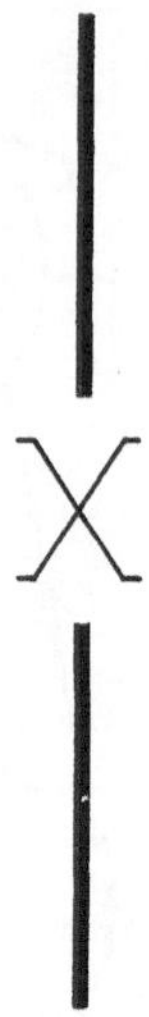

Fig. 37. — The correspondence is normal when the brushes are localized in the center of the after-image.

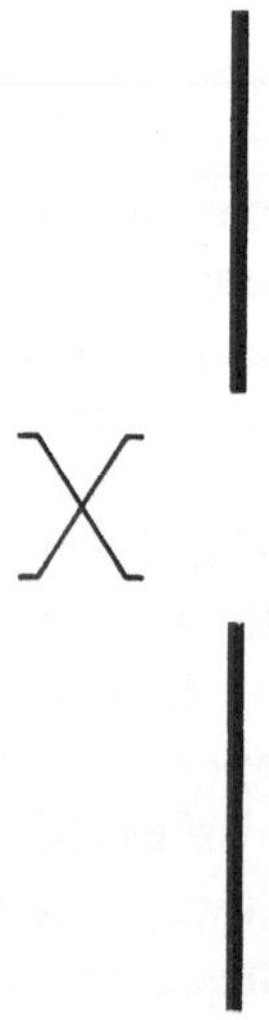

Fig. 38. — The correspondence is abnormal when the brushes appear displaced to one side.

XII. *Pre-operative examinations*

A. *The Prism-compensation test*

Indication: We perform this test, after the decision to operate has been taken (except in large angles) to see if the operation is indicated and as prognosis of the operative result.

Procedure: We have measured the objective angle with prisms and alternating cover (p. 220) and have controlled the sensorial reactions on this bifoveal stimulation (p. 228) (suppression, fusion, diplopia).

Since Woodward introduced the Fresnel prisms in 1965, the execution of this test has become much easier. As the value of a loose prism is not the same as of a Fresnel prism, we have to control by ourselves (at the Maddox scale) to which Fresnel prism the loose prism used to measure the angle of deviation corresponds. We attach this Fresnel prism (in esotropia naturally with base out) onto the glasses and we wait some minutes, after which we control with cover test type I if there are no fixation movements. If there are no fixation movements, we send the patient home for at least one day with this Fresnel prism on his glasses.

If on the first control with the cover test, there are again fixation movements, we increase the strength of the prism until there are no more fixation movements or even a slight overcorrection, the eyes coming from divergence under the cover test.

One or two days later we perform the same controls with prisms on.

1. Is there a change in the angle of deviation?
   - If there is no change: excellent operative prognosis.
   - If there is a decrease (rare) we repeat the prism compensation test with this smaller prism.
   - If there is a small increase: we repeat the prism compensation test with a stronger prism until a slight over-correction is obtained (cfr. conservative treatment).
2. Is there a change in sensorial reaction to the prism?
   Does the same diplopia exist or has suppression appeared? In some cases, especially in older patients (older than 9 years), we see the picture known as "horror fusionis".

B. *Tests to forecast post-operative diplopia*

Indication: In patients older than 8-9 years. The previously described prism compensation tests already gives us very useful information about what will possibly happen after an operation. If the test does not indicate diplopia, our chances of avoiding post-operative diplopia are fairly good but not absolute as postoperative diplopia can occur long after the operation, by change in the angle of deviation, or by diminution of the suppression in the deviating eye.

In cases where there is still diplopia after the prism compensation test is carried out for some days, we measure the extension of the suppression area on the synoptophore (p. 232) or with prisms before the Maddox scale and try to perform our operation so that diplopia is avoided. The value of the measurement of these suppression areas preoperatively remains subject to debate. Operating before the age of 9, avoiding overcorrections and unnecessary orthoptic anti-suppression therapy are better guides to prevent post-operative diplopia.

P.S. We are grateful to Prof. Dr. J. Lang for the permission to use the illustrations Nos. 2, 3, 7, 9, 12, 20, 23, 24, 27, 31 from his book: Strabisme, Ed. Hans Huber, Bern, and to Prof. Dr. G. Von Noorden for the permission to use the illustrations Nos. 4, 11, 13, 14, 15, 17, 18, 19, 21, 22, 36 from his "Atlas on Strabismus", C.V. Mosby Cy., St. Louis.

BIBLIOGRAPHY

(1) BADOCHE, J.M. and PINÇON, F. — Les secteurs dans le traitement du strabisme. Congrès de strabisme. Zermatt 1979.
(2) BAGOLINI, B. — Diagnostic et possibilité de traitement de l'état sensoriel du strabisme concomitant avec des instruments peu dissociants. *Ann. Ocul.*, 1961, *194*, 236-258.
(3) BREININ, G.M., CHIN N.B. and RIPPS, H. — A rationale for therapy of accommodative strabismus. *Amer. J. Ophthalmol.*, 1966, *61*, 1030-1037.
(4) BROWN, E.V.L. — Net average yearly changes in refraction of atropinized eyes from birth to beyond middle life. *Arch. Ophthalmol.*, 1938, *19*, 719-734.
(5) BROWN, H.W. — Srabismus Ophtalmic Symposium. The Mosby Company 1962.
(6) CHER, I. — Experiences with cyclogyl. *Trans. Opht. Soc. U.K.*, 1959, *79*, 665-671.
(7) CIANCIA, A.O. — Management of esodeviations under the age of two. *Int. Ophthalmol. Clin.*, 1967, *6*, 503-518.
(8) CRONE, R.A. — Alternating hyperphoria. *Brit. J. Ophthalmol.*, 1954, *38*, 591-604.
(9) CÜPPERS, C. and MÜHLENDYCK, H. — Erfahrungen mit der Penalisation. Schielbehandlung, B.V.A. Arbeitskreis, Schielbehandlung, Wiesbaden, 1976, Band 6, 87-104.
(10) CÜPPERS, C. and ADELSTEIN, F. — Zum Problem der echten und scheinbaren Abducenslähmung (das sogenannte Blockerungssyndrom), 46, Beiheft Klin. Mbl. Aug., Stuttgart, F. Enkeverlag, 1966, 270-278.
(11) DUKE-ELDER, St. and SCOTT, G.I. — System of Ophthalmology, Vol. 12, Neuro-Ophthalmology, London, H. Kimpton, 1971.
(12) DUKE-ELDER, St. and WYBAR, K. — System of Ophthalmology., Vol. 6, Ocular motility and strabismus, London, H. Kimpton, 1973.

(13) GETTES, B.C. — Dibutolinesulfate comparative clinical study of cycloplegia effect. *Arch. Ophthalmol.*, 1950, *43*, 446-453.
(14) HAASE, W. — Optische Penalisation als therapeutisches Hilfsmittel beim frühkindlichen Strabismus. Advances in Ophthal., Basel, Karger Verlag, 1978, 35, 26-44.
(15) INGRAM, R.M. and BARR, A. — Refraction of I-year-old children after cycloplegia with 1% cyclopentolate-comparison with findings after atropinisation. *Brit. J. Ophthalmol.*, 1979, *63*, 348-352.
(16) IRVINE, S.R. — A simple test for binocular vision. *Amer. J. Ophthalmol.*, 1944, *27*, 740-746.
(17) JAMPOLSKY, A. — A simplified approach to strabismus diagnosis, 34-92, Strabismus Ophthalmic symposium. The Mosby Co., 1971.
(18) JAMPOLSKY, A. — Some uses and abuses of orthoptics—the present status. Strabismus Ophthalmic Symposium. The Mosby Co., 1971.
(19) JAMPOLSKY, A. — Round table. Strabismus Ophthalmic Symposium. The Mosby Co., 1977.
(20) KNAPP, Ph. — The A and V patterns. Strabismus Ophthalmic Symposium. The Mosby Co., 1971.
(21) KNAPP, Ph. — Round table, Strabismus Ophthalmic Symposium. The Mosby Co., 1977.
(22) LAHAV-GUSS, Ch. and KAUFMANN, H. — Refraktionsänderungen im Kindesalter. *Klin. Mbl. Augenheilk.*, 1974, *164*, 274-278.
(23) LANG, J. — Strabisme - Diagnostic - Formes cliniques - Traitement. Bern, Ed. H. Huber, 1981.
(24) LAVAT, J., PRIGENT, G., DEBROUSSE, J.Y. and PARENT, B. — Mise au point actuelle d'une technique orthoptique dans le traitement de l'ésotropie. *Ann. Ocul.*, 1966, *7*, 641-667.
(25) MARRON, J. — Cycloplegia and Mydriasis by use of Atropine, scopolamine and homatropine-paredrine. *Arch. Ophthalmol.*, 1940, *23*, 340-350.
(26) MOLNAR, L. — Heredity features of strabismus. *Klin. Mbl. Augenheilk.*, 1967, *150*, 557-568.
(27) PARKS, M. — Round table. Strabismus Ophthalmic Symposium. The Mosby Co., 1977.
(28) PARKS, M. — Management of acquired esotropia. *Brit. J. Ophthalmol.*, 1974, *58*, 240-247.
(29) POULIQUEN, M.P. — Zum Problem der Penalisation. *Klin. Mbl. Augenheilk.*, 1972, *161*, 130-139.
(30) QUÉRÉ, M.A., CLERGEAU, G. et FONTENAILLE, N. — L'Hypermétrie de refixation. *Arch. Ophtal (Paris)*, 1975, *35*, 265-268.
(31) QUÉRÉ, M.A. — Die Methoden der Pénalisation in der Behandlung des Strabismus convergens. *Klin. Mbl. Augenheilk.*, 1972, *161*, 140-155.
(32) RÉTHY, I. and GAL, Zs. — Results and principles of a new method of optical correction of hypermetropia in cases of esotropia. *Acta Ophthalmol.*, 1968, *46*, 757-766.
(33) ROBB, R.M. and PETERSON, R.A. — Cycloplegic refraction in children. *J. Ped. Ophthalmol.*, 1968, *5*, 110-114.
(34) ROSENBAUM, A.L. and coll. — Cycloplegic refraction in esotropic children. Cyclogyl versus Atropine. Fourth Int. Orthopt. Congress Bern, 1979.
(35) SEPULCHRE DE CONDÉ, Ch. — L'insuffisance des cycloplégiques pour la détection de l'hypermétropie latente dans le strabisme convergent concomitant. Thèse Nancy, 1973.
(36) SLATAPER, F.J. — Age norms of refraction and vision. *Arch. Ophthalmol.*, 1950, *43*, 466-481.
(37) STANLEY, J.A. and BAISE, G. — The swinging flashlight test to detect minimal optic neuropathy. *Arch. Ophthalmol.*, 1968, *80*, 769-771.
(38) URIST, M.J. — Horizontal squint with secondary vertical deviations. *Arch. Ophthalmol.*, 1951, *46*, 245-267.
(39) URRETS-ZAVALIA, A. Jr. — Paralisis bilateral congenita del musculo oblicuo inferior. *Arch. Oftal. B. Air.*, 1948, *23*, 1-11.
(40) VEREECKEN, E. and ADELSTEIN, F. — Diagnostic et traitement de la «paralysie du droit externe». *Opthalmologica*, 1966, *151*, 465-476.

(41) VEREECKEN. E. and FERON, A. — Quelques considérations sur le strabisme paralytique. *Bull. Soc. Belge Opht.*, 1968, *150*, 682-693.
(42) WEISS, J.B. — Congrès strabologique, Zermatt 1979.
(43) WOLF, A.V. and HODGE, H.C. — Effects of atropinesulfate, methyl-atropine nitrate and homatropinehydrobromide on adult human eye. *Arch. Ophthalmol.*, 1946, *35*, 293-301.
(44) WORTHAM, C. — The Increase in Hypermetropia in children. *Brit. Orthopt. J.*, 1978, *35*, 83-90.

Bull. Soc. belge Ophtal., **195**, 245-267, 1981.

CHAPTER VII

AMBLYOPIA

A. Th. M. VAN BALEN (*)

I. *Introduction*

The definition of amblyopia is decreased vision without apparent organic defects or, in other words, purely functional disturbance of the visual acuity. The Dutch layman speaks of the lazy eye (lui oog), and in olden times the expression of visual obtusion (stompzichtigheid) was used. Although this was a more or less exact translation of the Greek word amblyopia, this could no longer be used because of the emotional connotation. The concept of amblyopia has changed in the course of time. Buffon in 1743 considered weakness of the eye as the primary cause of strabismus. Later on the concept of amblyopia ex anopsia was introduced. In 1788 the term amblyopia was used for very low visual acuity, next to amaurosis. This was of course more the indication of a sign and not a diagnosis. Bangerter in 1953 proposed the definition "decrease of visual acuity without organic defect". In 1960 Von Noorden and Burian added the reversibility by adequate therapy as a feature of amblyopia (41). The term functional amblyopia is a pleonasm (14) but we still have to use the adjective "functional", because in the ophthalmological literature (especially French literature) amblyopia is still used in general sense to indicate low visual acuity.

Twenty years ago Enoch used the Stiles-Crawford method (16) to demonstrate the existence of "amblyopia", caused by the oblique position of cones in the fovea. These cases have to be taken out of the

(*) Academisch Ziekenhuis der Vrije Universiteit, de Boelelaan 1117, 1081 HV Amsterdam.

concept of "amblyopia sensu strictiori". In view of the data of Hubel and Wiesel and Von Noorden concerning structural changes in the lateral geniculate body of visual deprived kittens and newborn monkeys, the definition of amblyopia as used in the first lines of this paragraph cannot be maintained, the more so because the structural changes in the lateral geniculate body have appeared to be reversible albeit in a limited period. Structural changes caused by defective function are well known in pathophysiology. To formulate an exact definition of amblyopia, the nature of the functional defect of amblyopia must be described.

On basis of practical experience different kinds of amblyopia have been discerned. Amblyopia that was found after treatment of congenital cataract, congenital corneal opacity and ptosis; amblyopia that was found as incorrectible low visual acuity in cases of ametropia (especially astigmatism) and anisometropia. The most frequently occurring amblyopia was the amblyopia found in the deviating eye of unilateral strabismus. On basis of theoretical considerations other differentiations were made; "amblyopia of arrest" in which the development of visual acuity was considered to be cut off; "amblyopia ex anopsia" in which visual acuity was lost by non-use and "suppression amblyopia" in which one supposed that the function of one eye was suppressed or inhibited by some higher neuronal mechanism to avoid diplopia.

The experiments on newborn kittens and monkeys, in which eyes were occluded or defocused or artificially deviated led Von Noorden to the hypothesis that all kinds of amblyopia were caused by the same disturbance i.e. a deprivation of normal visual experience in a sensitive period of life. In human beings this period was estimated (from clinical experience) to be from birth to approximately the age of 5 years (42). Von Noorden admitted the necessity of assuming some role of suppression in the genesis of amblyopia. Unilateral occlusion or defocusing always results in deeper amblyopia than bilateral deprivation. This can only be explained by some kind of binocular interaction, in which the function of the normal eye exerts some kind of inhibition on the deprived or deviated eye. In what measure deprivation and suppression are present in the genesis of different kinds of amblyopia is uncertain. It is to be expected that suppression is the main factor in strabismus amblyopia. Discrimination between strabismus amblyopia and deprivation amblyopia cannot always be made easily in individual cases. Strabismus amblyopia can be accompanied by anisometropia and nearly all cases of deprivation amblyopia are deviated.

A practical differentiation of amblyopia for the sake of treatment is the differentiation according to the fixation behaviour of the amblyopic eye:

1. amblyopia with centric fixation;
2. amblyopia with eccentric fixation; the last one with and without latent foveal principal visual direction;
3. amblyopia without fixation.

II. *Sensoric aspects*

A. *Psychophysics*

The essential feature of amblyopia is deficiency of visual acuity. The theories that describe amblyopia as a form of agnosia or as a defective "Gestaltauffassung" have been shown to be unfounded (9). On their own low level of visual acuity, amblyopes recognise any presented pattern.

When we speak of visual acuity, we do not only mean "minimum separabile", but also "minimum discriminabile" and to a far lesser extent "minimum visibile". In several situations of visual acuity examination, discrimination is more relevant than separation. Analysis leads to the conclusion that vision of a black object against a white background factually is a form of intensity discrimination. For instance, a single black line of 0.5 sec. in width can be discerned on a white field. Hecht and Mintz (21) and Byram (10) showed that such a line throws a shadow on the retina that contrasts only 1 % with the surrounding field.

As all factors influencing visual acuity (refraction, retinal mosaic, size of the pupil, illumination) are normal in amblyopic eyes, we can safely assume that the same contrast relations will reach the retina in amblyopic as in normal eyes; but we know that this contrast is poor.

Since Hering we also know that this poor (physical) contrast is increased by a subjective or, better, physiological contrast mechanism. In the literature several figures are given in which the effect of this mechanism is shown (fig. 1). Tschermak gives the following description of this phenomenon. "When an element of the visual system receives white stimulation, the stimulation of the surrounding elements is decreased and perhaps even a black stimulation of the surroundings occurs. This antagonistic relation of the surrounding elements occurs

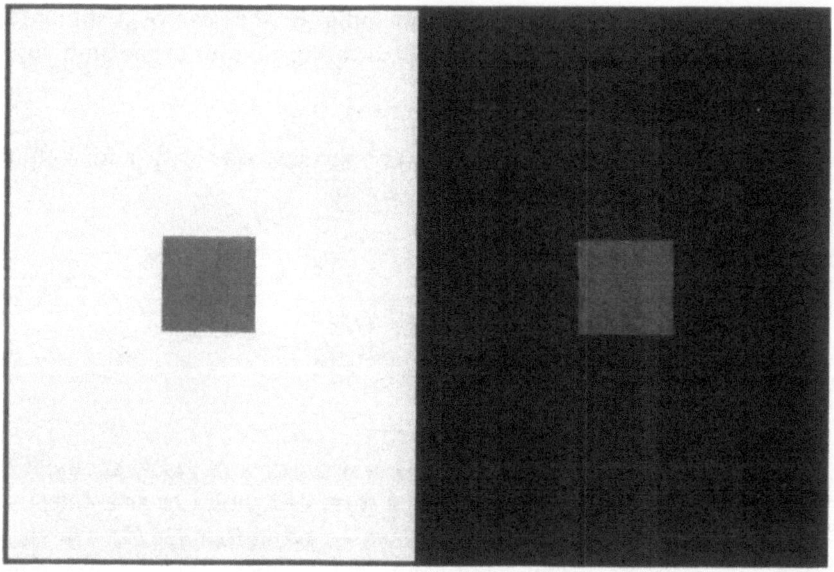

Fig. 1. — One of the figures that demonstrates the effect of physiological contrast. The brightness of the central quadrangle is influenced by the surrounding fields.

not exclusively in the retina, not on a psychophysical level but without doubt in that part of the visual system where both eyes are represented separately".

Per exclusionem we can state that disarrangement of this contrast mechanism must be the cause of the low visual acuity in amblyopia. In amblyopia we have to deal with a decrease of contrast or differential sensitivity and not of absolute sensitivity.

Wald and Burian (49) found a normal absolute sensitivity. Others found decreased sensitivity for small testlights in the fovea of the amblyopic eyes.

Oppel and Kranke (45) and Krzystkowa (28) tested this sensitivity in the earliest phase of dark adaptation. Lavergne (30), Weekers et al. (5), Loewer-Soeger (32) and Maraini and Peralta (37) tested the sensitivity for a small, red light in the Goldmann-Weekers adaptometer. They found lowered sensitivity especially in the fovea and not in relation with the decreased visual acuity. This also appeared in the static perimetry studies of Mackensen (35).

Since Lythgoe (34) (1940) we know that the sensitivity of the retina in different stages of adaptation not only depends on a certain equilibrium between rhodopsine and its decomposition products, but also on a change in neuronal organization in the retina. The size of the summation fields changes. Normally the summation fields measure 4-10 min. in the fovea and 15-30 min. in the periphery, according to Glezer (17). The summation fields grow in dark adaptation because of the decrease of inhibition in the receptive fields. The theory of Arden and Weale (1), implying equal sensitivity of single cones and rods, was confirmed. The differences in sensitivity are caused by neuronal organization. In light adaptation the rod field activity is taken over by the cone fields. Further increase of intensity causes reorganization of the cone receptive fields (17).

In conclusion, we can say that neuronal mechanisms in the retina are able to arrange an equilibrium of facilitation and inhibition adapted to the level of luminance of the test field and providing receptive fields of different size. This field organization must be the base of the subjective contrast mechanisms. The development of the visual acuity in the first months of life must be based on a development of the same field organisation. The receptive field of the immature retinal ganglion cell has a weak, widespread and ill-defined excitatory centre and a weak, wide-

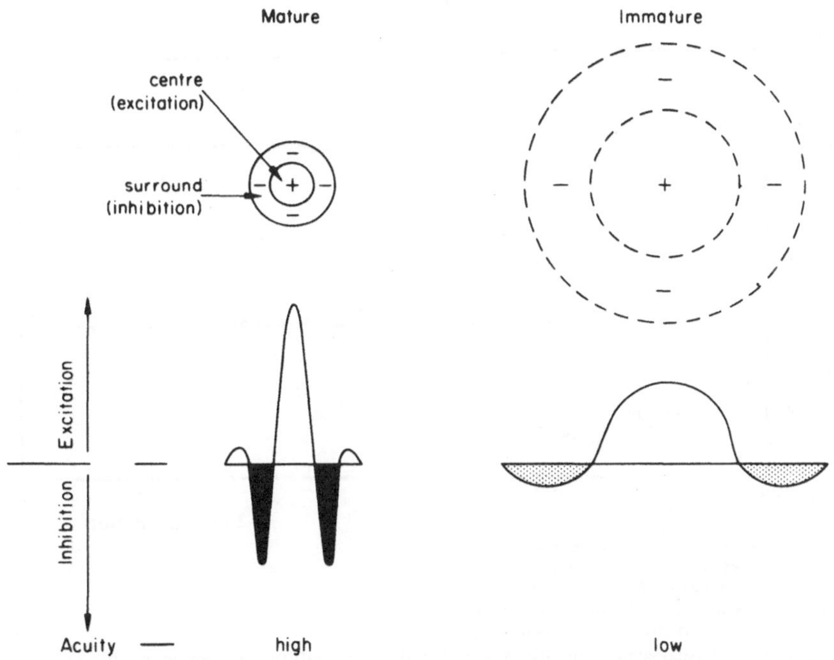

Fig. 2. — Comparison of mature and immature receptive field organisation shown schematically (from Ikeda H., 1979).

spread and ill-defined inhibitory surround. Such a receptive field gradually sharpens its excitatory and inhibitory profiles during development and becomes mature: this is characterized by a sharply-defined excitatory centre and a strong inhibitory surround. This is shown in figure 2 (26). The defect of this neuronal mechanism in amblyopia could be apparent in the phenomenon described by Ammann and later by Von Noorden and Burian (43), i.e., the decreasing visual acuity of amblyopic eyes during increasing light adaptation and the normal visual acuity at low levels of illumination (fig. 3). When the neuronal reorganization in the retina, which has to take place at high illumination levels, does not occur, the retina stays in the dark-adapted state with its relatively large summation fields and its correspondingly bad subjective contrast. Burian repeatedly emphasizes the dark-adapted behaviour of the amblyopic eye, and Meur (1964) (38) poses the following thesis after studying the summation coefficient in the fovea of amblyopic eyes: "The fovea in amblyopic eyes functions in photopic circumstances as if the cones remain dark adapted or, to put in other words, as if retina structures that are ruled by rods inhibit structures ruled by cones even in photopic circumstances". By using the grid of

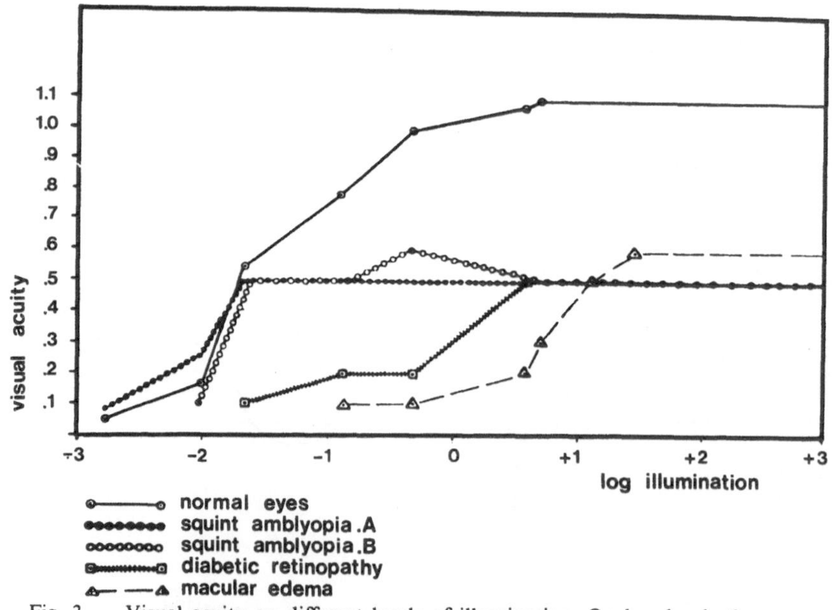

Fig. 3. — Visual acuity on different levels of illumination. On low levels the curve of visual acuity of the amblyopic eye concurs with that of the normal eye. From von Noorden and Burian, 1959.

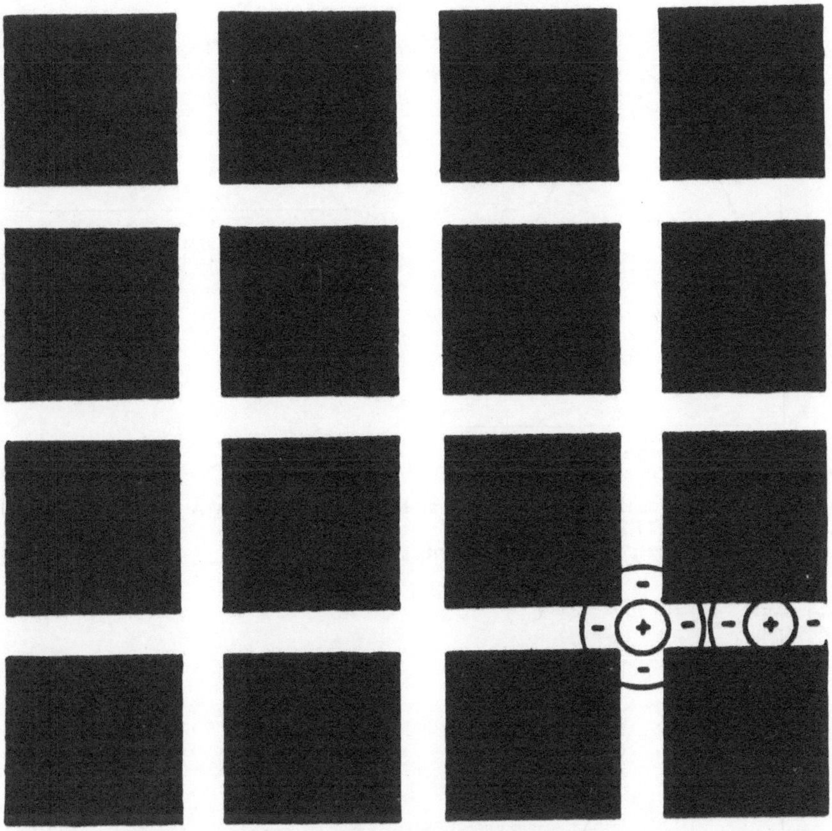

Fig. 4. — The grid of Hermann. Grayish spots on the intersections of the white bands indicating inhibition that is stronger at the crossings. By variation of the width of the white bands one can measure the diameter of the receptive fields.

Hermann, Meur (39) et al. (1968) found summation fields in the fovea of amblyopic eyes of 20-25 min. in diameter, i.e., in the range of size that normally is found in the periphery (fig. 4). The same was found by Grosvenor (18) and Miller (40). Lawwill and Burian (31) proved that the amblyopic eye needs more contrast than the normal eye. Hagemans (20) found abnormally high need of contrast in the high spatial frequency region of the contrast transfer function. The low spatial frequency region of modulated light was normally or even supernormally perceived by the amblyopic eye (fig. 5 and 6). Furthermore the amblyopic eye needs a larger test field than the normal eye.

The above described neuronal disorganization results in a decreased visual acuity and loss of physiological superiority of the fovea. This loss leads to sensoric and motoric disturbances. In general normalisation of

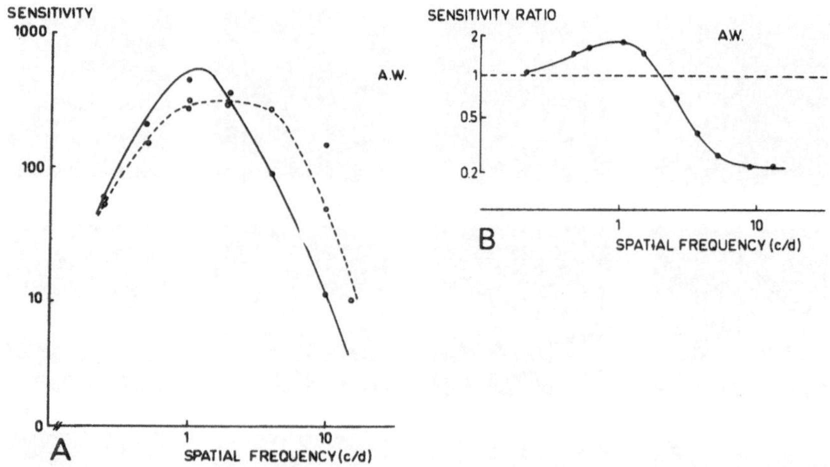

Fig. 5.
A. The contrast sensitivity arrives for the amblyopic eye (——) V.A. 0.4 and the normal eye (----) V.A. 1.25
B. The ratio between the contrast sensitivities shown in A.

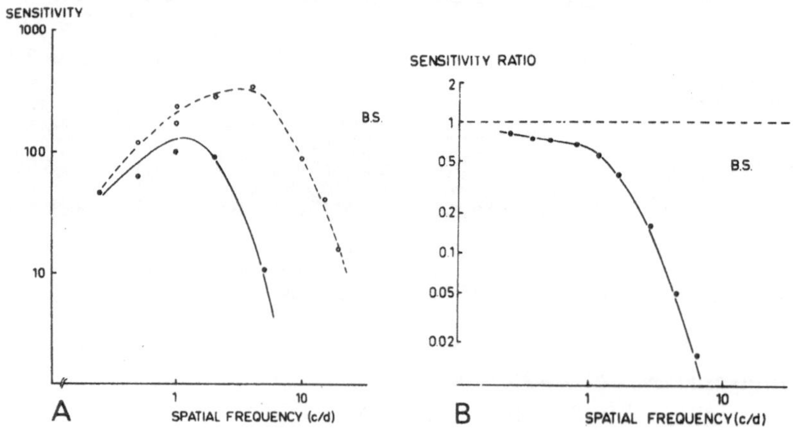

Fig. 6.
A. The contrast sensitivity curves for the amblyopic eye (——) V.A. 1.5/60 and the normal eye (----) V.A. 2.0.
B. The ratio between the contrast sensitivities shown in A.

functions of the amblyopic eye occurs in dark adaptation. This applies not only to visual acuity but also to the need of contrast and the fixation and following movements.

Some amblyopes have reduced visual acuity which is to be expected on the basis of their eccentric fixation, while others have much lower acuity than one would expect of the normal peripheral visual field. For some amblyopes contour interaction was normal, yet acuity was abnormal whereas for other amblyopes contour interaction was abnormal in the presence of normal as well as abnormal acuity. Contour interaction is called crowding effect or "Trennungsschwierigkeit" in clinical practice.

There are some indications that visual function may be affected differently in cases of strabismic amblyopia compared with cases in which anisometropia is involved. In the latter cases more of the visual field may be abnormal. The hint to difference in strabismic amblyopia and anisometropic amblyopia found in the contour interaction (crowding) effect on visual acuity is in accordance with recent findings of Hess that anisometropes do not "normalize" under reduced illumination as we know strabismus amblyopes do (22). Kiorpes and Boothe found a normal development of the acuity values for the deviated eyes in two experimentally esotropic infant monkeys for at least the first four weeks after surgery, while Crawford and Von Noorden reported that within 1 or 2 weeks there was already a shift in cortical ocular dominance away from the deviated eye. Thus the physiological changes in ocular dominance precede the emergence of behavorial amblyopia. A pattern such as this would be consistent with the clinical theory of suppression amblyopia which suggests that amblyopia is a carry over of suppression from binocular into monocular vision.

In the visual field of amblyopes the central scotomata are well known. The extent and the depth of the scotomata found with static perimetry do not correlate with the visual acuity. What is found is a decrease of lumination discrimination sensitivity in the central area. The extent and depth of the scotomata depend on the kind of stimulus used. Contrasts have more influence than unstructured luminous fields. In the binocular situation the scotoma in the amblyopic eye is larger than in the monocular situation.

B. *Electrophysiology*

The effects of deprivation and artificial strabismus were studied in the visual system of kittens (53, 24) and newborn monkeys (44). By study of behavior of these animals it is possible to ascertain the existence of amblyopia, but by electro-neurophysiological experiments it is possible to measure the resolving power of single neurons in the retina, lateral geniculate body (L.G.B.) and thus the effects of amblyopigenic factors on different parts of the visual system. The decrease of spatial resolving power is found in L.G.B. in monocular deprived kittens (36) (Blakemore and Vital 1980 did not find this in monkeys) and in monocular squinting kittens (25) in the sustained ganglion cells of the area centralis of the retina. The decrease of spatial resolution of the L.G.B. cells in artificially squinting kittens depends on the age at which the strabismus has been effectuated. Jacobson and Ikeda consider this kind of amblyopia as an arrest of development. In the primary visual cortex monocular deprivation causes a decrease in the proportion of cortical neurons that can be activated from both eyes. Nearly all neurons of the cortex striata are activated by stimulation of the non-occluded eye (52). In humans the ERG and even the foveal cone ERG is not affected in strabismic amblyopia. The defect in strabismic amblyopia does not involve a functional abnormality in the fovea distal to the ganglion cell layer (27).

Since van Balen (4) in 1960 described changes in the visual evoked cortical potentials on stimulation of the amblyopic eye, the interest in this kind of investigation has spread among the students of the visual system in man. Originally plain flash light stimulation was used, that resulted in very variable responses that were difficult to analyse. Only the comparison of the responses on stimulation of the normal eye and the amblyopic eye yielded results regarding amplitude and in some cases regarding waveform of the responses. Later investigations in which patterned light and more sophisticated averaging techniques were used showed an abnormal depression of the visual evoked responses when stimuli are presented to the amblyopic eye (33). In view of the basic defect of the amblyopic i.e. decreased contrast sensitivity the stimulus of choice would be the pure changes in spatial contrast of the counterphase checkerboard stimulation (48). The differences in amplitude between visual evoked responses after stimulation of the normal eye and the amblyopic eye are much more evident when using this kind of stimulus. The pattern evoked potential of the amblyopic eye appeared to consist mainly of a parafoveal component. This conclusion of Spekreyse et al. (48) also found by Arden (2), confirmed a hypothesis that was proposed by van Balen and Henkes (5) on base of data obtained in a different approach.

Sokol (47) advises the use of the VECP to monitor the occlusion treatment of amblyopia. He finds a quite good relation between the subjective visual acuity and the VECP that indicates the possibility to use the VECP in very young amblyopes. The differences in waveform of the VECP elicited by stimulation of the normal and the amblyopic eye, as originally described by van Balen (4) are seen in several of the registrations published by Sokol (47). The latter does not give an explanation for this phenomenon. The VECP gives an indication of lower visual acuity and decreased function of the fovea only. No specific features of the VECP by stimulation of the amblyopic eye are yet demonstrated. For that purpose the parameters of adaptation state and contour interaction have to be introduced in the experimental set-up of VECP in amblyopia.

C. *Neuroanatomy*

Experiments on kittens that had one palpebral fissure closed shortly after birth showed that cell growth in the L.G.B. can be influenced by competitive interaction between normal and deprived cells (19). At the beginning of the sensitive period unilateral lid closure and experimental strabismus of only 1-2 weeks duration cause a complete shift of cortical dominance, whereas histological changes in the LGN progress at a slower rate. Important is that the decrease in cell size appeared to be reversible after compulsive use of the deprived eye (11). The normalization of the functional changes in the cerebral cortex after compulsive use of the amblyopic eye precedes the normalization of cell size in the L.G.B. (13) Lid closure and experimental strabismus applied in monkeys towards the end of the first 3 months of life, cause no histological changes in the LGN and rather impredictable changes in cortical connections and visual acuity (Von Noorden and Crawford, 1979). The fact that bilateral occlusion of the palpebral fissure has little or no effect on the growth of cells in the L.G.B. (19) is another confirmation of the importance of binocular interaction for the genesis of amblyopia.

III. *Motoric aspects*

All the defects of amblyopic vision are sensoric or of sensoric origin. The motoric effects are secondary. For normal fixation, superiority of the fovea is necessary. In amblyopia one of two systems of ocular motility drops out, i.e., foveal vision with its fixation and fusion reflexes that are symmetrical in regard to the fovea. What is left is spatial orientation (ambiant vision) with its optokinetic reflex and conjugated movement that are asymmetrical in regard to the fovea. Thus the existence in amblyopia of asymmetric optokinetic nystagmus, occlusion nystagmus, eccentric fixation, and monocular nystagmus is explained (14). In eccentric fixation the fixation region is usually more extended than that of normal centric fixation (100 μ). Very seldom the different fixation points are limited to such a small area that one could speak of a pseudo fovea. Cases of total lack of fixation are also very rare. With different kinds of ophthalmoscopes different fixation behaviour can be observed. Fixation also changes with direction of gaze. In temporal direction the fixation is more eccentric than in the direction straight ahead. With electro-oculography the unsteady fixation of amblyopia can be registered, whereas the normal small fixation movements of central fixation cannot be registered. The frequently occurring jerk nystagmus of amblyopia can also be registered by this method. The unsteadiness of fixation is apparent especially in following movements and after gaze movements. The defects of the following movements become more apparent when the velocity is increased. The motoric disturbances are found in all kinds of amblyopia. They are coordinated when the amblyopic eye leads the gaze. In general the disturbances are more serious in deep amblyopia, but the correlation is not strict (35).

IV. *Conclusion*

The essence of amblyopia is the loss of the sensoric superiority of the fovea and of the zero-point function of the fovea for the motoric behaviour. Clinically this results in decrease of visual acuity and disturbance of fixation and fixation movements. The decreased visual acuity is not a defective form vision but essentially a decreased contrast sensitivity. Amblyopia is caused by deprivation of normal visual experience in the period of development of the visual system, by abnormal binocular interaction, or by both. There are several experimental and clinical indications that deprivation amblyopia and squint amblyopia are not exactly the same. It seems reasonable to assume that in squint amblyopia abnormal binocular interaction (suppression) is the main cause. It is still in discussion where in the visual system amblyopia is effectuated.

The incidence of amblyopia in congenital esotropia is approximately 40%. In all convergent strabismus concomitans the incidence of amblyopia is estimated to be 50-55%. There is no correlation with the angle of squint. The earlier notion that suppression has to be stronger in small angles of squint is not supported by clinical data.

But the more recent notion that in large angles of squint the foveal image is more defocused also does not hold. The focusing of the foveal image in the deviated eye is accidental and depends only on the distance of an object that happens to be in the direction of the visual axis of the deviated eye. In my opinion defocusing is not the cause but the result of amblyopia.

V. *The diagnosis of amblyopia*

For adequate treatment early detection is necessary. In unilateral esotropia one can safely assume that the deviated eye is amblyopic. In less apparent heterotropia one needs the covertest for diagnosis. When on covering one eye the child starts to make movements of fending off and shows signs of displeasure in a greater degree than on covering the other eye, the latter very probably is amblyopic, the more so when it is evident that fixation is not taken over by that eye; that the eye makes roving movements and that on uncovering the other eye takes over fixation immediately.

It is very important to keep in mind that not all deviated eyes are amblyopic. Unilateral organic or structural defects can cause strabismus. One has to do a thorough examination of the eye to exclude retinoblastoma, scars of toxoplasmaretinochorioiditis and optic atrophy, but also small cataracts like cataracta polaris. In most of these cases the normal office ophthalmological examination suffices but in cases of cone dysfunctions or early optic neuropathy one needs electro-ophthalmological examination.

In examination with the visuscope or any other funduscope with projection of a fixation object, one can find unsteady fixation in the fovea, parafoveal, paramacular or far eccentric. In general one can say that the more eccentric the more unsteady fixation is. In esotropia eccentric fixation is nearly always nasally of the fovea. As already mentioned in part I several kinds of fixation can be discerned.

A. foveolar fixation: on asking to look at the star of the visuscope the patient immediately focusses his fovea and the star remains on the fovea.
B. unsteady foveolar: the fixation is momentarily picked up by the fovea, but the star moves from the fovea in all directions.
C. nystagmiform foveolar: pendular movements from a point nasally of the fovea to the fovea.
D. eccentric fixation with latent foveal principal visual direction.
E. eccentric fixation without foveal principal visual direction.

Some authors call only "E" real eccentric fixation. The other intermediate cases of non-foveal fixation were important for the prognosis of pleioptic treatment, but have less significance now that occlusion is the treatment of choice.

Amblyopia can be differentiated according to the measure of decrease of visual acuity but, although there is some correlation with the measure of eccentricity, results of treatment cannot be predicted from these measures.

Up to the age of four years the above mentioned features of amblyopia are the ones upon which you have to build your diagnosis. From four years on, but usually not before 7-8 years, the possibility of psychophysical examination exists that enables us to detect features of amblyopic vision in cases of low visual acuity of uncertain origin.

A. *The "Ammann" effect*

In the paragraph "Sensoric aspects" the Ammann defect is discussed and the experiments done by Burian and Von Noorden are mentioned. The visual acuity of the amblyopic eye does not increase when the luminance of the test field is increased. It stays on its low level while the visual acuity of the normal eye increases. The luminance/visual acuity relation is much to elaborate and demanding to use as a test method in the out patient department. By use of a neutral density filter however, it is possible to decrease the luminance of the V.A.-test, untill the V.A. of the normal eye is approximately 0.5. In the amblyopic eye the use of this filter does not influence the V.A. (fig. 7). In this way one defines one (arbitrarily chosen) point on the curve of Von Noorden and Burian. This is not a very accurate test. In deep amblyopia (V.A. <0.2) the test is undecisive. In anisometropia-amblyopia the Ammann effect is reported not to be present. In strabismus-amblyopia however the neutral density filter test has enabled us to distinguish between amblyopia and very slight organic disturbances (6).

B. *The „Trennschwierigkeit" or „crowding effect".* Single optotypes are always easier to read than optotypes in rows, but the "crowding" has more influence on the visual acuity of the amblyopic eye than on the visual acuity of the normal eye. Ducam Jouveaux (15) found a correlation between the influence of crowding and the age of children below the age of 7 years. Others say that the crowding effect is found in any kind of decreased visual acuity. Cüppers supposed that "Trennschwierigkeit" was caused by eccentric fixation. This hypothesis found some confirmation in an investigation in which the crowding of horizontal rows of optotypi was more effectual on visual acuity than the crowding of vertical rows of optotypi (7). In practice the test of

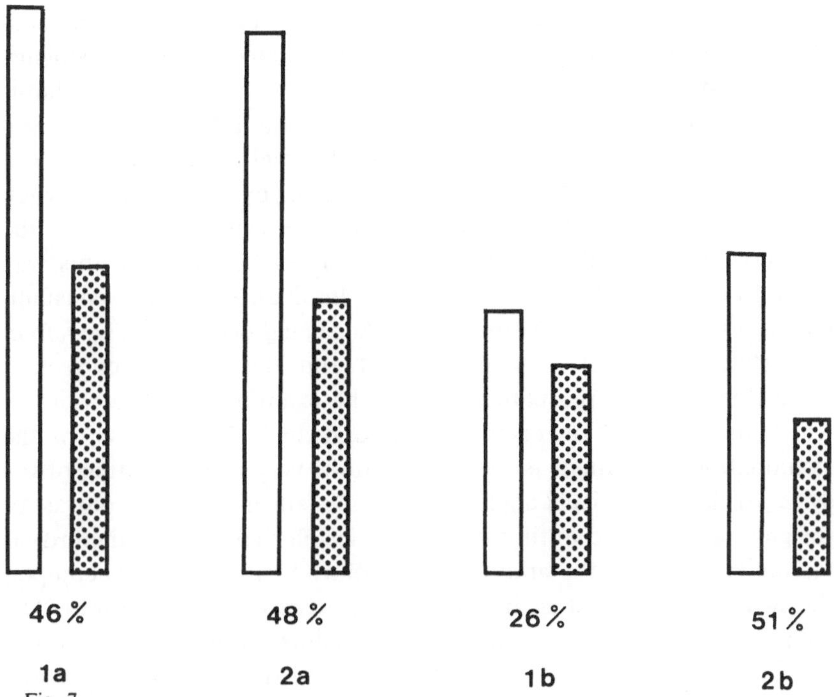

Fig. 7.
1a: normal eye of amblyopic group.
2a: normal eye of organic lesion group.
1b: affected eye of amblyopic group.
2b: affected eye of organic lesion group.
White columns represent the average visual acuity of 50 eyes. Shaded columns represent the average visual acuity of 50 eyes reduced by a neutral density filter.

"Trennschwierigkeit" is difficult. A great number of acuity tests have to be performed and especially in children decreased attention plays an important role in the crowding effect (15).

C. The visual acuity of the amblyopic eye is reduced in direct proportion to the intensity of stimulation received by the sound eye (3). In dichoptic situations (for instance phasendifferenzhaploscope) the suppression effect of the normal eye on the amblyopic eye is even stronger especially in esotropia and hypermetropic anisometropia (3). This test has diagnostic value and possibly also prognostic value as regards occlusion therapy. This test can also be used in latent nystagmus to detemine whether true amblyopia is present or not.

D. The contrastsensitivity, being the basis function that is impaired in amblyopia, should be the target of diagnostic procedures. A method of examination had to be found that was feasible for clinical use. Hagemans describes an automated registration of the contrast transfer function (20). The stimulus, a sinusoidally modulated vertical frequency grating superimposed on a predetermined average background luminance (100 lux), is presented to the patient on a T.V. monitor screen. The size of the screen has a height of 5° of visual angle and a width of 12°. The contrast can be varied by the patient by depressing a switch (to diminish the contrast) or by releasing the switch (to increase the contrast). The modulation depth (contrast) can be varied in this way from 100 to 0% while the background luminance remains constant. One eye is examined at a time—the other being occluded. The refractory state is accurately predetermined and the optimal correction should be worn by the patient during the examination. The room in which the examination takes place is darkened. At the onset of the examination the patient is presented with a very coarse grating of 0.1 cycle per degree of visual angle. By depressing the switch the contrast of the grating is reduced until it becomes invisible. The patient then releases the switch until the grating just becomes visible again, whereupon the switch is depressed again. This process is repeated eight times. The values of the last eight contrast reversal points are then averaged in a microprocessor system and the result plotted on an X-Y against the frequency. The next grating, with a spatial frequency twice that of the former grating, is automatically presented on the screen and the whole process is repeated. In this way nine spatial frequencies are presented spanning the visual spectrum, and the contrast sensitivity of the eye is plotted against the frequency on a chart. When the first eye has been examined in this way, the whole system is reset (by depressing one switch) and the other eye is examined. The results of this eye are plotted on the same chart (for easy comparison), whereby the difference in sensitivity of the two eyes is also plotted (from data stored in the system's memory from the first examination), taking the normal eye as reference. With this automated method of examination, recording nine frequencies per eye, the examination takes about 25 minutes for both eyes. When more data become available it may be possible to make a diagnosis of amblyopia using only two or three frequencies, greatly reducing the examination time. We have found that this system can be used from an age of about eight years upwards. At lower ages an electrodiagnostic method is perhaps a more suitable method, because of easy distraction, loss of interest, and difficulty in instruction of the patient. In about 80% of the cases of amblyopia examined to date, we found a significant characteristic not found in any other disease with impaired vision. In the low frequency range the contrastsensitivity of the amblyopic eye is increased in comparison to the fellow normal eye. In cases of deep amblyopia (vision less than 1/10) this does not always occur. The contrastsensitivity for the higher frequencies is always impaired in amblyopia as can be expected (fig. 5 and fig. 6). The screen size was determined from other experiments, where we found that if a greater area than 10-12° of the retina was stimulated (comparing to the macular area), no further information at any frequency (greater contrast sensitivity) could be elicited.

E. In the paragraph on electrophysiology we already discussed the use of the VECP in the investigation of amblyopia. Because the VECP's in amblyopia, even those elicited by patterned stimuli, do not show specific features, they cannot as yet be used as a diagnostic tool.

When different spatial frequencies, different adaptation levels and contour interactions will be used in the stimuli, the VECP's probably will become the objective diagnostic tool we need. In the course of occlusion treatment the VER reflects more or less the change in dominance. The latency of the VER of the occluded (better) eye increases and the amplitude decreases. The VER changes do not correlate to clinical assessment of visual acuity (Arden and Barnard, 1980).

VI. *The treatment of amblyopia*

As soon as the diagnosis of amblyopia is established and the necessary optical correction of the refraction anomaly is given, total occlusion of the fixating eye is given during 24 hours a day. Every compromise like partial or intermittent occlusion is futile in the beginning of the treatment. The same applies to the atropinisation of the fixating eye. Of course one has to be cautious, occlusion itself can be the cause of amblyopia of the fixating eye: amblyopia à bascule. The younger the child, the shorter the period of total occlusion has to be; the frequency of control has to be adapted to the age of the patient. Hugonnier (46) advises a period of two days for a child of two years old; three days for a child of three and so on. Roper Hall found amblyopia with eccentric fixation of the originally fixating eye of children of three already after 4 days occlusion. Parks is of the opinion that occlusion is prohibited in children of less than 6 months old. Our management of occlusion is control after 2 days in a 1 year old, after 4 days in a two year old and so on. The risk of "amblyopia à bascule" should not be exaggerated, where it occurs it is easily reversible. The majority of amblyopes of less than 4 years old benefit by occlusion therapy. In children older than 4 year when eccentric fixation is present, occlusion therapy is considered to be less successful but it is always worthwhile giving it a trial (12) even in 9 year old children. Vereecken does not occlude amblyopes of more than 6 year old. When under the influence of a well-managed occlusion therapy the originally roving eccentric fixation becomes fixated to a limited eccentric area, we stop the occlusion therapy.

The so-called inverse occlusion i.e. occlusion of the amblyopic eye was used to loosen an eccentric fixation thereby causing amblyopia without fixation that can be treated by ortho-occlusion or occlusion of the fixating eye.

Occlusion is best executed by applying an eyepad that is light-thight but not airthight (e.g. Poroplast eyepads). At the control visit the visual acuity is measured, if possible, but always the behaviour of fixation is the main indicator of result of the therapy. As long as fixation is taken over by the occluded eye immediately after removing the occlusion pad, the dominance of that eye is still evident. Complete success of occlusion therapy is spontaneously alternating fixation. In between these two extremes one sees a hesitating take-over of fixation that best can be met by alternating occlusion, starting with 6 days occlusion of the dominating eye and 1 day occlusion of the amblyopic eye. The alternation changes according to the fixation behaviour in 5:2, 3:2, 2:1 to reach ultimately 1:1.

It is important to give full information about the scope of occlusion therapy to the parents of the amblyopic child. One has to warn the parents that the squint is not cured by occlusion therapy, indeed the angle of squint may increase. Some parents feel that alternating squint is more serious than unilateral squint.

Sometimes one has to perform surgical correction of strabismus before amblyopia treatment is possible, especially in large convergent angles and cases with pseudoparalysis of abduction. In these cases central fixation is mechanically inhibited. Presenting the visuscopestar from the temporal side one finds increasing eccentricity of fixation or coarse fixation nystagmus as a sign of this mechanical impediment. Occlusion therapy is certainly not contraindicated in the absence of central fixation. The result depends more on the duration of amblyopia: 80% favorable result in amblyopia of 0-2 year duration, 40% in amblyopia of 2-4 year duration, and 20% in amblyopia of more than 4 year duration. Connatal amblyopia is an exception, the maximum admittable duration being 3 months. The longer the duration of amblyopia the more eccentric fixation will be found; no fixation or "roving fixation" is more frequent in cases of short duration (51, 29).

In general, occlusion therapy (strictly executed) is to be prefered to the method of Bangerter (8) in amblyopes younger than 7 year. After that the results of both methods are more or less equal. The method of Cüppers (after image) is demanding and has good but transient results. The method of Bangerter relies principally on stimulation of the fovea whereas the method of Cüppers uses a foveal afterimage to teach the patient to use his fovea as fixation point and to value this point as straight ahead. In view of these methods, Cüppers discerned several kinds of amblyopia that are already mentioned on page 247. A useful, not too expensive instrument for pleioptic therapy—active therapy of amblyopia according to the method of Bangerter or Cüppers—is the projectoscope by Keeler.

It is my opinion that amblyopia with eccentric fixation in patients older than 8 or 9 year should not be treated, because the moderate and transient success does not counterbalance the expenses and the trouble of the method. Only in amblyopia of monoculi pleioptic therapy may be given consideration, but the end result of parafoveal fixation with a visual acuity of 0.3 is attained also spontaneously in these cases. Perhaps a recently described method of control of unsteady, eccentric fixation in amblyopic eyes by auditory feedback of the eye position can be used in amblyopia of monoculi. I have no experience with this method (Flom e.a., 1980).

The red filter (Wratten 93 Kodak) treatment of eccentric fixation has known only a very short period of popularity. The occlusion of the normal eye and the red filter in front of the amblyopic eye leaves the patient in a dark and indistinct world. The heavy burden of this therapy lies totally on the shoulders of the patient and also the therapy does not give sufficient result to justify the trouble.

After elimination of the amblyopia the problem arises of maintaining the visual acuity depending on the age of the patient, the state of monocular vision and the type of amblyopia before treatment. Of a group of 75 amblyopes of which 93% got normal visual acuity after treatment, 5 years later only 65% had normal visual acuity and after stopping occlusion during one year only 40% still had normal visual acuity.

After the age of 5 years a difference in prognosis between amblyopia with foveal and with extrafoveal fixation becomes evident, the latter leads more to relapses but also the treated amblyopia with central fixation can gradually lose visual acuity after apparent cure. The cause probably is an inferior binocular cooperation that frequently exists in these cases. This applies also for the cases of microstrabismus that are the result of operation and of treatment of anisometropic amblyopia.

A method to maintain the visual acuity after occlusion therapy is needed. Several methods have been proposed like periodical occlusion and "Ausschleichender Schichtocclusion" (29). In our experience, however, the optical penalisation of Pouliquen and Quéré is the method of choice. We have insufficient experience with the pure drug penalisation, i.e. pilocarpine in the amblyopic eye and atropine in the normal eye. The optical penalisation is the least bothersome to the child and does not demand any control by the parents apart from the control of wearing the glasses. When the visual acuity is lower than 0.3 the so-called near penalisation is given, i.e. atropinisation and exact correction of the fixating eye and 2-3 diopters overcorrection of the amblyopic eye. When the visual acuity is more than 0.5, the so-called far penalisation can be started, i.e. three diopters overcorrection and atropinisation of the good eye and normal correction of the amblyopic eye. In the long run atropinisation of the normal eye can be stopped. This is what Weiss advised under the name of light penalisation. The advantage of penalisation is that any degree of binocular cooperation that might exist is less disturbed than is the case in periodical occlusion or Schichtocclusion. Some authors (e.g. Vereecken) advise optical penalisation not only for maintaining the achieved visual acuity after occlusion therapy (especially in micro strabismus) but also for

a. amblyopia treatment in nystagmus latens cases;
b. slight amblyopia in children of less than six years old;
c. amblyopia in children of more than six years old;
d. hypermetropic anisometropic amblyopia. This situation can optically be favorable for the so called far penalisation.

Recently a new method of amblyopia treatment has been proposed by a group of investigators from Cambridge who were studying the contrast transference function of normal and amblyopic eyes. Campbell invented a device on which sharp edged, high contrast gratings were placed and rotated so as to occupy all orientation positions. A series of discs with different spatial frequencies and different contrast is shown to the patient. The treatment is commenced using the finest stripes he can see. This disc is placed on the central spindle of the apparatus and the patient is asked to draw or play games on the perspex plate that is covering the rotating disc. The treatment lasts 7 minutes and during this time all the gratings which are narrower than the one the patient started with should be used. The average number of treatments required to achieve maximum improvement is five. The treatments are repeated at intervals which can be as short as a day or as long as a month. The authors (50) claim an amazingly high rate of success in a group of 37 patients (age group 2½-11 years). These results have not yet been confirmed by an independent investigation. The initiators of this method admit that they do not know how or why this therapy works. The relative fast and easily attained results of this therapy as compared with the occlusion therapy tended to make this method very popular even before real assessment had been made.

Several recent reports on this kind of therapy were not favorable.

BIBLIOGRAPHY

(1) ARDEN, G.B. and WEALE, R.A. — Nervous mechanisms and dark adaptation. *J. Physiol.*, 1954, *125*, 417-426.
(2) ARDEN, G.B. — Amblyopia. *Docum. Ophthal. Proc. Ser.*, 1977, *11*, 31-38.
(3) AWAYA, S. and NOORDEN, G.K. VON — Visual acuity of amblyopic eyes under monocular and binocular conditions: further observations. *J. Pediat. Ophthal.*, 1972, *9*, 8-13.
(4) BALEN, A.Th.M. VAN — De electro-encephalografische reactie op lichtprikkeling en zijn betekenis voor de oogheelkundige diagnostiek. Thesis, Rotterdam, Klomp en Bosman, 1960.
(5) BALEN, A.Th.M. VAN and HENKES, H.E. — Attention and amblyopia. *Brit. J. Ophthal.*, 1962, *46*, 12-20.
(6) BALEN, A.Th.M. VAN — Theoretical aspects of amblyopia. Perspectives in Ophthalmology. Amsterdam, Excerpta Medica, 1970, 122-129.
(7) BALEN, A.Th.M. VAN — The evaluation of visual acuity. Orthoptics; Proceedings of the Second International Orthoptic Congress, Amsterdam, May 11-13, 1971. Amsterdam, Excerpta Medica, 1972, 139-145.
(8) BANGERTER, A. — Amblyopiebehandlung, Basel, S. Karger, 1953.
(9) BURIAN, H.M., BENTON, A.L. & LIPSIUS, R.C. — Visual cognitive functions in patients with strabismic amblyopia. *Arch. Ophthal.*, 1962, *68*, 785-791.
(10) BYRAM, G.M. — The physical and photochemical basis of visual resolving power. II. Visual acuity and photochemistry of the retina. *J. Opt. Soc. Amer.*, 1944, *34*, 718-738.
(11) CHOW, K.L. and STEWART, D.L. — Reversal of structural and functional effects of long-term visual deprivation in cats. *Exp. Neurol.*, 1972, *34*, 409-433.
(12) CORTE, H. DE — Effet de l'occlusion directe sur le mode de fixation de l'œil strabique et amblyope. *Bull. Soc. Belge Ophtal.*, 1968, *149*, 559-570.
(13) CRAWFORD, M.L.J. and NOORDEN, G.K. VON — The effects of short-term experimental strabismus on the visual system in macaca mulatta. *Invest. Ophthalmol. Vis. Sci.*, 1979, *18*, 496-505.
(14) CRONE, R.A. — Amblyopia: the pathology of motor disorders in amblyopic eyes. *Docum. Ophthal. Proc. Ser.*, 1977, *11*, 9-18.
(15) DUCAM JUVEAUX — Étude de l'acuité visuelle des enfants et des problèmes posés par sa mesure. Thesis Sorbonne, Paris, 1968.
(16) ENOCH, J.M. — Receptor amblyopia. *Amer. J. Ophthal.*, 1959, *48*, 262-274.
(17) GLEZER, V.D. — The receptive fields of the retina. *Vision Res.*, 1965, *5*, 497-525.

(18) GROSVENOR, T. — The effects of duration and background luminance upon the brightness discrimination of an amblyope. *Amer. J. Optom.*, 1957, *34*, 639-663.
(19) GUILLERY, R.W. — The effects of lid suture upon the growth of cells in the dorsal lateral geniculate nucleus of kittens. *J. Comp. Neurol.*, 1973, *148*, 417-422.
(20) HAGEMANS, K.H. and VAN BALEN, A.Th.M. — A new test for the diagnosis of amblyopia. Orthoptics, Research and Practise. Transactions of the fourth international orthoptic congress, London, Kimpton, 1981, 50-61.
(21) HECHT, S. and MINTZ, F.U. — The visibility of single lines at various illuminations and the retinal basis of visual resolution. *J. Gen. Physiol.*, 1939, *22*, 593-612.
(22) HESS, R.F., CAMPBELL, F.W. and ZIMMERN, R. — Differences in the neural basis of human amblyopias: the effect of mean luminance. *Vision Research*, 1980, *20*, 295-305.
(23) HUGONNIER, R. — Strabismes; hétérophories paralysies oculomotrices (les déséquilibres oculo-moteurs en clinique). Paris, Masson, 1959.
(24) IKEDA, H. and WRIGHT, M.J. — Properties of LGN cells in kittens reared with convergent squint: a neurophysiological demonstration of amblyopia. *Exp. Brain Res.*, 1976, *25*, 63-77.
(25) IKEDA, H. and TREMAIN, K.E. — Amblyopia occurs in retinal ganglion cells in cats reared with convergent squint without alternating fixation. *Exp. Brain Res.*, 1979, *35*, 559-582.
(26) IDEKA, H. — Physiological basis of visual acuity and its development in kittens. *Child: care, health and development*, 1970, *5*, 375-383.
(27) JACOBSON, S.G., SANDBERG, M.A., EFFRON, H. and BERSON, E.L. — Foveal cone electroretinograms in strabismic amblyopia. *Trans. ophthal. Soc. U.K.*, 1979, *99*, 353-356.
(28) KRZYSTKOWA, K. — Investigations on dark adaptation in amblyopia. *Klin. Oczna*, 1967, *37*, 73-78.
(29) LANG, J. — Strabismus; Diagnostik, Schielformen, Therapie. Bern, Huber, 1971.
(30) LAVERGNE, G. — Étude de l'adaptation à l'obscurité des cônes de l'œil amblyope. *Bull. Soc. Belge Ophtal.*, 1961, *126*, 1121-1130.
(31) LAWWILL, T. and BURIAN, H.M. — Luminance, contrast function and visual acuity in functional amblyopia. *Amer. J. Ophthal.*, 1966, *62*, 511-520.
(32) LOEWER-SIEGER, D.H. — Amblyopie; een studie over de kenmerken en de behandeling. Thesis, Amsterdam, J. Ruysendaal, 1962.
(33) LOMBROSO, C.T., DUFFY, F.H. and ROBB, R.M. — Selective suppression of cerebral evoked potentials to patterned light in amblyopia ex anopsia. *Electroenceph. Clin. Neurophysiol.*, 1969, *27*, 238-247.
(34) LYTHGOE, R.J. — The mechanism of dark adaptation. *Brit. J. Ophthal.*, 1940, *24*, 21-43.
(35) MACKENSEN, G. — Die Untersuchung des schwachsichtigen Auges: Fixation, Sehschärfe und Gesichtsfeld. In: Hollwich, F. (ed.), Schielen; Pleoptik, Orthoptik, Operation. Stuttgart, F. Enke, 1961, 185-213.
(36) MAFFEI, L. and FIORENTINI, A. — Monocular deprivation in kittens impairs the spatial geniculate neurons. *Nature*, 1976, *264*, 754-755.
(37) MARAINI, G. and PERALTA, S. — Il comportamento della retina centrale nell'amblyopia durante l'adattamento all'oscurita. *Ann. Ottal.*, 1962, *88*, 267-273.
(38) MEUR, G. — Étude des sommations spatiales rétiniennes dans les amblyopies fonctionnelles. *Bull. Soc. Belge Ophthal.*, 1964, *137*, 377-383.
(39) MEUR, G., PAYAN, M. and VOLA, J. — Détermination indirecte de la dimension des champs réceptifs rétiniens de l'amblyope au moyen des grilles de Hermann. *Bull. Soc. Belge Ophthal.*, *150*, 615-622.
(40) MILLER, E.F. — Investigations of the nature and cause of impaired acuity in amblyopia. *Amer. J. Optom.*, 1955, *32*, 10-29.
(41) NOORDEN, G.K. VON and BURIAN, H.M. — Perceptual blanking in normal and amblyopic eyes. *Arch. Ophthal.*, 1960, *64*, 817-822.
(42) NOORDEN, G.K. VON — Factors involved in the production of amblyopia. *Brit. J. Ophthal.*, 1974, *58*, 158-164.
(43) NOORDEN, G.K. VON and BURIAN, H.M. — Visual acuity in normal and amblyopic patients under reduced illumination. *Arch. Ophthal.*, 1959, *61*, 533-535 / 1959, *62*, 396-399.

(44) NOORDEN, G.K. VON and MIDDLEDITCH, P.R. — Histology of the monkey lateral geniculate nucleus after unilateral lid closure and experimental strabismus: further observations. *Invest. Ophthal.*, 1975, *14*, 674-683.
(45) OPPEL, O. and KRANKE, D. — Vergleichende Untersuchungen über das Verhalten der Dunkeladaptation normaler und schielamblyoper Augen. *Graefes Arch. Ophthal.*, 1958, *159*, 486-501.
(46) PARKS, M.M. and FRIENDLY, D.S. — Treatment of eccentric fixation in children under four years of age. *Amer. J. Ophthal.*, 1966, *61*, 395-399.
(47) SOKOL, S. — Pattern visual evoked potentials: their use in pediatric ophthalmology. *Int. Ophthal. Clin.*, 1980, *1*, 251-268.
(48) SPEKREIJSE, H., KHOE, LEE, H. and TWEEL, L.H. VANDER — A case of amblyopia; electrophysiology and psychophysics of luminance and contrast. In: The visual system. Neurophysiology, Biophysics and Their Clinical Applications. Ed. G.B. Arden, New York, Plenum Press, 1972. *Adv. Exp. Med. Biol.*, 1972, *24*, 141-156.
(49) WALD, G. and BURIAN, H.M. — The dissociation of form vision and light perception in strabismic amblyopia. *Amer. J. Ophthal.*, 1944, *27*, 950-963.
(50) WATSON, P.G., BANKS, R.V., CAMPBELL, F.W. and HESS, R.F. — Clinical assessment of a new treatment for amblyopia. *Trans. Ophthal. Soc. U.K.*, 1978, *98*, 201.
(51) WEEKERS, R., LAVERGNE, G. THOMAS-DECORTIS, G. and URY, M. — Contribution à l'étude des fonctions maculaires et paramaculaires dans l'amblyopie. *Docum. Ophthal.*, 1962, *16*, 253-275.
(52) WIESEL, T.N. and HUBEL, D.H. — Effects of visual deprivation on morphology and physiology of cells in the cat's lateral geniculate body. *J. Neurophysiol.*, 1963, *26*, 978-993.

Bull. Soc. belge Ophtal., **195**, 269-299, 1981.

CHAPTER VIII

THE CONSERVATIVE TREATMENT OF SQUINT

E. VEREECKEN (*)

Introduction

The ideal purpose of squint treatment is threefold: to obtain a normal and equal vision in both eyes, orthophoria in all directions of gaze and a good binocular cooperation between both eyes; this means bifoveal fusion and a good fusional range. It is often not possible to obtain this ideal. Therefore the practical aims we look for in all-day practice are to obtain a normal vision in both eyes, a cosmetically acceptable strabismus (with an angle of deviation as near to 0° as possible) and a binocular cooperation as good as possible, often limited to peripheral fusion with a little foveal suppression scotoma in the slightly deviating eye.

There are two main ways to achieve this goal; first the conservative way and second the operative one (chapter IX). We practically always first try the different possibilities of conservative treatment. When there is no further improvement with and when the strabismus is esthetically disturbing, then we proceed to operative treatment.

A first question to be answered is: how soon should the treatment of a child with strabismus be started? The answer is very simple: as soon as possible after the onset of the squint (this depends upon good information of the public) and certainly directly after the diagnosis has been made (this depends only upon the doctor). No squinting child is too young to receive treatment.

The age of onset—a very important fact for prognosis—is dealt with in chapter V. Still more important for us is the time that has elapsed

Park Ryvissche 66, 9710 Zwijnaarde (Belgium).

between the onset of strabismus and the first consultation (60). The fact that this lapse of time has been remarkably shortened especially during the two last decades is the most important therapeutical progress we have made. This is especially true for amblyopia, which exists in approximately 60% of esotropia cases. We know that the percentage of amblyopia and the percentage of eccentric fixation increases with age and everyone agrees that the results of amblyopia treatment are the better, the earlier the treatment is performed (60). The same applies for the correction of the refractive error with spectacles and for the improvement of motor and sensorial disturbances.

So we postulate our therapeutical guide-lines as follows:

1. The result of every conservative treatment is the better, the earlier the treatment is started.

2. Every conservative treatment should be applied continuously. Establishing the diagnosis and performing the treatment as early as possible is, in our opinion, the main strabismus problem. What can we do for further improvement? First, the public should be better informed; an earlier and more consequent treatment by the eye doctor is also required. Nevertheless, the chief problem lies in the diagnostic field. If we analyse those who have postponed consultation, we see that the lack of an "alarm symptom" is the main reason (61). In more than 50% of all esotropias the manifest angle of deviation was less than 8° (17). That is the reason why we perform an examination on presumptive squint as described (chapter VI) in all children of whom one parent, brother or sister, squints (the so-called "high-risk children"). In these children we always perform a cyclopentolate 1% retinoscopy, because the association of refractive errors with esotropia is more significant as the association of esotropia with positive family history (29). If we do not find a squint in these children, but on the contrary we find refractive errors greater than +2.5 D hyperopia in the more emmetropic eye, anisometropia (defined as a difference of more than 1 D between both eyes) or astigmatism of more than 1.5 D, we prescribe the full optical correction of these refractive errors, if these "high-risk children" are in their critical years for visual development.

Ingram demonstrated that such hyperopia is significantly associated with esotropia ($P<0.001$) and the presence of amblyopia ($P<0.01$) (29). Prophylactic investigation and even prophylactic treatment is advisable in these cases.

I. *Basic treatments*

A. *Optical treatment*

In a great many cases the state of refraction is the primary cause of squint, and provided the patient is seen sufficiently early, the primary treatment is the correction of the refractive error (Keith Lyle) (35).

Some very important new viewpoints have been reported:

1. The variability of the refraction in children

Recent research (26-43) indicates that infants show ten times the incidence and considerably greater amounts of clinically significant astigmatism than school children. The amount begins to decrease in the second semester of life and the incidence declines during the third year (30). In the first year of life Howland (26) finds 12% astigmatism greater than 2 D. 13.23% of the children examined by Ingram at the age of 1 year had +1.5 D or more astigmatism in one or both eyes (31).

Anisometropia may appear at any age. 6.5% of the children examined by Ingram (31) at the age of 1 year showed anisometropia. The anisometropia was significantly associated with bilateral hyperopia, but even more significantly associated with astigmatism of +1.5 D or more in one or both eyes.

Most strabologists accept that anisometropia plays an important role in the development of amblyopia; some authors (Keiner, Fletcher) believe that anisometropia is the result of amblyopia (18, 34). Others (18, 41, 42) maintain that in cases with unilateral strabismus, anisometropia occurs. The emmetropization or myopisation in the non-fixing eye clearly lagged behind that in the fixing eye, and this long after cessation of therapy. We found the same anisometropia sometimes in cases where strabismus had been completely cured.

The conceptions about hyperopia have considerably changed. According to a widespread opinion (35), the normal eyes show at birth up to 5 D of hyperopia and this amount, decreasing as the age progresses, is regarded as physiological. It has now generally been accepted that the mean hyperopia in newborn babies is approximately +0.6 D (21, 22, 31). The refraction studies done on the same children in different ages clearly indicate that hyperopia increases until the age of 6 to 7 years (5, 37, 56).

2. The early discovery of accommodation

In 1956 Themen (58) reported that in 98% of 457 normal babies, examined at the age of 2 weeks to 1 year, accommodation is discovered by the child between the sixth and fifteenth week of life; it is first monocular than binocular. In 1965 Haynes and collaborators (25) published exactly the same results; they were not familiar with the work of Themen and they used a different method. This research has since been confirmed by multiple clinical data (3, 8, 32, 51).

3. The importance of small refractive errors

In the examination of Themen, 72 mothers complained of periodical esotropia of their child while looking at their hands or while feeding. The moment of this complaint was always in accordance with the period of the discovery of the unilateral accommodation. Themen could verify this complaint in 28 babies. In 20 of them the hyperopia was 0-1 D, in 6 others the hyperopia was 1-2 D, and in 2 babies the hyperopia was 2-4 D. The periodical squint disappeared spontaneously in 18 of these children, 10 remained manifestly squinting. The squint in these cases never developed at an other moment.

In opposition to the since Donders well known opinion (14) that accommodative strabismus occurs after the second year of life and exclusively in moderate or high hypermetropia, Themen showed evidence that accommodative strabismus may occur with low refraction anomalies and in the first months of life. This opinion has since been largely confirmed by clinical data (3, 7). Parks states that 49% of accommodative esotropias have a hyperopia less than 3 D (47).

4. Repeated atropine retinoscopy is necessary in esotropes under 6 (chapter VI).

It is of utmost importance to take these new viewpoints into consideration because the most frequently committed mistake in strabismus-therapy is, in our opinion without doubt, the undercorrection of the refractive error. In 1976 Cüppers and Muhlendyck (10) declared that 65% of all spectacles, prescribed by other eye doctors in cases of esotropia, were undercorrected by more than +0.5 D and this control was done only under cyclopentolate. Controlled with atropine it would probably have been still more.

Therefore we propose the following guidelines of optical treatment:

1. We prescribe the full correction of all refractive errors found in

our retinoscopy done under atropine ointment 1%. The full correction of astigmatism is important for the visual acuity of these children: if the child sees better, it readily accepts the glasses. From our refraction practice in adults we all know that adding a small cylinder often greatly increases the visual acuity and comfort. If in the course of amblyopia treatment, there is no further improvement in visual acuity, we should always consider the possibility that astigmatism has been insufficiently corrected. Clinical experience sometimes shows influence of exact cylinder correction on the angle of deviation and on the quality of binocular cooperation. The exact correction of astigmatism is often difficult because cycloplegia, especially with atropine, less with cyclopentolate, does not always reveal the total astigmatism nor the exact axis (15, 20, 31) and subjective cooperation at that age is often unreliable.

In myopia with esotropia we prescribe the minimal negative glass giving full vision in the distance. Even in cases of myopia the refraction must be done under atropine, because these cases often present a pronounced accommodative tonus (23, 36) and under atropine we often find less myopia.

Anisometropia, especially hypermetropic astigmatism in children is fully corrected. Young children easily support great differences in glasses. Early correction is certainly necessary in anisometropia.

The opinion about the full correction of hyperopia has considerably changed the last ten years. First of all, the retinoscopy must be done under atropine 1% ointment. The generally accepted theory says that if we find neutralisation of the reflection in each meridian with a +4 D, we have to subtract +1.5 D for the working distance of 60 cm and a+1 D to allow for the tone of the ciliary muscle (Duke Elder) (15). The required glass would then be +1.5 D. This subtraction of +1 D for the tone of the ciliary muscle is no longer accepted (10, 48); we now always prescribe +3 D, which from the theoretical point of view is a slight overcorrection, but is never refused in practice, especially if we take the precaution to continue atropine application once a day for three to four days to facilitate the acceptance of the glasses.

Subjective estimation of the refraction should follow the objective measurement in a child who is sufficiently cooperative. We verify if the lenses found by the retinoscopy give full visual acuity or at least a visual acuity as good as without glasses. We do this test if possible immediately after the retinoscopy and we repeat it later when the cycloplegic effect has worn off. This subjective test, when the cycloplegia effect has worn off, is most useful in the final adjustment of the precise axis and of the amount of the cylindrical lens in cases of astigmatism.

2. This full correction should be prescribed as soon as possible after the onset of the squint. This early correction is very important for the prevention of amblyopia, as the percentage of amblyopia increases with age and as refractive errors and especially anisometropia play an important role in the development of amblyopia. The most ametropic eye always has an unsharp foveal image and, as accommodation is always equal in both eyes, and directed by the dominant eye (law of Hering), this gives use to a diminished and unsuitable accommodation in the amblyopic eye (1, 46, 59). This early correction is equally important for the treatment of amblyopia; let us think only of the bilateral amblyopia where full vision is easily reached as full optical correction is given early. Neurophysiological research (28) confirms the necessity of early and adequate correction of refractive errors for the therapy of amblyopia. The influence of early correction on the motor status is already evident from the fact that the disappearance of the strabismus by glasses is much easier to obtain when the strabismus is still intermittent, than when the strabismus becomes permanent. It is evident that retinal images of equal sharpness in both eyes are a necessary basis for the possible development of binocular cooperation. The spectacles allow us other kinds of treatment (occlusion, penalisation, prisms) which influence the sensorial status too.

3. It is worthless to prescribe the full correction of refractive errors, if the spectacles are not worn constantly. This is very important and we always take plenty of time to explain this to the parents by telling them that as soon as the child opens his eyes, the spectacles must be worn until he goes to bed at night. Even, if while bathing or for cleaning the spectacles should be taken off, the child must be instructed to close his eyes. When the spectacles are correct, we do not have difficulties with the children to accept the glasses; if difficulties arise, it usually is because of the parents.

4. The measurement of refraction must be repeated regularly.

— An exact measurement of refraction in children is technically difficult; even an experienced refractionist often feels insecure about his measurement. In cases of amblyopia or gross adduction of one eye it is often impossible to know the exact refraction as fixation is not foveal. Astigmatism is less under cycloplegia than wihout cycloplegia.

— The refraction of young children often varies as already described.

— Last but not least: it is a certitude now that the cycloplegia with cyclopentolate certainly and even with atropine is often (especially in esotropia in young children and with dark irides) not complete (chapter VI). As in normal people the hyperopia increases until the age of 6-7 years, the only possibility to liberate the total hyperopia is by repeating the retinoscopy and adapt the glasses every time we find higher values of hypermetropia. Knapp (36) states: "I do not believe in a single refraction, the leading cause of my bad operative results was that I believed the original refraction. A great many of them had been listed as having +0.50 D or a +1 D and ended up with a +5 D".

Some points of discussion are left:

1) What is the smallest hypermetropic correction worth being prescribed?

There is no relation between the amount of uncorrected hypermetropia and the amount of deviation (7, 65). A small correction can merely lessen a great deal or even abolish the angle of deviation, a high correction can cause only a small lessening of the angle. As the effect of spectacles on the angle of deviation is not predictable and as spectacles are a necessary pre-requisite for further treatment (penalisation, sector, occlusion and prisms) the prescription of glasses is advisable, especially in the somewhat older children. In cases with large angles of deviation and small refractive errors (early squint) some people prefer to operate directly and to prescribe spectacles if there is still an esodeviation postoperatively.

2) Earliest age at which glasses can be ordered for a child?

Until recently, glasses were generally not prescribed before the age of 1½ years. This limit has decreased until the age of 4-6 months, by better knowledge of the importance of optical correction at the earliest possible age and by technical advances in fitting spectacles for so young children (fig. 1 and 2).

These spectacles are characterized by a very low bridge, they do not have pads fitting on the sides of the nose, the lenses are big, to avoid looking above or beside the spectacles, the side-pieces are fitted with spring hinges; at the end of the side-pieces a perforation permits to pass an elastic band behind the head, an effective method of tying-on spectacles in very young children. There are different models adapted to the age: babycoque model (less than 4 months); from 4 to 8 months spectacles with optical center at 34 mm; from 8 to 18 months with the optical centre at 36 mm; from 18 months to 5 years there are three different models with optical centre from 36 to 42 mm.

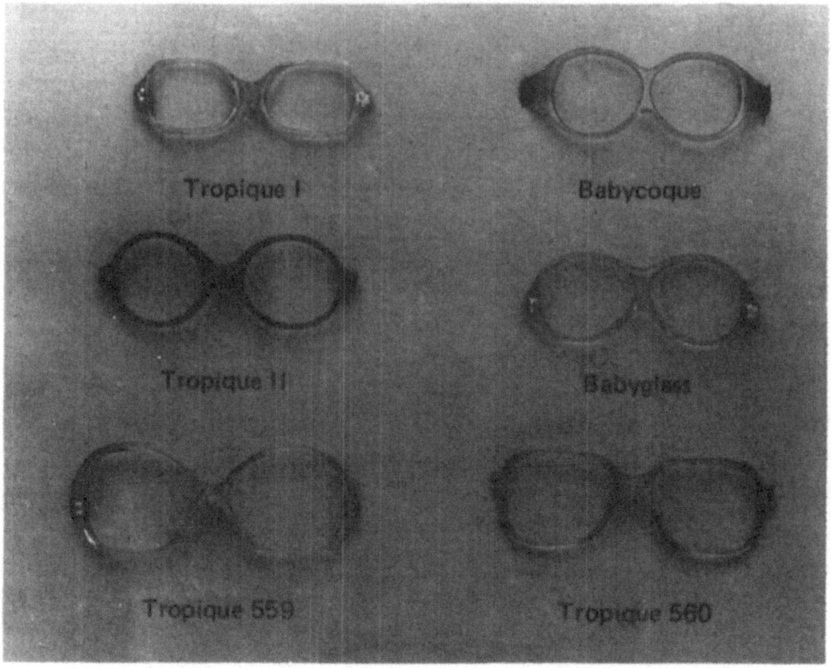

Fig. 1. — Special spectacles for young children.

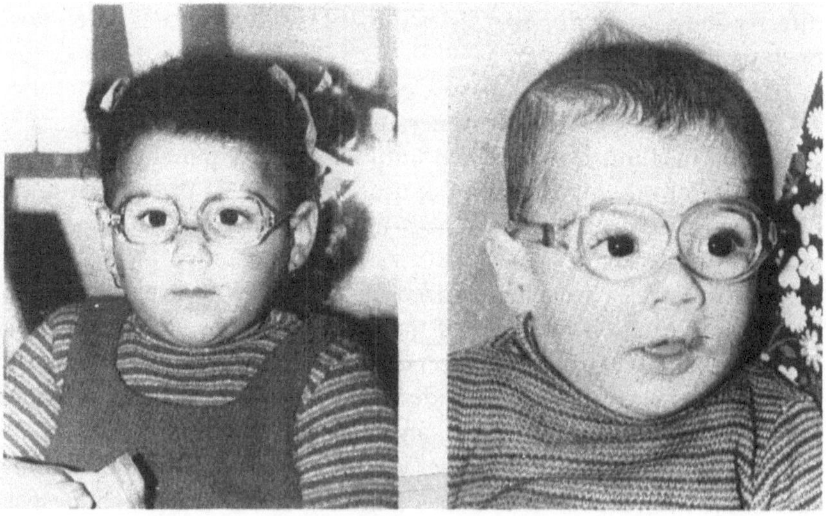

A B

Fig. 2. — The right child with a babycoque frame, the left child with a tropique 1 frame.

A. Babycoque glasses.
B. Tropique 1 glasses.

3) The making and fitting of glasses.

It is essential that the patient should look through the optical centre of his lenses, otherwise a prismatic effect is produced.

As in esotropia the glasses are often of high power, it is necessary to measure the interpupillary distance, and to mention it on the spectacle prescription.

In these high power glasses, the centre and the periphery of a lens can show a marked refractional difference; this constitutes another reason for exact centering of the glasses and for prescribing big spectacles, thus avoiding the danger that the child adopts a slight torticollis position to look through the border of the lens (a good sign to detect overcorrection: we have to look for it and to ask the parents).

The tilting of the glasses is important too: they should be as nearly as possible perpendicular to the visual axis. If any tilt is introduced the spherical power is slightly increased and a cylindrical effect is added.

The distance at which the spectacles are worn is of considerable importance for the effective strength of the lens (normally 13 to 14 mm in front of the cornea). A convex lens situated farther away increases in strength; a wrong distance in marked anisometropia can also cause some annoyance. Plastic lenses of high power have the great advantage of their lightness and they do not fog-up so quickly as glass in changing temperatures, but they suffer from the disadvantage of susceptibility to scratching.

Conclusion:

Refraction plays a predominant role in origin, type and course of strabismus. Hamburger (24) states that the refraction determines the sensorial status and Jampolsky (32) does not believe in an equal refraction in a child with unilateral strabismus.

In our opinion the full correction of the refractive error by glasses, prescribed at the earliest possible age and worn constantly, is the basic treatment of the majority of strabismus cases. This treatment can be done by anyone; it is the unique treatment of our rich therapeutical arsenal, active on all three objectives of strabismus treatment. It is often an essential step in establishing an etiological diagnosis.

B. *Occlusion*

1. Total occlusion

Total occlusion should be performed:

1) for the treatment of amblyopia (chapter VII).

2) for the influence on the sensorial status.

Occlusion, if performed early enough, prevents or refrains the further development of anomalous retinal correspondence, which is generally accepted as an adaptation of the sensorial status to a motor disturbance, although research on heredity (55) seems to indicate that sensorial disturbances can exist without motor disturbances (microstrabismus). The influence of occlusion on correspondence is demonstrated (17) by the fact that after successful amblyopia treatment, correspondence tested in free space was normal in about 60% of cases especially in children under five years of age and in cases where dominance could be switched.

3) for the influence on the motor status.

Occlusion, performed as soon as possible, preserves or obtains normal muscle action in all directions of gaze, by avoiding the effect of paresis, overaction or contracture. In practically all cases the "pseudo-abducens palsy" in young children disappears by occlusion (62). If secondary muscle and Tenon's capsula changes have already developed the occlusion often can no longer obtain this normal muscle action and early operation is then indicated. The duration of the occlusion may be dependent upon the motor status and not only upon the amblyopia cure.

4) For the influence on the angle of deviation.

The angle of deviation can decrease under occlusion, but as occlusion is practically always coupled to the wearing of glasses, it is difficult to say if it is the occlusion or the spectacles which cause this decrease in angle of deviation. In some cases the angle of deviation increases with occlusion, possibly by disruption of previously existing peripheral fusion, by transforming the pre-existing heterophoria into an esotropia (manifest and latent deviation) as especially happens in microstrabismus, or by blockage of nystagmus in adduction with increase of the angle of deviation (12).

Conclusion: Total occlusion is a very effective form of treatment; it is active on the four levels described. There are some disadvantages: if wrongly practiced there is the danger of occlusion amblyopia in very young children, the possible increase of the angle of deviation and the appearance of dissociated vertical divergence.

2. Sector occlusion

This special form of occlusion is very popular in France (2). This very cheap and cosmetically acceptable (Venilia damier blanc model can be found in any drugstore) occlusion has the great advantage that it can be cut easily into the most different forms. It is used as a diagnostic tool in very young children (fig. 3).

It is also used in the prevention and the treatment of amblyopia and motor disturbances (fig. 4).

The results are optimal if the application is early and continuous.

For the treatment of amblyopia we prefer total occlusion or penalisation, but we often use sector-occlusion as consolidation of amblyopia treatment, as treatment of underactions of certain muscles (e.g. the binasal sector—occlusion in pseudo-abducens palsy in the young child), as prevention of abnormal binocular cooperation, or in cases where the "spastic" factor is pronounced. To be effective, these binasal sectors must be so big that with either eye straight the outer limit of the sector touches the inner pupillary border. The control of effectivity of these sector-occlusions is easy. We walk around the child and observe if, when we are to his right, he looks with his right eye, when we are to his left side that he looks with his left eye, or if by turning his head, he tries to continue to fix always with the same eye. Sectors are easily adaptable

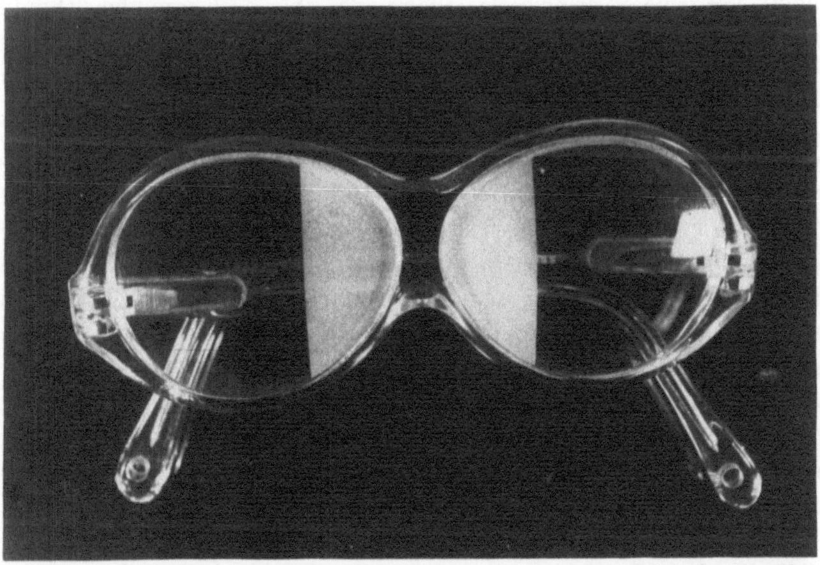

Fig. 3. — Spectacles with binasal sector occlusion to detect squint in young children.

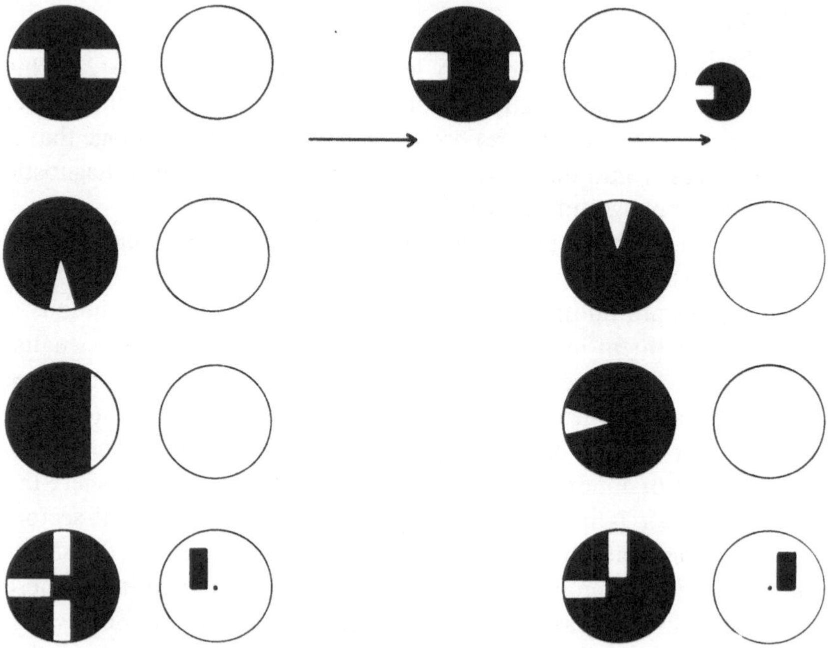

Fig. 4. — Different forms of sector occlusion used as treatmemt of amblyopia and of motor disturbances.

and changeable from case to case, each case should be judged individually, the general principle is that under this occlusion they should alternate and show a normal ocular motility.

C. *Penalisation*

In 1958 at the International Congress of Brussels, Pfandl (50) described six cases of concomitant esotropia with anisometropia (a moderate unilateral myopia) characterized by absence of amblyopia and presence of normal correspondence. In this communication of two pages all the important features of this new therapeutical method are described: a) to try to obtain an alternation between distance and near vision by means of a consciously inexact optical correction for one eye (optical penalisation). One eye is exclusively used for near vision, the other for distant vision (balance spatiale of the French authors). b) To prevent—if performed early by this alternation—the development of amblyopia and anomalous correspondence.

This treatment became popular especially in France and Germany; different forms of penalisation were described with different indications (10, 23, 52, 53) but the result of penalisation treatment is better the earlier it is applied. The treatment must be permanent. The forms of penalisation we use most are the near penalisation (atropinisation and exact correction of the fixating eye and 2 to 3 diopters overcorrection of the amblyopic eye) and the slight penalisation (an overcorrection of +1.5 D on the fixating eye). The indications of penalisation are:

1. The amblyopia treatment (cfr. chapter VII).

2. In unilateral esotropia, after amblyopia treatment by total occlusion, or in cases without amblyopia, penalisation is often used as an intermediate stage in the treatment, especially for its marked effect on relaxation of accommodation (10, 23, 52, 53). In cases of near penalisation this can be measured easily through the continuous use of atropine in the fixating eye (easy refraction control at every visit) but also by the amelioration of the distant vision of the amblyopic eye through its +2 or +3 D overcorrection.

3. All authors (10, 23, 52, 53) agree that by penalisation a decrease in the angle of deviation is frequent and especially a very pronounced decrease in the so-called "convergence excess". It is not sure if this decrease in angle of deviation is due only to the accommodative relaxation or if other factors also play a role here (23).

4. Penalisation performed early should avoid in a great majority of cases the appearance of motor incomitances (53).

5. Optical penalisation in the beginning seemed to offer an adequate way of treatment of anomalous retinal correspondence (50, 53). Experience and careful observation taught us that normalisation of correspondence happens rarely and when it happens, it is only if the angle of deviation becomes zero. That the influence of penalisation on correspondence is only slight is not amazing, because penalisation only lessens the binocular vision but does not abolish it in normal persons. In microstrabismus and in cases of amblyopia without strabismus, the existence of binocular vision is shown, principally in the zone between 30 cm and 2 m, notwithstanding penalisation (23).

Conclusion: Occlusion and optical penalisation are important remedies in conservative strabismus treatment. Early and permanent application is essential. The main difference between both is that in total occlusion one eye is completely closed, in penalisation it is not; here "la balance spatiale" is essential: one eye is used for distant vision, the other for near vision. We should control at every examination if this alternation is continued; this is often difficult to observe in young children when the angle of deviation becomes minimal by our treatment, as measuring the visual acuity is not yet possible. In cases of slight penalisation, it often occurs that the "overcorrection" of + 1.5 D no longer remains an overcorrection.

A disturbance of the pupil reactions, pupil size, and accommodation range has not been observed even after this sometimes long lasting use of atropine (10, 48).

Occlusion and optical penalisation are links in the whole strabismus treatment. As they are both dissociative methods, they should be used only as long as necessary for the amblyopia treatment, to obtain normal motility and maximal relaxation of accommodation.

II. *Treatment adapted to the strabismus groups*

A. *Early onset strabismus group*

This is certainly a very mixed group linked together by the date of onset of the squint. We mention only:

1) the esotropia of very early onset with bilateral limitation of abduction, large angle of deviation, jerk nystagmus, torticollis, and low hyperopia (9, 34);
2) alternating esotropia with rather large angle of deviation and low hyperopia (cross-fixation);
3) cases of pure accommodative squint or intermittent esotropia;
4) the so-called "spastic" cases with a variable angle of deviation whereby early optical correction and occlusion give remarkable results;
5) some cases of nystagmus blocked in convergence, in which the eyes are apparently straight with nystagmus or one eye is strongly adducted without nystagmus (12).

It is obvious that in such a mixture there is no common therapeutical approach. Everyone agrees that if amblyopia is present, it should first be eliminated by total occlusion of the good eye (cave occlusion amblyopia) carried out preferentially until free alternation is obtained. In some cases when motor factors constitute an obstacle to amblyopia treatment, it is indicated to operate first. Once amblyopia is eradicated or when the esotropia is alternating, the opinions about the ensuing therapeutics are quite different. Some authors (49, 64) strongly advocate early operation (between six months and one year) in cases with large angles and low refractive errors, since by early alignment the chances to obtain sensory fusion would be greater and since in their opinion the low refractive error cannot play a significant role in this large angle. For the advocates of this early surgery the real problems start after this operation is realised. In 55% of these early operated cases an accommodative esotropia appears at the age of 2½ years; there is also a 90% possibility of the appearance of a dissociated vertical divergence, and a 65% chance of developing overacting inferior obliques (49). According to Von Noorden, correcting operations for under- or over-corrections are often necessary (64).

The tendency in these cases to first treat with conservative methods is more generally accepted. First of all, the incidence of amblyopia in this group is considerably higher than generally thought, and there are very often limitations of abduction. In cases of amblyopia total occlusion is to be preferred, to avoid that the child looks with his good eye between the border of his spectacles and nose by turning his head. This occlusion should last a long time, otherwise the majority goes back preferring the originally fixating eye. The occlusion is necessary too for ocular motility. The occlusion should be carried out until free alternation and free motility are obtained. Limitation of abduction without amblyopia is a nice indication for sector-occlusion together with abduction exercices.

Secondly, an examination at that age may not show us the real picture (36) and a good examination of ocular motility is practically impossible. Still more important is the fact that repeated refraction controls are mandatory because the refraction error in children may change significantly, may not have developed at the time of the initial examination, and one single refraction does not show the total hypermetropia. Our conservative treatment eliminates the amblyopia, egalizes the dominance, prevents or diminishes the depth of anomalous retinal correspondence and suppression and normalizes the ocular motility. Since the early application of continuous conservative treatment, there is a marked decrease in vertical incomitances which otherwise appear so frequently at about 1½ years of age (32, 49).

If after this conservative treatment there is still a cosmetically disturbing angle of deviation, an operation is indicated, but the children have then reached an age where an exact motor examination is possible, and where we can be sure about refraction and amblyopia. This conservative treatment is in reality not lasting longer than the early operation method because re-operations are seldom necessary and most of all because, even when the early operation shows a good result, this is practically always a microstrabismus, very often with amblyopia. Experience tells us that the parents, even when informed about the necessity of regular post-operative controls, neglect these when the cosmetic appearance is good. This amblyopia of microstrabismus is detected late, and its treatment is very difficult.

B. *Late onset strabismus group*

This late onset strabismus is characterized in chapter V as often unilateral, normosensorial and intermittent. Hypermetropia plays a cardinal role.

This group is subdivided into:

- pure accommodative esotropia,
- atypical accommodative esotropia,
- partially accommodative esotropia.

Here certainly it is true that early treatment, as long as the strabismus is intermittent, results in a much higher percentage of cure, that is to say in a much higher percentage of pure accommodative strabismus. The only way to determine to which subdivision a patient belongs, is to liberate the total hyperopia.

The first visit serves for establishing the diagnosis of esotropia and for prescribing atropine ointment 1%. At the second visit the atropine retinoscopy is performed and the full correction of the refractive error is prescribed. The glasses should be worn continuously. We should not admit prejudices such as: "An accommodative squint in a child under one year of age is impossible; a large angle of deviation cannot be of accommodative nature; the refractive error is too moderate to explain that angle of deviation (3, 7, 47, 58); orthophorisation by spectacles is impossible as the esotropia has been lasting for weeks (48).". Our experience proves the contrary, but it is true that the chance of obtaining orthophorisation by spectacles diminishes and the time necessary to reach orthophorisation increases, the longer a constant squint existed.

The first control examination after the prescription of glasses is three weeks later. We ask the parents if there were difficulties in accepting the glasses: does the child take off his glasses frequently, does he look over his glasses, does he adopt a torticollis position to look through the border of his glasses?

Then we examine with fully accommodative targets for distance and near if at the cover test there is still an angle of deviation. There are two possibilities:

– There is an angle of deviation

Some people accept directly the fact that the strabismus is only partially accommodative. Other people, especially in America, try miotics for 4 to 6 weeks to eliminate further the accommodation (4, 36). An extreme way is followed by Rethy (54) who prescribes daily instillations of atropine, alternate occlusion and overcorrections of +0.75 D or more to relax accommodation. This kind of treatment is rejected by most authors because this long lasting atropinisation and overcorrection should hinder emmetropisation and should give rise to accommodation paresis. We believe that these arguments are wrong because in our opinion, at this age emmetropisation does not happen anymore, to the contrary, hypermetropia increases normally (5, 37, 56), and it is shown that there is no change in accommodation range after long lasting atropinisation or wearing of glasses (10).

For us, this treatment is impracticable in daily practice. We follow another way adapted to the situation and the age of the child. If there is a tendency to unilaterality, which often happens, we prescribe a slight penalisation (overcorrection of +1 D on the dominant eye). If the squint is really alternating, our treatment depends upon the age of the patient. If he is old enough to permit testing of visual acuity for distance, we add +0.5 D to 1 D as "clip-on" to the ordinary frame and if the visual acuity for distance is full, we prescribe this addition. If the child is too young to test visual acuity, we look if he easily accepted his first (11) "overcorrection", if the angle of deviation is variable, and we add the same "clip-on" to the ordinary frame and let him go for a while asking the accompanying parent to observe if the child accepts this overcorrection.

When the child does not accept the overcorrection or if there is a limitation of abduction, we add a binasal sector-occlusion, which sometimes has an amazing effect on the angle of deviation (spastic factors).

– There is no angle of deviation

When there is no angle for distance and near with accommodative fixation targets, the strabismus is purely accommodative. When there is orthophoria for distance, and esotropia for near, we have an atypical accommodative strabismus.

In subsequent control examinations these same two possibilities occur. In cases, with manifest esotropia, we carefully observe and ask the parents if the angle of deviation is variable. This variability of the angle is for us the sign that accommodation is not yet completely eliminated. We try again with slight penalisation, slight overcorrection and repeated refractions under cycloplegia to do this. If after six months a manifest angle of deviation remains, we have to do with a partially accommodative squint.

1. Pure accommodative strabismus

In a pure accommodative squint the wearing of spectacles eliminates the squint for distance and near. The incidence of pure accommodative strabismus is on the increase, since we do really all that is possible to eliminate accommodation completely. Since Themen (58) we know that accommodative strabismus is possible in the first year of life. The term "late onset" is therefore no longer appropriate.

But orthophoria is not the end stage of the treatment. We have to be sure of the binocular vision and of the visual acuity. As soon as orthophoria is obtained,the sensorial status is examined with less-dissociating examination methods (chapter VI). We cannot assume that normal binocular vision exists merely from the fact that the eyes are made straight by the glasses. As in cases of microtropia the answers to these sensorial tests can be normal, control by cover test type I is necessary to detect if this is real orthophoria or small angle esotropia.

The tendency to suppression or amblyopia is particularly strong in accommodative strabismus. Therefore, testing the visual acuity as early as possible is always necessary. In cases of slight amblyopia we perform a slight penalisation.

Unless the glasses are required for reasons apart from strabismus, e.g. astigmatism, anisometropia or high hypermetropia, we always try to reduce the convex spherical correction to the weakest which keeps the squint controlled. This should be done gradually or at the beginning the children may remove their glasses for certain outdoor activities, and at the end they may remove them altogether. In some cases this is never possible. Orthoptic exercises may be helpful.

High hypermetropia (5 D and more) demands frequent controls because in these cases the tendency to divergence is strong (6, 36). On binocular examination most of these patients show very weak binocular functions. The near point of convergence is first to recede (developing an exodeviation for near and then soon the eyes start going out for distance). Again it is better and easier to prevent than to cure. Once the divergence has started it is difficult to stay ahead off the process, the eyes keep going out. The minimal + glass which procures orthophoria for near and distance is prescribed from the beginning, the convergence and the strength of the binocular function is always tested. Orthoptic exercices to increase the strength of the binocular functions are indicated.

2. Atypical accommodative strabismus

In Chapter V this form of strabismus is defined as follows: the eyes are straight for distance (if necessary with correction of the hypermetropia) but there is an esodeviation for near even with glasses. The AC/A ratio is greater than 1.

There is controversy whether the distance/near relationship in strabismus can be considered synonymous to the AC/A ratio. In our opinion all the discussions about AC/A ratio do not apport anything of clinical value in the treatment of squint. Therefore we limit ourselves to the very simple measurement of the angle of deviation for near and distance.

Classically the treatment of an atypical accommodative strabismus consists in the full correction of the refractive error by glasses, the prescription of bifocals or the use of miotics.

Bifocals

The only indication for bifocals is when there is orthophoria and normal binocular vision for distance and not for near. The strength of the bifocal segment must be determined by measurement in every case (prism and cover test) and the minimum additional plus power is chosen which will keep the eyes straight. The bifocal segment must be taken large enough and set high enough so that the top of the bifocal segment bisects the pupil when the child looks straight ahead. It is easy to control if the child uses his bifocal segment to read, by observing if it spontaneously raises its chin and lowers its eyes to look through the bifocal segment. If the child does not do so, we oblige it to do so by instillations of atropine. Since the application of our systematic accommodation relaxation method we do not prescribe bifocals any more. Jampolsky could remove 80% of his bifocals by prescribing the really full correction of hypermetropia for distant vision (32).

Miotics

Miotics are drugs which stimulate accommodation peripherally by contraction of the ciliary muscle and they also constrict the pupil. Therefore the central accommodation stimulus decreases as well as the accommodative convergence. Javal (33) was the first to use miotics in strabismus, but it was Abraham (1949) who introduced and popularized (especially in America) miotic therapy (1, 4, 36).

The miotics most commonly used are pilocarpine 1%, D.F.P. 0.025%, phospholine iodide 0.06% and 0.125%. The latter is now by far the most used; once a day, preferably in the morning, unless the subjective disturbances as trouble vision or headache which are frequent in the first days of instillation, oblige us to give it at night the first days. To judge if the instillation is well done, the reactivity of the pupil to light is more important than the size of the pupil. A good therapeutic effect is possible with relatively large pupils which react slowly to light.

The "classic" indications for miotic therapy are:

1) first of all the treatment of "convergence excess". Miotics and bifocals are correlated in the treatment of "convergence excess"; if the "convergence excess" disappears with bifocals, it will disappear with miotics too.
2) Miotics are used especially in America as a diagnostic tool to see if there is still residual accommodation after full correction of the refractive error by glasses.
3) Some people use miotics to eliminate accommodation if the hyperopia is not more than 4 D (27). Miotics are sometimes used in young children instead of spectacles and in high hypermetropia to permit the prescription of weaker positive glasses.
4) Miotics are used post-operatively if there is a residual angle of convergence, to diminish this convergence and this independently of the fact that the strabismus before surgery was accommodative or not (57).

Unfortunately miotics present multiple side-effects:

Local side-effects

A child on miotics should be examined regularly at the slit lamp to see if there is any appearance of cysts of the pupillary border of the iris, possibly leading to pupil occlusion. These cysts always disappear at the end of the treatment and can be strongly prevented by adding phenylephrine 5% to the miotic. Diminution of visual acuity by pupil constriction and frontal headache in the beginning of the administration are possible. Lens opacities as described in glaucoma patients do not occur in children. A closed-angle glaucoma is described in a 7 year old boy with esotropia after 7 weeks administration of 0.125% phospholine iodide, once a day. Von Noorden mentions a retinal detachment in a 20-year-old girl with esotropia (63).

General side effects

The general side effects are those of cholinergic intoxication: diarrhoea, profuse sweating, sialorrhoe and apathia. When a child on miotic therapy must be operated on with succinylcholine as muscle relaxans, the treatment must be stopped at least four weeks before the operation. The anaesthesiologist should always be informed of this. Therefore the weakest solution giving sufficient result is used. The patients should be seen regularly and the frequency of administration should be gradually reduced to a minimum necessary to obtain a good result.

We never use miotics as diagnostic tool or in place of glasses. The efficacy of miotics to eliminate accommodation is clearly less than glasses or penalisation. Parks (49) states that miotic treatment is harder and less reliable in the management of the accommodative component than the optical system of spectacles; miotics have too many local and general side-effects to be used for a long time. Miotics are certainly effective in the treatment of "convergence excess" but we use them only as a temporary measure. In our opinion it are accommodative and innervational factors which play the dominant role in "convergence excess". This is made clear by the fact that penalisation eliminates "convergence excess" in the great majority of cases (23), and that Jampolsky could remove 80% of his bifocals by prescribing a really full correction for distant vision. The incidence of "convergence excess" in our practice is far less than indicated in the literature (Parks in 60% of his accommodative strabismus (47), Quere (53) in 40% of all convergent strabismus) since the application of our systematic accommodation relaxation method. In these cases patience is a sound therapeutical principle. As "convergence excess" is a self-limiting disease, it is advisable to await the effect of passage of time upon the over-convergence at near. If, despite a full correction of the refractive error, a disturbing "convergence excess" is present, we use phopholine iodide in the weakest solution together with orthoptic exercises to strengthen the binocular functions, and this for the shortest period possible. As moderate unilateral amblyopia is frequent in "convergence excess", visual acuity should always be tested carefully. The amblyopia should be treated with occlusion, slight penalisation or "Ausschleichokklusiv". If there is a postoperative residual angle in convergence, miotics are tried in the immediate postoperative period, as some authors pretend that accommodation is set free by operation (57).

3. Partially accommodative strabismus

This is an esotropia of which the angle of deviation is only reduced in extent by the wearing of spectacles which correct the hypermetropia. With our treatment method we have practically always obtained alternating esotropia with a constant angle of deviation and free ocular motility. In some selected cases prism treatment (p.291) is possible. Surgical treatment is nearly always required for cosmetically disturbing cases (angle of deviation greater than 6°) but with precaution. We know from the literature (6, 18, 44) that in approximately 2/3 of moderate esotropias (an angle of deviation which does not exceed 12° to 15°) a spontaneous decrease of this angle occurs, and that in 10 to 20% of these cases the strabismus becomes divergent (this especially in high hypermetropia).

C. *Microstrabismus*

An angle of deviation of less than 6° and anomalous binocular vision, often fairly well developed, characterize microstrabismus. This can be a primary microstrabismus or secondary to our treatment (conservative or operative).

The only treatment to execute is the amblyopia treatment. This amblyopia treatment is often hard and long lasting as microstrabismus and amblyopia are often diagnosed very late (38) and as the rivalry between both eyes in microstrabismus is pronounced. It is practically impossible to obtain a change in dominance and there often exists a discrepancy between fixation and visual acuity; even with normalized visual acuity, fixation cannot be held by this eye, as can be done in other cases of strabismus.

In microstrabismus the visual acuity is often worse for near than for distance, especially in reading texts (39). There is a strong tendency to recurrence of amblyopia in microstrabismus. The amblyopia treatment consists in adequate correction of the refractive error (as anisometropia is particularly frequent in microstrabismus) and in occlusion or optical penalisation, because most of these cases are school children where a total occlusion is psychologically difficult to accept.

III. *Complementary treatment*

A. *Prism treatment*

The use of prisms is easy since the introduction in 1965 by Woodward of press-on prisms (Fresnel) (fig. 5). These prisms cause some

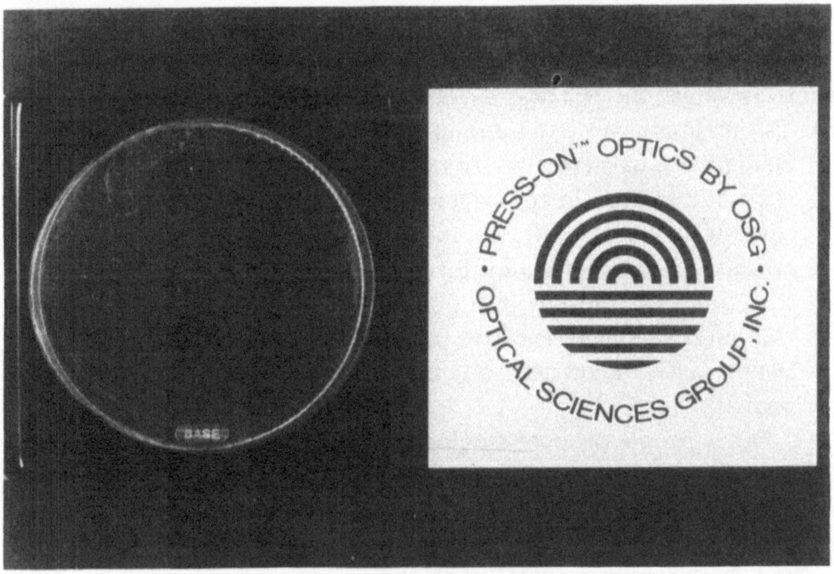

Fig. 5. — The Fresnel prisms.

reduction and distortion in visual acuity, especially for the higher values; the maximal reduction is 1 or 2 lines at the visual acuity chart. A Fresnel prism of 20 pD is not the same as a loose prism of 20 pD, the easiest way is to compare both ourselves at the Maddox scale. If the residual angle is less than 6°, after the possibilities of conservative treatment are exhausted, we are confronted with a microstrabismus.

If the residual angle is greater than 6°, we perform a prism compensation test (chap. VI, XII).

The following possibilities may occur:

1. There is no increase in the angle of deviation. When the angle of deviation is maximally 20 pD, we incorporate in the spectacles the prisms which compensate the angle. This constitutes a permanent bifoveal stimulation for the patient, he exercises his binocular vision all the day. In the course of time we try to diminish the prisms. When the angle of deviation is greater than 20 pD we are obliged to use the Fresnel prisms. These diminish the visual acuity of 1 or 2 lines on the test

chart, which is often not tolerated very well by the child. Therefore we prefer surgical treatment based on this angle of deviation; the prognosis of the operation is very good.

2. There is a decrease in the angle of deviation (rare). Surgical treatment is indicated on the minimum angle under prisms, unless the angle of deviation is less than 6°.

3. There is an increase in the angle of deviation.

The angle of deviation found after the prism compensation test is the same as before the test was carried out or less.

a) The prismatic overcorrection (11).

Here prisms of increasing strength are put before the eyes until there is no more return in convergence of the eyes behind the prisms. On cover test type II both eyes make fixation movements from divergence. This overcorrection by prisms is left continuously in place, sometimes for months, waiting until the prism can be diminished without returning of the eyes in convergence. This treatment is long lasting and difficult for patient and doctor. The results are disappointing.

Other people propose surgical treatment based on the angle with no return in convergence. This results in frequent large divergences. A trend now in vogue in Europe is to operate the originally existing angle (= the static angle of deviation) with recess-resect operation, and the "dynamic angle" with the Faden operation of Cüppers.

b) We do it our way.

If the angle of deviation is e.g. 30 pD and an overcorrection of 10 pD is sufficient to prevent a further return in convergence, we operate based on these 40 pD; this also constitutes a consciously slight surgical overcorrection. If the eyes return under this slight prismatic overcorrection to an angle of deviation of +10 pD, we operate based on these 40 pD; we know that the result will be a slight residual angle. If the eyes return under prism to the original angle of deviation, we refuse surgical treatment and explain it to the patient.

B. *Orthoptic treatment*

The exercises for treating anomalies of binocular vision, for overcoming deviation of the visual axes and for helping to restore comfortable binocular single vision, are called orthoptics. This term also embraces the methods of examination (chap. VI). Javal (33) introduced the conception of training the eyes to work together by means of exercises and put this therapeutic approach upon a sound basis.

The essential objectives of orthoptics are:

1) to overcome suppression;
2) to facilitate the return to a normal localisation;
3) to increase the range of fusion.

As diagnosis and treatment of strabismus is done much earlier than before, so that in most cases strabismus treatment is finished before the "orthoptic age" is attained, the golden age of orthoptic exercises is passed and the accent lies more and more on orthoptics as diagnostic method (13, 16).

The active orthoptical treatment of anomalous retinal correspondence is completely abandoned. As the time between the onset of strabismus and the first consultation has been greatly shortened, incidence and depth of anomalous retinal correspondence has been strongly reduced, and by our conservative treatment correspondence is often normalized (especially in cases where the originally suppressed or amblyopic eye becomes the dominant eye).

Contrary to the opinion of some people, who completely reject orthoptics, these exercises continue to have their indications, limited surely, in our therapeutical arsenal (13, 16).

These indications are:

1. The "convergence insufficiency": this is the triumph of orthoptic exercises. Convergence exercises can be practised at home provided physiological diplopia can be demonstrated.
2. Heterophoria with subjective symptoms.
3. "Convergence excess": anti-suppression exercises, here with the eyes focused for near vision, relaxation of accommodation exercises and stereogram cards (fig. 6).
4. Orthophoria with weak binocular functions: anti-suppression and fusion exercises.

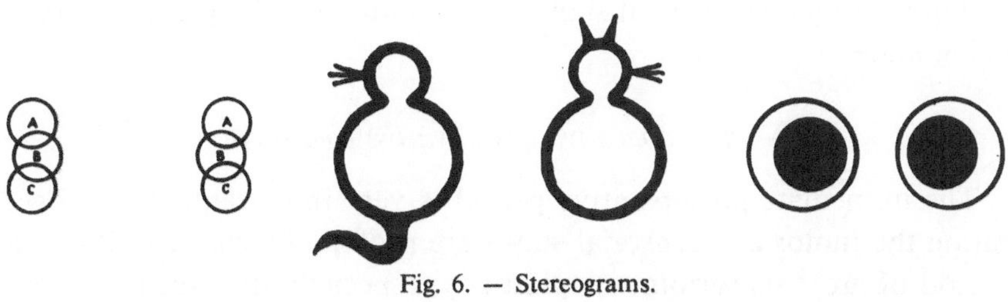

Fig. 6. — Stereograms.

5. Pure accommodative strabismus: anti-suppression exercises and exercises to teach the patient relaxation of accommodation with consequent relaxation of convergence, and to teach dissociation of accommodation and convergence.
6. The immediate postoperative period: exercises to enhance the often very weak normal binocular functions and to overcome the unilateral suppression.

Lavat and coll. proposed orthoptic exercises in free space (40) at the angle of deviation (fig. 7).

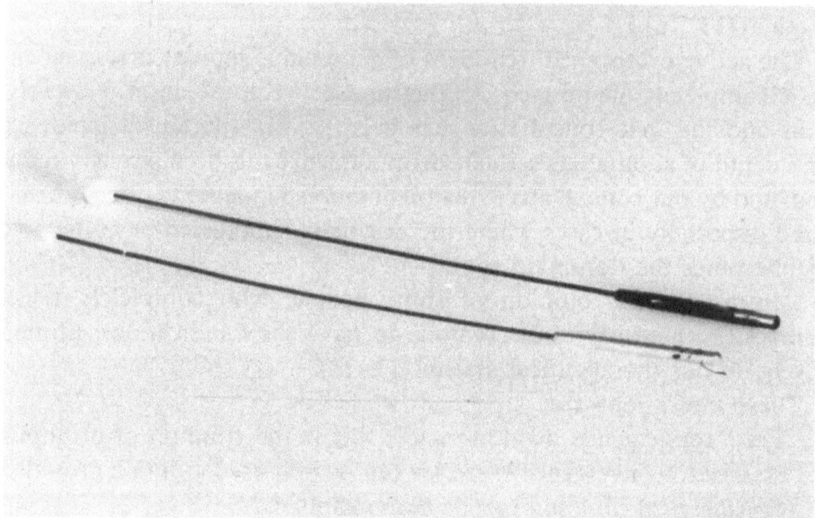

Fig. 7. — Instruments for orthoptic exercises in free space at the objective angle (Lavat-Prigent).

The main instruments for these orthoptic exercises are, in addition to the synoptophore, prism bars, red and green glasses, stereograms and stereogram cards. The phasendifferenzhaploskop of Aulhorn is certainly very appropriated for orthoptical diagnosis and exercises (chap. VI, XI). We give these exercises in a series of stages in 30 minute sessions and our orthoptic treatment should only continue as long as progress is being made.

IV. *Postoperative conservative treatment*

The immediate postoperative period is very important. By the operation the motor and sensorial status are profoundly changed, this is a period of great sensoriomotor plasticity, especially in cases of surgery

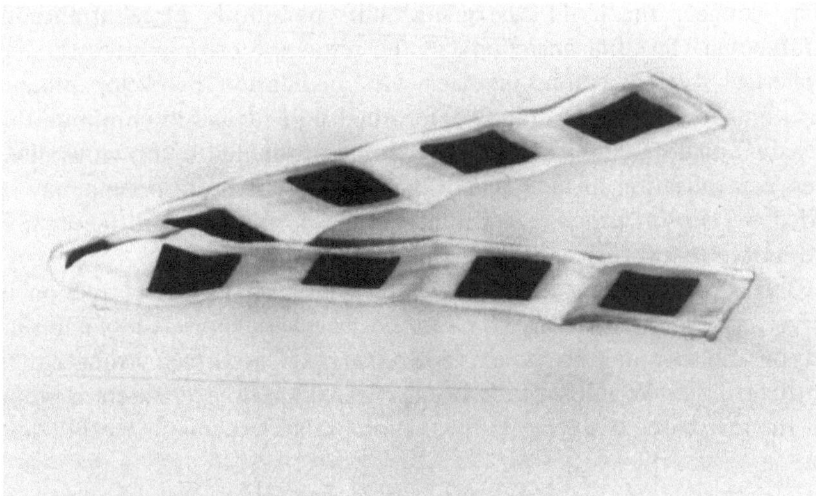

Fig. 8. — An excellent and cheap help for post-operative motility exercises.
Device to elicit optokinetic nystagmus.

on the dominant eye. Several times a day the parents should perform motility exercises in all directions of gaze (fig. 8).

On the sensorial plan, there are different possibilities:

1. Orthophoria: an examination of the binocular status with less-dissociating methods is strictly indicated (chap. VI, XI), a normal correspondence with more or less fusion or an anomalous correspondence (paradoxical diplopia) can be found. In both cases frequent controls are necessary and in every examination we should control if orthophoria persists, if there is no recurrence of amblyopia, if there is no danger of unilateral suppression and if binocular functions develop in the desired direction. Orthoptic exercises to execute preferentially in normal surroundings are indicated to fight neutralisation and to enhance normal binocular cooperation. We usually propose a trial of 5 exercises, in this period it is possible to judge the motivation and cooperation of the patient and the progress in binocular cooperation.

2. There is a slight residual angle in convergence. In this case diplopia is rare or fugitive as the fixated object falls on the deviated eye on a previously suppressed part of the nasal retina. This means that there is no signal to appeal fusion, divergent fusional movements are already extremely limited. The first thing to do is to prevent the recurrence of amblyopia using an "Ausschleichokklusiv" or a slight penalisation.

The younger the child, the greater this possibility of recurrence of amblyopia. The full correction of the refractive error is necessary. A spherical overcorrection together with instillation of cyclopentolate, and on the other hand miotics are proposed as trials to eliminate this residual angle. If the residual angle is not eliminated by previous devices, neutralisation of the angle of deviation by base-out prisms may be tried by clip-on prisms. Since the perfect correction is difficult, it is advisable to overcorrect the residual deviation.

3. There is a slight angle in divergence. A slight overcorrection in divergence is preferred by some authors because there is less neutralisation and fusional movements in convergence are much stronger than in divergence. Wo do not exactly agree. Orthoptic exercises are useful in the rare cases with spontaneous diplopia and normal correspondence.

The glasses may be discontinued or a weaker convex spherical correction prescribed as long as the visual acuity of the patient permits. The glasses should be of sufficient strength to prevent a relapse into convergent squint. "Clip-on" concave spherical glasses may be useful as a temporary measure. If the divergence is incomitant in the horizontal sense, we have to think of a "tight lateral rectus syndrome" by an excessive resection of the lateral rectus. The forced duction test is indicated for the diagnosis.

4. If there is a large post-operative residual angle or if there are disturbing vertical incomitances, a second surgical treatment is necessary. If the residual angle is in convergence, we wait with reoperation for at least six months, to see if there is not a spontaneous decrease in the angle of deviation.

Treatment of post-operative diplopia

The best treatment of post-operative diplopia is prevention (chap. VI, XII). When the correspondence is normal (exceptional) orthoptic exercises are useful, except in older children or adults with "horror fusionis". When the correspondence is anomalous as it practically always is, there is no treatment. We can try to diminish the angle of deviation by prescribing weaker spherical glasses and by doing so fall back in a suppression zone, or we prescribe an "Ausschleichokklusiv" for the deviating eye to decrease the strength of the double image and to clearly show the patient which image is "false" and to facilitate the suppression or at least the neglect of this "false" image.

BIBLIOGRAPHY

(1) ABRAHAM, S.V. — Accommodation in the amblyopic eye. *Amer. J. Ophthalmol.*, 1961, *52*, 197.

(2) BADOCHE, J.M. et PINÇON, F. — Les secteurs dans le traitement de strabisme. Congrès de strabisme, Zermatt 1979.

(3) BAKER, J.D. and PARKS, M.M. — Accommodative esotropia. *Amer. J. Ophthalmol.*, 1980, *90*, 11-19.

(4) BREININ, G.W., CHIN, N.B. and RIPPS, H. — A rationale for therapy of accommodative strabismus. *Amer. J. Ophthalmol.*, 1966, *61*, 1030-1037.

(5) BROWN, E.V.L. — Net average yearly changes in refraction of atropinized eyes from birth to beyond middle life. *Arch. Ophthalmol.*, 1938, *19*, 719-734.

(6) BURIAN, H.M. — Hypermetropia and Esotropia. *J. Ped. Ophthalmol.*, 1972, *9*, 135-143.

(7) BURIAN, H.M. — Comitant Strabismus. *The Ohio State Med. J.*, 1958, *54*, 173-181.

(8) BURIAN, H.M. and VON NOORDEN, G.K. — Binocular vision and ocular motility. St. Louis, The C.V. Mosby Company, 1974.

(9) CIANCIA, A.O. — Management of esodeviations under the age of two. *Int. Opht. Clin.*, 1967, *6*, 503-518.

(10) CÜPPERS, C. and MÜHLENDYCK, H. — Erfahrungen mit der Penalisation. BVA Arbeitskreis Schielbehandlung, Wiesbaden 1976, Band 6, 87-104.

(11) CÜPPERS, C. and ADELSTEIN, F. — Le traitement de la correspondance rétinienne anormale à l'aide de prismes. *Ann. Ocul. (Paris)*, 1970, *203*, 445-457.

(12) CÜPPERS, C. and ADELSTEIN, F. — Zum problem der echten und scheinbaren Abducenslähmung (das sogenannte Blockierungssyndrom). *46. Beiheft Klin. Mbl. Aug.*, 1966, 270-278. F. Enke Verlag, Stuttgart.

(13) CRONE, R.A. and VAN DEN BOSCH, J.G. — The sweet and bitter fruits of orthoptic exercises. Perspectives in Opht., Vol. II, Amsterdam, Excerpta Medica, 171-178, 1970.

(14) DONDERS, F.C. — Accommodation and Refraction of the eye. London, The New Sydenham Society, 1864.

(15) DUKE-ELDER, S. — Ophtalmic Optics and refraction. Volume V, System of Ophtalmology, vol. V, p. 285. 1970, H. Kimpton, London.

(16) DOUGLAS, A.A. — The centenary of orthoptics. *Trans. Opht. Soc. U.K.*, 1963, *83*, 559-572.

(17) FERON, A. and VEREECKEN, E. — L'amblyopie dans la pratique privée. *Bull. Soc. Belge d'Opht.*, 1969, *151*, 363-372.

(18) FLETCHER, M. — Strabismus Symposium Giessen. 1966, Karger Verlag Basel.

(19) FLETCHER, M. — Strabismus Ophthalmic Symposium New Orleans, 1971; The C.V. Mosby Co.

(20) FULTON, A.B. and coll. — Cycloplegic refractions in infants and young children. *Amer. J. Ophthalmol.*, 1980, *90*, 239-247.

(21) GOLDSCHMIDT, E. — Refraction in the newborn. *Acta Ophthalmol.*, 1969, *47*, 570-578.

(22) GRIGNOLO, A. and RIVARA, A. — Observations biométriques sur l'œil des enfants nés à terme et des prématures au cours de la première année. *Ann. Ocul.*, 1968, *201*, 817-826.

(23) HAASE, W. — Optische Penalisation als therapeutisches Hilfsmittel beim frühkindlichen Strabismus. *Advances in Opht.*, 1978, *35*, 26-44. S. Karger Basel.

(24) HAMBURGER, F.A. — Die Phorie im Dienste der Verträglichkeit von Brillen gläsern. 1976 BVA, Arbeitskreis Schielbehandlung, Band 6, 167-173, 1976, Wiesbaden.

(25) HAYNES, H., WHITE, B.L. and HELD, R. — Visual Accommodation in Human Infants. *Science*, 1965, *148*, 528-530.

(26) HOWLAND, H.C., ATKINSON, J., BRADDICK, O. and FRENCH, J. — Infant astigmatism measured by photorefraction. *Science*, 1978, *202*, 331-332.

(27) HUBER, A. — Die Miotika in der Behandlung des Strabismus concomitans convergens. *Klin. Mbl. Augenheilk.*, 1968, *153*, 476-485.

(28) IKEDA, I. and WRIGHT, M.J. — Neurophysiological basis for amblyopia. *Brit. Orth. J.*, 1975, *32*, 2-13.

(29) INGRAM, R.M. — Refraction as a basis for screening children for squint and amblyopia. *Brit. J. Ophthalmol.*, 1977, *61*, 8-15.
(30) INGRAM, R.M. and BAR, A. — Changes in refraction between the ages of 1 and 3.5 years. *Brit. J. Ophthalmol.*, 1979, *63*, 339-342.
(31) INGRAM, R.M. — Refraction of 1 year old children after atropine cycloplegia. *Brit. J. Ophthalmol.*, 1979, *63*, 343-347.
(32) JAMPOLSKY, A. — Strabismic Ophthalmic Symposium, New Orleans, The C.V. Mosby Co., 1977.
(33) JAVAL, E. — Manuel théorique et pratique du strabisme. Masson, Paris 1896.
(34) KEINER, G.G. — New viewpoints on the origin of squint. The Hague, Martinus Nyhoff, 1951.
(35) KEITH LYLE, T.K. and BRIDGEMAN, G.J. — Worth and Chavasse's squint. Baillière, Tindall and Cox, London 1959.
(36) KNAPP, P. — Strabismus Ophthalmic Symposium, New Orleans. The C.V. Mosby Co., 1977.
(37) LAHAV-GUSS, Ch. and KAUFMANN, H. — Refraktionsänderungen im Kindesalter: Hyperopie. *Kl. Mbl. Augenheilk.*, 1974, *164*, 274-278.
(38) LANG, J. — Mikrostrabismus. Bücherei des Augenarztes. Stuttgart, F. Enkeverlag, 1973.
(39) LANG, J. — Strabisme. Diagnostic - Formes cliniques - Traitement. Bern, Ed. H. Huber, 1981.
(40) LAVAT, J., PRIGENT, G., DEBROUSSE, J.Y. et PARENT, B. — Mise au point actuelle d'une technique orthoptique dans le traitement de l'ésotropie. *Ann. Ocul.*, 1966, *7*, 641-667.
(41) LEFFERTSTRA, L.J. — Vergleichende Untersuchungen auf unterschiedliche Refraktionsänderungen beider Augen bei Patienten mit Strabismus convergens. *Kl. Mbl. Augenheilk.*, 1977, *170*, 74-79.
(42) LEPARD, C.W. — Comparative changes in the error of refraction between fixing and amblyopic eyes during growth and development. *Amer. J. Ophthalmol.*, 1975, *80*, 485.
(43) MOHINDRA, J. — Astigmatism in Infants. *Science*, 1978, *202*, 329-330.
(44) MOORE, S. — The natural course of esotropia. *Amer. Orth. J.*, 1971, *21*, 80.
(45) OTTO — Lehrbuch und Atlas der Orthoptik. Bern, H. Huber Verlag, 1975.
(46) OTTO J. and SAFRA, D. — Methods and results of quantitative determination of accommodation in amblyopia und strabismus. Orthopt. Past, present, Future, 1976.
(47) PARKS, M.M. — Strabismus Ophthalmic Symposium New Orleans. The C.V. Mosby Co., 1962.
(48) PARKS, M.M. — Management of acquired esotropia. *Brit. J. Ophthalmol.*, 1974, *58*, 240-247.
(49) PARKS, M.M. — Strabismus Ophthalmic Symposium New Orleans, The C.V. Mosby Co., 1977.
(50) PFANDL, E. — Ein Neuer Weg zur Verhinderhung der Ausbildung einer anomalen retinalen Korrespondenz bei Strabismus convergens. Acta XVIII Conc. Opht. Belgica, 1958, Vol. I, 202-203.
(51) POLLARD, Z.F. — Accommodative esotropia during the first year of life. *Arch. Ophthalmol.*, 1976, *94*, 1912-1913.
(52) POULIQUEN, M.P. — Zum Problem der Penalisation. *Kl. Mbl. Augenheilk.*, 1972, *161*, 130-139.
(53) QUÉRÉ, M.A. — Die Methoden der Penalisation in der Behandlung des Strabismus convergens. *Kl. Mbl. Augenheilk.*, 1972, *161*, 140-155.
(54) RÉTHY, I. and GAL, Zs. — Results and principles of a new method of optical correction of hypermetropia in cases of esotropia. *Acta Opht.*, 1968, *46*, 757-766.
(55) RICHTER, S. — Untersuchungen über die Heredität des Strabismus concomitans. Abh. Geb. Aug. Thieme Verlag, Leipzig 1967, Band 35.
(56) SLATAPER, F.J. — Age norms of refraction and vision. *Arch. Ophthalmol.*, 1950, *43*, 466-481.
(57) SÉPULCHRE DE CONDÉ, Ch. — L'Insuffisance des cycloplégiques pour la détection de l'hypermétropie latente dans le strabisme convergent. Thèse Nancy 1973.
(58) THEMEN, C.G.W. — De ontwikkeling van het accommodatievermogen in de eerste levensmaanden. Leiden, E. IJdo N.V., 1956.

(59) THOMAS, Ch. and SPIELMANN, A. — Accommodation et amblyopie. *Bull. et Mém. Soc. Fr. Opht.*, 1970, *83*, 196-202.
(60) VEREECKEN, E. — Le traitement de l'amblyopie par l'occlusion. *Bull. Soc. Belge Opht.*, 1965, *140*, 432-444.
(61) VEREECKEN, E., FERON, A. and EVENS, L. — Importance de la détection précoce du strabisme et de l'amblyopie. *Bull. Soc. Belge Opht.*, 1966, *143*, 729-737.
(62) VEREECKEN, E. and ADELSTEIN, F. — Diagnostic et traitement de la «paralysie» du droit externe. *Ophthalmologica*, 1966, *151*, 465-476.
(63) VON NOORDEN, G.K. — Strabismus Ophthalmic Symposium New Orleans, The Mosby Co., 1977.
(64) VON NOORDEN, G.K. — Congrès de strabisme, Zermatt 1980.
(65) WORTHAM, C. — The Increase in Hypermetropia in children? *Brit. Orth. J.*, 1978, *35*, 83-90.

Bull. Soc. belge Ophtal., **195**, 301-358, 1981.

CHAPTER IX

SURGICAL MANAGEMENT OF ESOTROPIA

M.H. GOBIN (*)

INTRODUCTION

It is not our intention to give a survey of the existing surgical techniques and indications; we rather want to give practical hints with regard to the techniques and to discuss the conventional indications in general terms. Special attention is paid to the complications as they can cause real trouble to both the patient and the ophthalmologist.

We devoted a chapter to our own surgical approach. We think that a sagittalization of the oblique muscles plays an important role in the pathogenesis of strabismus and we thus systematically perform a combined oblique and horizontal muscle surgery. As surgery to measure is impossible, we rather aim at an overcorrection which is easier to compensate than an undercorrection. Because the accommodative element of the squint disappears when our surgery is successful, we take the horizontal deviation into account as measured without wearing spectacles.

SURGICAL TECHNIQUES

A. *General directives*

In order to fix the eyeball we place a curved and toothless Pean forceps right on the limbus. We prefer this instrument to a traction suture because it allows the assistant to move the eye in any direction required. It is of great importance to place this instrument at the correct place; for a rectus muscle this means just in front of its insertion

(*) Orthoptic Department, University Eye Clinic of Leiden, The Netherlands.
Centre of Strabology, 44 Karel Oomsstreet, 2000 Antwerp, Belgium.

and for an oblique muscle just between the two neighbouring rectus muscles. The ciliary vessels can serve as a landmark. On placing the Pean forceps at the right place one can use it as a point of reference when a turning of the eye during the operation interferes with a good orientation.

The place of the conjunctival incision needs some comment: one must avoid cutting too far away from the limbus: the greater the distance from the cornea the greater the risk of bleeding because of increased vascularization. Besides, as the conjunctival wound has a tendency to adhere to the sclera, a localization near the fornix can impede the eye movements by traction on the eyelids. Personally we make the incision at 1 cm from and parallel to the limbus.

In order to operate on a rectus muscle the conjunctiva is incised in front of the muscle's insertion. The capsule of Tenon has to be opened laterally to this insertion in order to avoid damaging the ciliary vessels. The latter, two or three in number, run along the surface of the muscle and, crossing the insertion, they continue their course towards the limbus. They often bend towards the insertion of the neighbouring rectus muscles so that, in order to avoid bleeding, one must lift up the capsule whilst cutting it and avoid touching the sclera with the points of the scissors.

Once the capsule of Tenon is opened a squint hook is placed underneath the tendon of the rectus muscle. One should not make a giant sweep, in order not to grasp the deeper lying tissues. This is especially true for the lateral rectus where the inferior oblique muscle can be hooked and for the superior rectus where the tendon of the superior oblique is adjacent.

To obtain a clean white canthus we remove the capsule of Tenon in front of the insertion of the rectus muscle (fig. 1); this prevents the

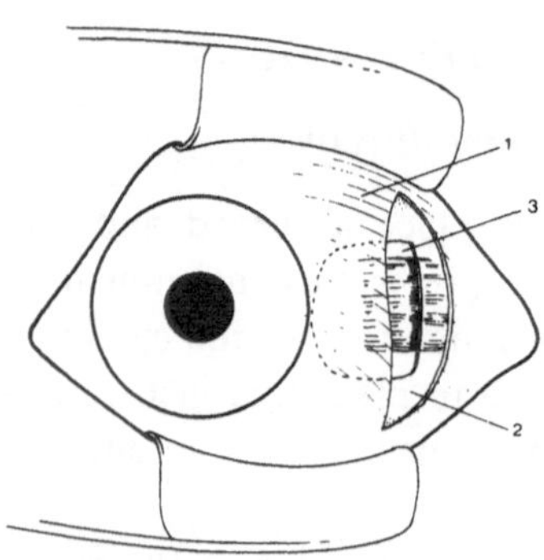

1. Conjunctiva
2. Tenon's capsule
3. Sclera

Fig. 1. — Excision of Tenon's capsule in front of the muscle (dotted line).

capsule from retracting towards the limbus and from becoming a vascularized thickness which gives the canthus an unaesthetic reddish aspect (fig. 27a). Concerning the lateral rectus we carefully cut away the remnant tendon at the original insertion in order not to attract attention to the blue area behind it.

The suture we use is 6/0 Vicryl but other sutures may be good as well on the condition that they are thin and non irritant; therefore we strongly advise against the use of catgut which may produce an allergic reaction, especially if it was already used before. On the rectus muscles we use two sutures, one on each side of the tendon. We never knot the thread over the tendon itself because we want to reduce the amount of foreign material as much as possible; if one takes a firm bite on the tendon the muscle will not slip. Notwithstanding all precautions the suture may tear out of the tendon and remain suspended in the perimysium; the slackness of the grip makes one aware of this and a look at the inner surface of the muscle will show the tendon which may be retracted several millimeters (fig. 2).

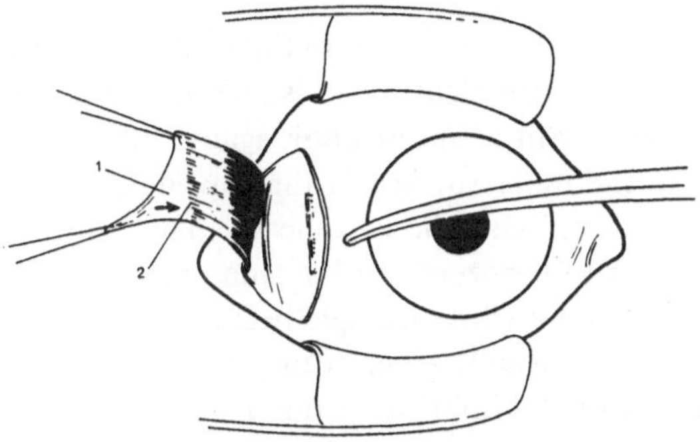

1. Perimysium
2. Retracted tendon

Fig. 2. — The tendon is torn out and retracts into the perimysium (arrow).

The check ligaments of a rectus muscle will be stretched by a recession especially when it is a large one and this could result in a duction limitation; in case of a resection, the check ligaments will be pulled forwards dragging the surrounding tissues with them. To avoid this, one can cut these check ligaments but the remedy risks to be worse than the disease if traumatism results in adhesions. Where the horizontal recti are concerned we advise cutting the check ligaments only in older children and in reoperations. The check ligaments of the vertical recti however always need to be cut in order to avoid traction upon the tarsus; this is especially true with the inferior rectus.

We can avoid bleeding by saving the ciliary vessels until the last possible moment. The largest ciliary vessels fortunately lie free on the tendon and can be picked up in the suture. Once the tendon is cut the vessels will of course start bleeding but, as the muscle retracts, they are twisted with a slackening of the blood flow as a result. Bleeding can be stopped by squeezing the tendon between the conjunctiva and the sclera by means of a squint hook whilst sticking the needle into the sclera (fig. 3).

It is not always that easy to localize the correct place of reinsertion; therefore attention must be paid to the blue area behind the original insertion which can serve as a guide.

Before closing the wound it is very important to check if no surrounding tissue is gripped in the sutures of the muscle. The conjunctival incision is closed with one or more sutures, say one every 5 mm.

In order to operate on the inferior oblique muscle the conjunctival incision is made in the temporal under quadrant at 1 cm from and parallel to the limbus; care must be taken to cut through the capsule of Tenon, the temporal portion of the muscle lying inside the capsule (fig. 4).

After having opened the capsule of Tenon the oblique muscle must be brought out at sight. The muscle can clearly be visualised by pulling up the capsule and by pressing it with a squint hook against the lower tarsus. The muscle adheres to the inner surface of the capsule and not to the sclera and it will be lifted up with the capsule so that it can be easily gripped by means of a pair of tweezers. With a small squint hook the muscle is *pulled caudally* so that a white triangle becomes visible in the depth (fig. 5). A vorticose vein usually runs in the nasal tip of this triangle, at the temporal border of the inferior rectus. It is worthwhile having a look at this vorticose vein because it sometimes lies very close to the posterior border of the inferior oblique; in some cases it even penetrates into the muscle body. If one does not pay attention the vorticose vein can easily be hooked up and cut together with the inferior oblique.

The squint hook is carefully put in in the temporal tip of the white triangle and the muscle is hooked up before the pair of tweezers releases its grasp. During this manoeuvre the squint hook must remain pointed straight temporalwards in order not to pick up the fibrous extensions of Lockwood's ligament. Once the muscle is lifted one must check the white triangle again to make sure that the muscle did not slip. It is unnecessary to pass the squint hook between the muscle and the capsule of Tenon.

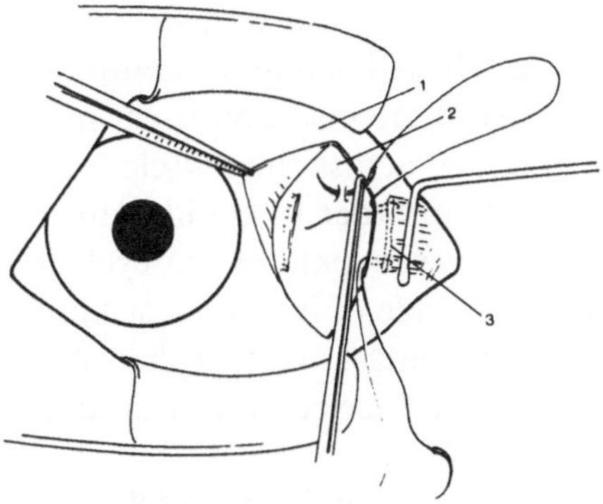

1. Conjunctiva
2. Sclera
3. Muscle stump

Fig. 3. — Compression of the muscle stump by means of a squint hook in order to stop bleeding whilst inserting the needle into the sclera.

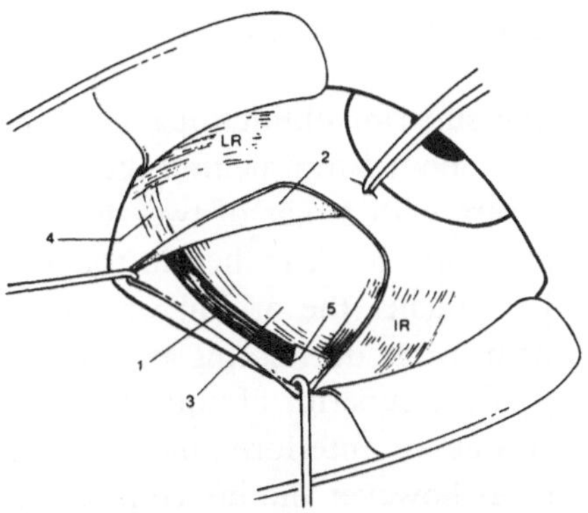

1. Inferior oblique muscle
2. Tenon's capsule
3. Bulbus
4. Inferior oblique disappearing underneath the lateral rectus
5. Aperture through which the inferior oblique penetrates Tenon's capsule.

Fig. 4. — The temporal part of the inferior oblique muscle lying inside Tenon's capsule.

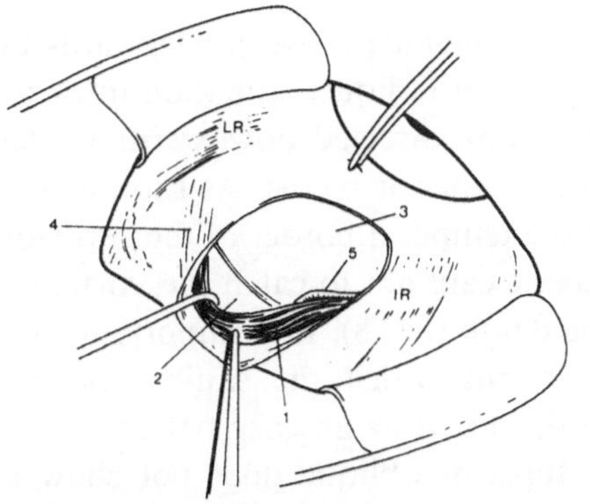

1. Inferior oblique muscle
2. Posterior part of Tenon's capsule forming the white triangle
3. Bulbus
4. Inferior oblique running towards the lateral rectus
5. Vorticose vein

Fig. 5. — The white triangle.

In case the inferior oblique has to be displaced the suture is placed before the muscle is cut because a bleeding muscle stump can impede a good view; then the anterior part of the insertion is cut near the sclera whilst the posterior part is sectioned across the muscle fibres, the scissors being pointed temporalwards in order to avoid damaging the ciliary vessels and nerves of the posterior pole of the eyeball. Once the muscle is severed an inspection is made of its posterior border in order to make sure that the perimysium is intact and that the whole muscle is detached (fig. 6). Indeed any uncut posterior fibres can undo the effect of the operation.

In order to operate on the superior oblique muscle an incision is made through the conjunctiva and the capsule of Tenon in the temporal upper quadrant. A squint hook is placed under the superior rectus in order to pull the eye downwards. A long spatula of 5 mm width and 15 mm length is introduced in the wound and lifted up; in this way the sclera is clearly exposed (fig. 7).

The anterior tip of the tendon of the superior oblique lies near the temporal border of the superior rectus at about 5 mm behind the insertion of this muscle. On grasping the sclera with a pair of tweezers one can easily pick up the tendon. A small squint hook is then introduced underneath and pushed nasally until it touches the orbital wall. Care must be taken to remain as anterior as possible during this manoeuvre because otherwise the posterior fibres of the superior oblique could be perforated; indeed the latter sometimes curve anteriorly and insert at the nasal upper quadrant of the sclera. If however the insertion of the superior oblique cannot be gripped the squint hook may be introduced underneath the tendon of the superior rectus with the point being directed anteriorly. Once the nasal orbital wall is reached the point is turned backwards.

The following step of the procedure is making a sweep backwards in order to pull out the tendon of the superior oblique. Attention must be paid to keep the point of the squint hook directed downwards to the sclera in order to avoid picking up the superior rectus. As soon as the point of the squint hook appears at the temporal border of the superior rectus it must be turned upwards taking care not to catch the vorticose vein which can easily be seen in the depth (fig. 8). It is important that the assistant releases the superior rectus whilst the squint hook is passed underneath the muscle in order to allow an easy passage.

Unlike the inferior oblique, the superior oblique does not show a white triangle in the depth. Therefore, after having cut the tendon, one

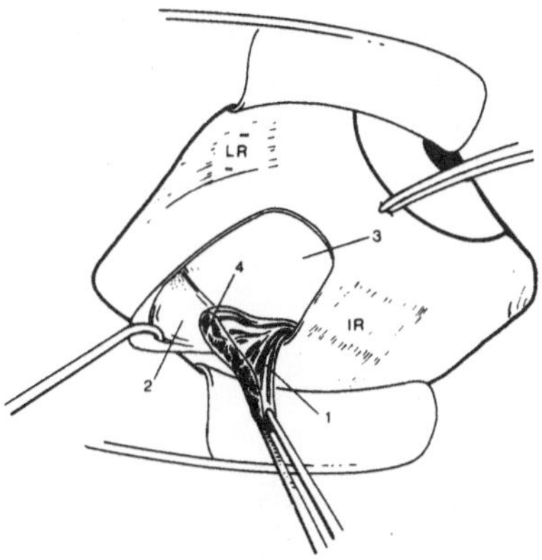

1. Inferior oblique muscle
2. Capsule of Tenon
3. Bulbus
4. Posterior border of the muscle

Fig. 6. — Control of the perimysium of the posterior border of the inferior oblique.

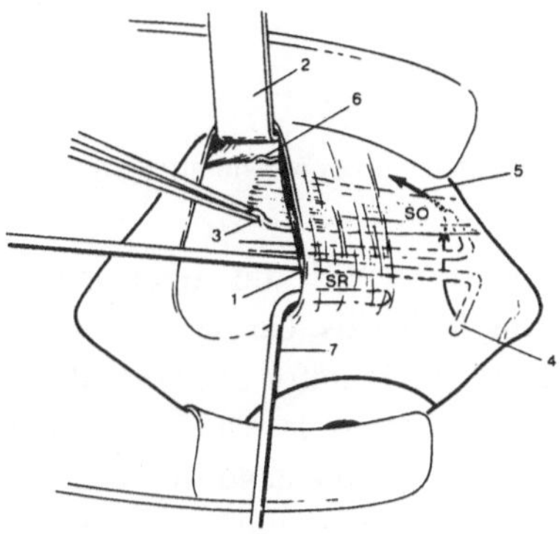

1. Temporal border of the superior rectus
2. Opening the wound with a long spatula
3. The anterior tip of the superior oblique's tendon
4. The point of the squint hook which is pushed underneath the superior rectus is turned backwards (arrow) once the nasal orbital wall is touched
5. Sweeping the squint hook backwards (arrow)
6. Vorticose vein
7. Squint hook pulling the eye downwards

Fig. 7. — Catching the superior oblique muscle of the right eye.

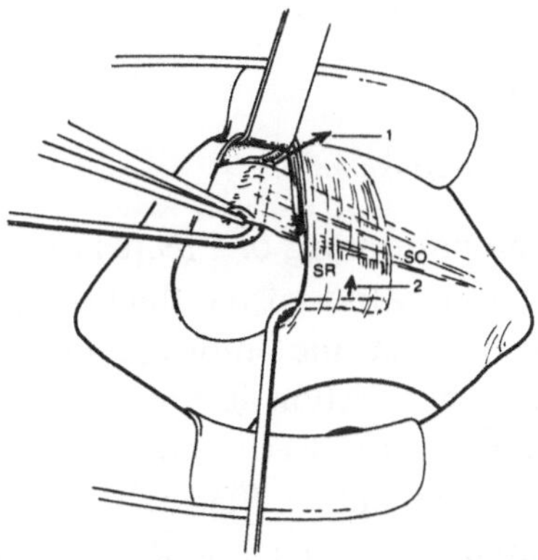

Fig. 8. — Turning upwards the point of the squint hook (arrow 1) after it appears at the temporal border of the superior rectus which is released during this manoeuvre (arrow 2).

must push the squint hook backwards along the original insertion to make sure that no posterior fibres remain attached to the sclera (fig. 9). In case the tendon is not completely severed the squint hook bumps against the remaining fibres producing an intorsion and an abduction of the eye.

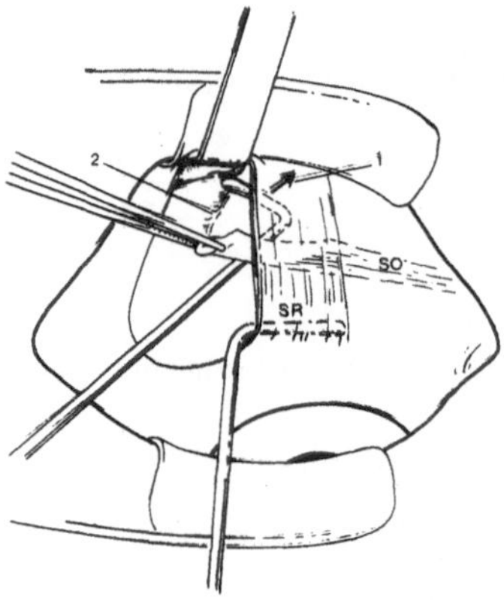

1. Direction in which the squint hook is pushed
2. The original insertion

Fig. 9. — The final control to make sure that no posterior fibres remain attached to the sclera.

The superior oblique has no firm connections with the superior rectus so that it is not prevented from slipping forwards. Consequently the tendon can reattach to the sclera anterior to the equatorial plane of the eye thus inverting the secondary actions of the muscle which becomes an adductor instead of an abductor and an elevator instead of a depressor. In order to prevent this complication one must push the tendon backwards before closing the wound.

B. *Specific directives*

1. *Strengthening procedures*

Strengthening of a rectus muscle

A tucking or an anteropositioning of a rectus muscle is to be avoided because of esthetical reasons. Indeed the thickening of the tendon will result in a reddish swelling near the limbus giving the aspect of a pseudostrabismus. Therefore a resection is the procedure of choice. The capsule of Tenon in front of the insertion must be excised to prevent it from curling up towards the limbus (fig. 27b).

After a muscle clamp has been fixed on the tendon a suture is placed near each border of the muscle and at the given distance of the insertion. After having cut the tendon the sutures are inserted in the sclera at

1 mm of each end of the insertion. This way the tendon will be spread so that the middle part cannot retract.

Before closing the wound special care must be given to keep the plica semilunaris in place. After a resection of the medial rectus muscle the eye will remain in an adducted position during the anaesthesia and the following sleep. The conjunctival wound lying near to the muscle stump will adhere to it, thus fixing the plica near the limbus and folding the conjunctiva over the cornea. When the eye regains a straight position the plica is pulled with it resulting in an unaesthetic aspect of pseudostrabismus (fig. 10). To avoid this complication one must fix the conjunctiva to the muscle's insertion. Therefore a suture is passed through the conjunctiva at about 5 mm from the limbus and knotted after the middle of the tendon and of the scleral insertion is picked up (fig. 11). In this way, the conjunctiva is shoved between the wound and

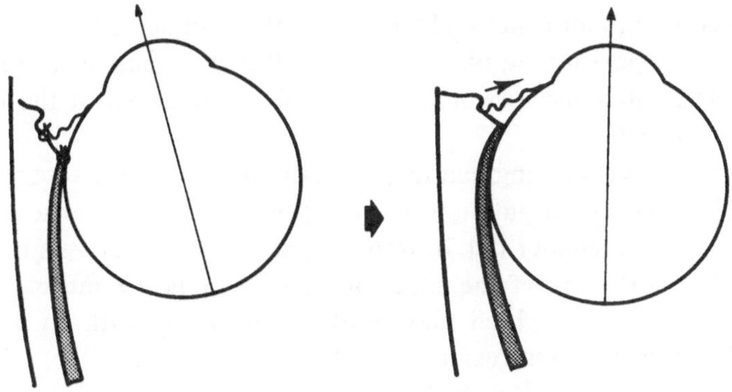

Fig. 10. — Attraction of the plica semilunaris towards the limbus: if the muscle stump touches the conjunctival wound they will adhere and when the eye regains a straight position the plica is pulled with it (arrow).

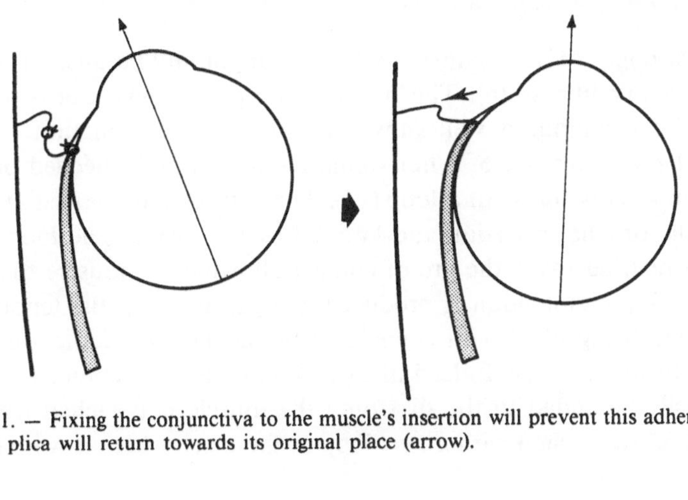

Fig. 11. — Fixing the conjunctiva to the muscle's insertion will prevent this adherence so that the plica will return towards its original place (arrow).

the muscle stump preventing them from adhering. Once the swelling has disappeared the plica will retract towards the internal canthus.

Strengthening of an oblique muscle

A strengthening of the inferior oblique is always carried out at the temporal side of the inferior rectus. A shortening of the tendon of the superior oblique can be done on the nasal as well as on the temporal side of the superior rectus. We prefer not to strengthen the tendon at the nasal side because the fold can bump against the trochlea limiting the action of the muscle. In our opinion the best technique of strengthening the superior oblique is a tuck at the temporal side attaching the fold to the sclera in order to prevent the tendon from slipping back to its original place.

In practice the difficulties of a good exposure of the deep lying operation area makes an exact realignment of the muscle rather illusive. A certain anteropositioning of the line of pull of the muscle seems to be inevitable so that the torsional action will be enhanced at the cost of the vertical one.

We do not like a strengthening procedure of an oblique muscle. This surgery implies a manipulation in the depth and near the posterior pole of the eye with a greater risk of traumatism and consecutive adhesions. Besides, a shortening of the superior oblique pulls the muscle's body towards the trochlea which may limit the elevation with an acquired Brown's syndrome as a result.

2. *Weakening procedures*

Weakening of a rectus muscle

We strongly advise against any form of myotomy because of the risk of secondary fibrosis (6). The best and simplest weakening is a recession. The technique is well-known and needs no explanation.

If a larger recession of a horizontal rectus muscle is needed one can perform a recession with a loop (14). The sutures are inserted at 5 mm from the original insertion and knotted over a probe. The loop which thus is realised saves the arc of contact allowing the muscle to retract further. A pseudotendon is produced, the gap between the tendon and the sclera being filled with connective tissue. This pseudotendon even allows further surgery. Indeed in case of an undercorrection a new loop can easily be added to the first one: the muscle is detached from the sclera and reattached with a new loop at the place where it was sutured at the first instance (fig. 12). We thus can distinguish a primary loop which is placed on a muscle that has not yet been recessed and a secondary one which is placed on an already recessed muscle. We also make a distinction between a small loop which is made by means of a probe with a diametre of $1\frac{1}{2}$ mm and a large one that is obtained by means of a 2 mm probe.

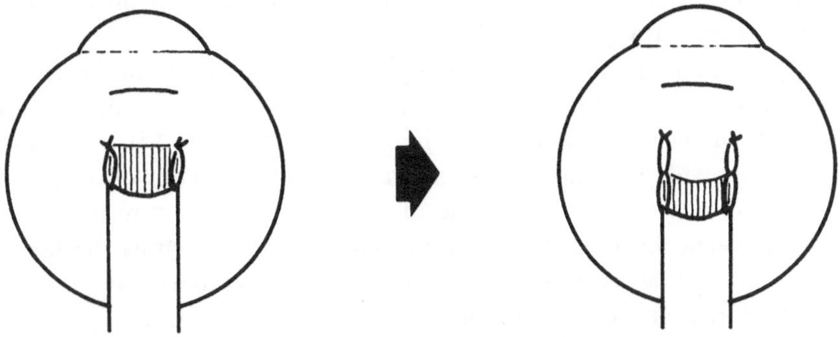

Fig. 12. — Primary and secondary loop recession: the gap between the tendon and the sclera is filled up with connective tissue (left); the pseudotendon thus produced can be hung in a new loop (right).

A slanted recession of a rectus muscle is advocated by some surgeons (25). One extremity of the tendon is recessed more than the other. In this way, the effect of the recession varies with the vertical position of the eye.

A central tenotomy of a rectus muscle can be performed if one needs to perform less than a recession. The middle part of the tendon is cut near the sclera and a small part of 1 mm width is left attached at each extremity of the insertion so that the middle of the muscle can retract (fig. 13). This procedure results in a weakening which is of temporary

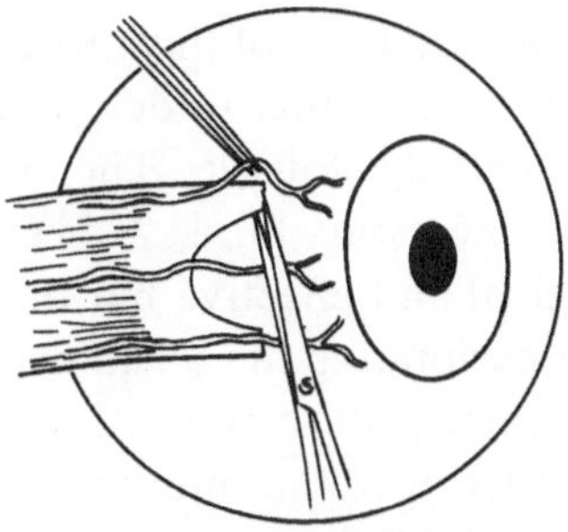

Fig. 13. — Central tenotomy of a rectus muscle: the middle part of the tendon is cut near the sclera while the scissors are passed underneath the ciliary vessels.

nature in many cases, the tendon creeping back to the original insertion. While cutting the tendon the ciliary vessels should be avoided if possible by passing the scissors underneath; in this way other rectus muscles can be operated on if necessary without a risk of anterior segment ischemia. Care must be also be taken to cut any foot plate insertions present; these can easily be missed as they run several millimeters behind the original insertion. If left unsevered they will prevent the muscle from retracting.

A particular method of weakening a rectus muscle is the posterior fixation suture (9). This procedure reduces the muscular response to an excessive innervation by limiting the arc of contact (fig. 14). Therefore the muscle body is sutured to the sclera behind the equator of the globe by placing one stitch at each side of the muscle; the suture is passed twice through the muscle leaving its border free. Care must be taken not to damage the vorticose veins nor the posterior ciliary artery which has its intrascleral course just in between.

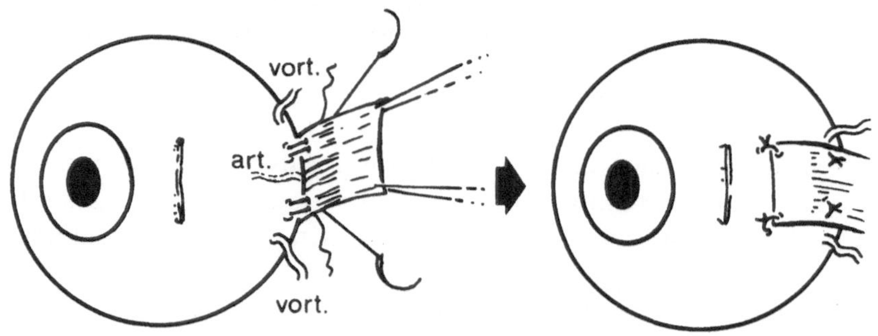

Fig. 14. — Posterior fixation suture (Faden operation). The muscle is fixed to the sclera behind the equator of the globe, the sutures being placed between the vorticose veins and the posterior ciliary artery.

In order to facilitate the approach one can temporarily disinsert the rectus muscle but the disadvantages of this procedure are the number of sutures lying about and the difficulty to determine the correct place of passing the suture through the muscle. Therefore it is better not to detach the muscle if not necessary (3, 4, 7, 11).

The operation is original and effective but there are some disadvantages. There is a risk of perforating the sclera near to the macula and of damaging the neurovascular pedicle behind the eye (31). Furthermore, the part of the muscle anterior to the suture may atrophy and extensive adhesions may arise in the depth.

A way of avoiding a perforation is to put the needle in the upper layers of the sclera compensating the depth of the stitch by its length (2 mm). A good exposure of the operation area is also helpful but the excessive traction on the eye which is required enhances the risk of damaging the neurovascular pedicle. Therefore a frequent control of the pupil is necessary and if mydriasis shows up traction on the eyeball must be released for a while.

Atrophy of the muscle can be avoided by girding instead of fixing the muscle (33). The thread is not passed through but over the muscle taking care not to strangulate it when tying (fig. 15).

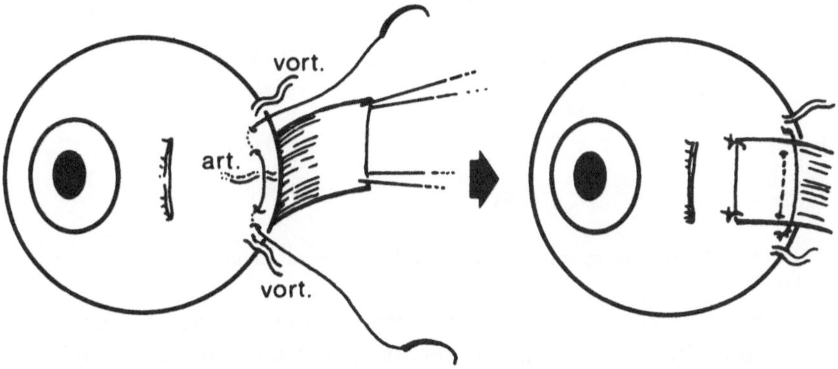

Fig. 15. — The posterior fixation can also be realised by girding instead of fixing the muscle.

Extensive adhesions in the depth are probably the most frequent complications (34). Personally we have encountered adhesions which were so strong that it became impossible to detach the muscle from the sclera and to restore the arc of contact. In that event the operation creates an irreversible situation.

Weakening of an oblique muscle

We advise against a myotomy in the muscle's body because of the bleeding and the risk of adhesions which can induce a recurrence of the elevation in adduction. A recession is the best method of weakening an inferior oblique. The muscle is detached from its insertion and reattached to the sclera along its course. We reattach the anterior tip of the muscle halfway between the lateral and the inferior rectus and *as far back as possible* without taking a risk of perforation. A second stitch in the dept is superfluous as the muscle lies smoothly against the sclera and is kept in place by the capsule of Tenon. The posterior fibres are allowed to retract as they are responsible for the vertical action of the muscle.

In order to obtain a maximal weakening a disinsertion of the inferior oblique can be done. The muscle is cut at its insertion so that it can retract freely towards the inferior rectus. To prevent the muscle stump from readhering to its original insertion we close the aperture through which it penetrates the capsule of Tenon (fig. 16).

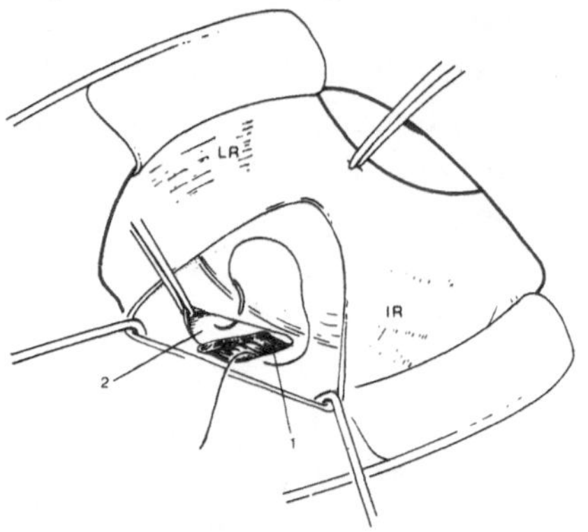

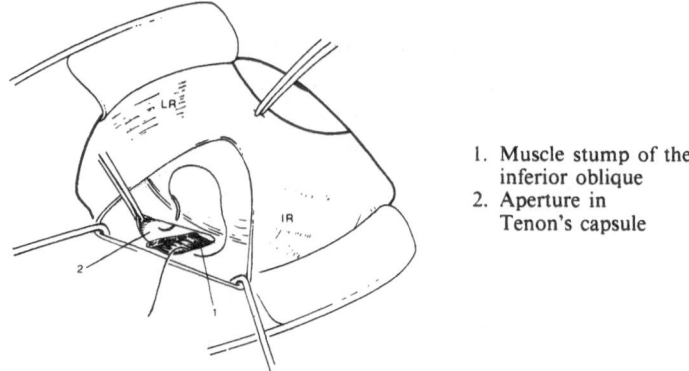

1. Muscle stump of the inferior oblique
2. Aperture in Tenon's capsule

Fig. 16. — Closing the aperture through which the inferior oblique penetrates the capsule of Tenon.

In order to weaken the superior oblique muscle one can perform a recession with a loop (19). The tendon is cut near the sclera and reattached to the original insertion by means of a loop of about 5 mm length and *as far back as possible.* Care must be taken to put the knot at the height of the insertion in order not to place it underneath the superior rectus.

A disinsertion may be carried out in extreme cases. The tendon of the superior oblique is cut at the scleral insertion without being reattached. This procedure gives excellent results but can lead to a paresis of the muscle.

3. *Transpositioning procedures*

Transpositioning of a rectus muscle

The horizontal rectus muscles may be displaced up or downwards (24) and the vertical recti nasal or temporalwards (28). Half measures are of little value: one has to displace the muscle at least 5 mm. Our transpositions equalize the width of the insertion; we fix one tip of the tendon at the height of the opposite end of the scleral insertion and we stretch the tendon parallel to the limbus. In this way, the second stitch will be placed near to the insertion of the neighboring rectus muscle so that attention must be paid not to damage the ciliary vessels of the latter.

A transpositioning of the horizonal recti will be combined with a resection or a recession. Combined with a recession it could lead to a duction limitation so that either the recession or the vertical displacement has to be reduced. A transpositioning of the vertical recti is rarely combined with a strengthening or a weakening procedure so that the tendon can be displaced full width; this can be done without any noticeable influence on the vertical movements. Concerning the inferior rectus the connections with the inferior oblique should be cut in order to avoid a limitation of depression by traction on Lockwood's ligament.

Transpositioning of an oblique muscle

The point of attachment of an oblique muscle can be displaced forwards so that the line of pull becomes less sagittal (16). Concerning the inferior oblique this sagittalisation is obtained by means of a posterior myectomy, an anteropositioning or a disinsertion (fig. 17).

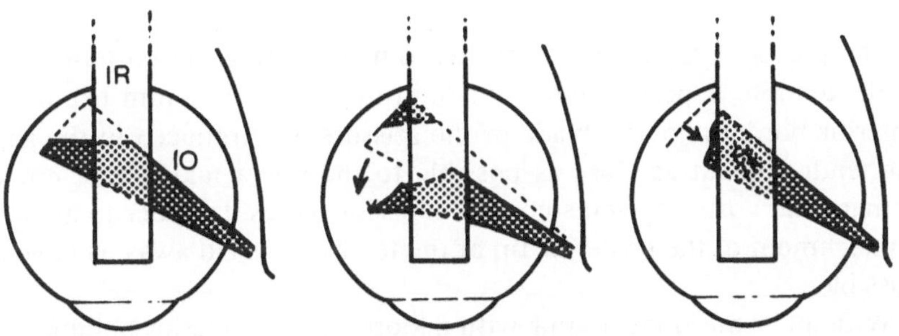

Fig. 17. — Desagittalization of the inferior oblique muscle; from left to right: posterior myectomy, anteropositioning and disinsertion.

The posterior myectomy is carried out by cutting the posterior part of the muscle's insertion leaving it attached to the sclera by a strand of 2 mm. After having pulled the muscle up and caudalwards we grip the anterior tip of the insertion and we place one scissor blade just behind the tweezers and the other one in the white triangle which appears in the depth. We then cut the posterior part of the muscle keeping the scissors pointed temporalwards.

In order to perform an anteropositioning we detach the muscle from the sclera after having placed a suture *at the equator of the globe*, halfway between the inferior and the lateral rectus. We reattach the anterior tip of the muscle allowing the posterior part to retract freely (15).

With a disinsertion we cut the whole muscle so that it can retract towards the inferior rectus where it is held by means of the connections between both muscles.

A transpositioning of the superior oblique consists of a posterior tenectomy, an anteropositioning with a loop or a disinsertion (fig. 18).

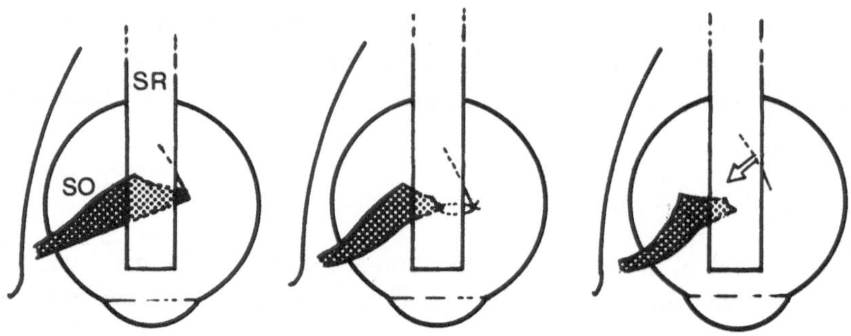

Fig. 18. — Desagittalization of the superior oblique muscle; from left to right: posterior tenectomy, anteropositioning with a loop and disinsertion.

The posterior tenectomy is carried out by cutting the posterior part of the tendon. A perforation is made in the tendon at 2 mm behind its anterior border and one blade of the scissors is introduced in the gap; the tendon is cut as close as possible to the sclera taking care not to damage the vorticose veins nor the superior rectus. In order to avoid a reattachment of the posterior tip of the tendon it is cut away as large as possible.

With an "anteropositioning with a loop" of the superior oblique, the whole tendon is cut and the anterior tip is reattached to the *anterior extremity of the insertion.* The thread is pulled forwards and knotted over the squint hook which is placed under the superior rectus: the length of the loop thus produced equalizes the distance between the insertion of both muscles. The knot must be pushed against the scleral insertion so that it cannot induce adhesions underneath the superior rectus.

A disinsertion of the superior oblique consists of a free retraction of the tendon towards the trochlea. After the tendon has been cut close to the sclera the posterior part is removed in order to prevent it from readhering to the posterior pole of the globe.

In some cases the anterior part of the tendon of the superior oblique is strengthened selectively in order to enhance the torsional action of the muscle leaving its vertical action unaffected (18). The anterior third of the tendon is pulled forwards and temporalwards and is attached to the sclera with a single stitch (fig. 19); the same procedure can be applied to the inferior oblique as it is possible to divide the muscle along its anteroposterior axis. A recession of the anterior part of the antagonist is added. We could also consider however performing a tenotomy of the anterior part of one oblique muscle and of the posterior part of its antagonist.

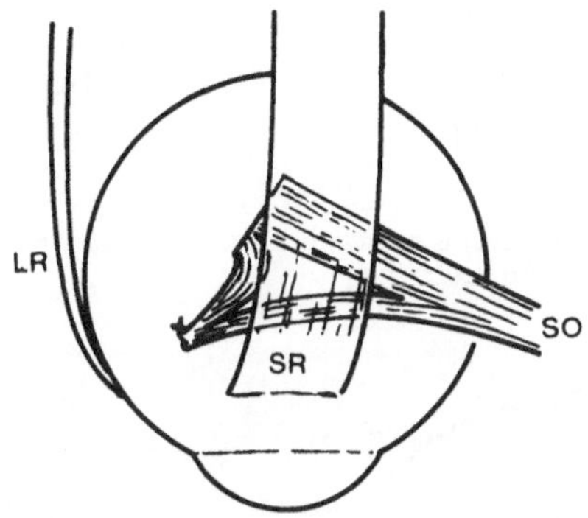

Fig. 19. — Strengthening of the anterior part of the tendon of the superior oblique.

SURGICAL EFFECTS

1. *Surgery of the horizontal rectus muscles*

A muscle is not strengthened by a shortening, it is tightened; thus a resection of a muscle does not enhance its force, it only changes the position of the eye supposing the innervation reaching the muscles remains unchanged before and after the operation. In addition a large shortening can be effective by means of the mechanical resistance against the eye movements it introduces. In this way a large resection of a lateral rectus acts as a progressive brake against the adduction excess: the more the eye is adducted the more the shortened lateral rectus is stretched and the more resistance the muscle will offer (fig. 20). This progressive brake of course depends on both the amount of shortening and the elasticity of the muscle. As a consequence an excessive resection can exceed the limits of this elasticity and thus create such a powerful brake that the adduction is limited, resulting in a "tight lateral rectus syndrome" (21).

In the same way a recession of a muscle within the normal limits does not weaken but it releases the muscle. In addition to the change of

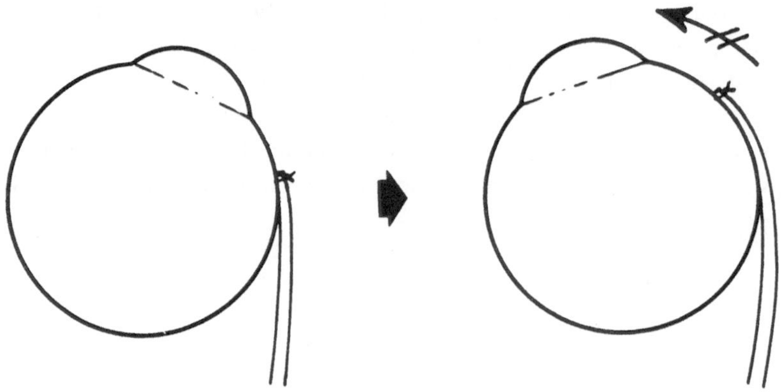

Fig. 20. — A resection of a rectus muscle induces a progressive brake against the duction towards the opposite side (crossed arrow).

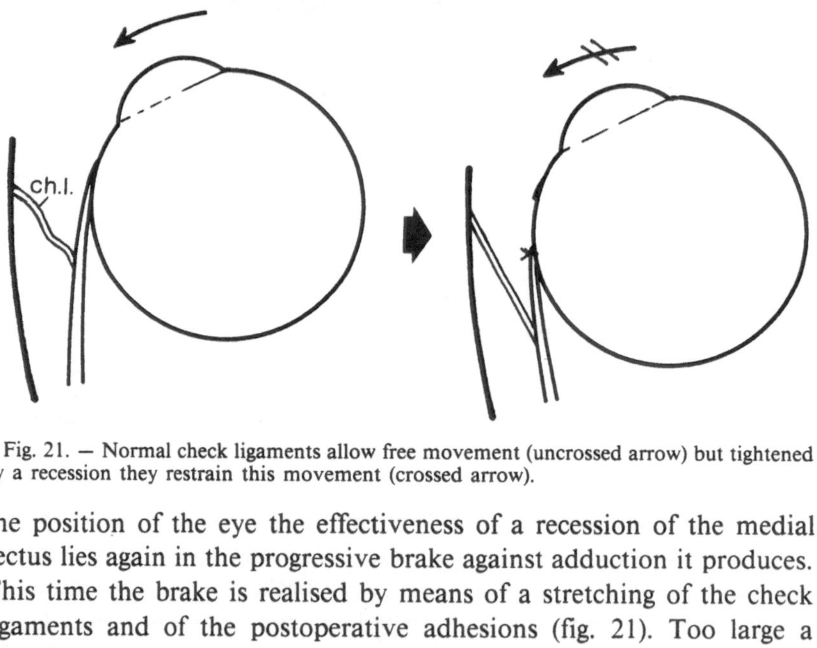

Fig. 21. — Normal check ligaments allow free movement (uncrossed arrow) but tightened by a recession they restrain this movement (crossed arrow).

the position of the eye the effectiveness of a recession of the medial rectus lies again in the progressive brake against adduction it produces. This time the brake is realised by means of a stretching of the check ligaments and of the postoperative adhesions (fig. 21). Too large a recession or too strong an adhesion will create such a powerful brake that the adduction becomes limited.

The force of the progressive brake depends for a great deal on the immediate postoperative position of the operated eye. If the latter presents a large divergent position during the first days after surgery the brake will be stronger: if the adhesions are formed with the eye in an abducted position they will be more tightened on adduction indeed than if they were formed with the eye in a straight position (fig. 22).

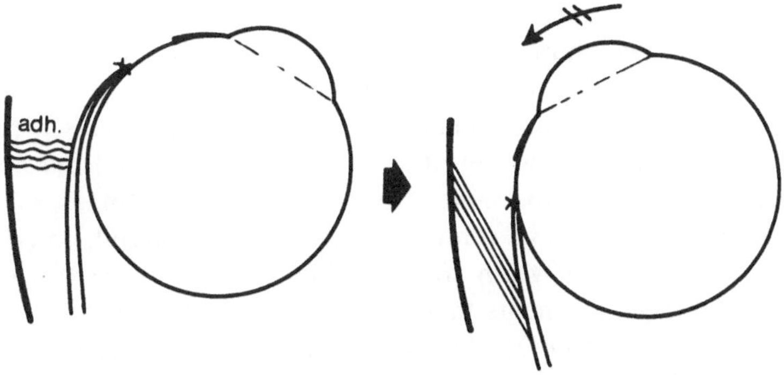

Fig. 22. — Adhesions can act as a progressive brake (crossed arrow) especially when formed with the eye being turned to the opposite side.

A combination of a recession of a medial rectus with a resection of the homolateral antagonist undoubtedly enhances the effect of the operation and, when combined, these procedures have a greater effect as when performed separately. We think that the explanation can be found in the fact that a combined surgery puts the eye in a more abducted position in the immediate postoperative period thus resulting in a stronger progressive brake against adduction.

A combination of a recession of a medial rectus with a recession of the contralateral medial rectus also increases the effect of surgery. The cause lies again in the fact that the squinting eye will present a greater abducted position postoperatively with a stronger brake as a consequence. This time the greater abducted position of the squinting eye is obtained by an increase of contraction of the lateral rectus which is induced by the recession of the medial rectus of the fixing eye (Hering's law).

It is very important to put the progressive brake on the squinting eye as it has to compensate for the adduction excess of this eye. The effect of monocular surgery is maximum indeed when the non operated eye is fixing but is reduced considerably when the operated eye is fixing.

The posterior fixation suture reduces the rotating power of the muscle without influencing the position of the eye in the primary position (9). The intervention is essentially a surgery of the arc of contact (30). The arc of contact of the medial rectus covers 30° and within this limit the muscle has a maximum rotating effect as it does not unroll completely. Behind this limit the rotating effect of the muscle decreases and the retraction effect increases. The posterior fixation suture reduces the arc of contact and the further back the muscle is fixed the more it becomes a retractor bulbi.

If the muscle is not recessed at the same time the operation of Cüppers gives a maximum strength reduction with a minimum length reduction (10). However, in many instances the strength reduction will not only be due to the abolition of the arc of contact: the muscle part in front of the suture is put out of action and can even undergo fibrosis which practically has the same effect as a large myectomy.

The posterior fixation suture also acts as a powerful progressive brake. The adhesions which are formed and which can be very extensive act as check ligaments thus impeding the adduction.

A slanted recession of the horizontal rectus muscles makes the action of the muscle dependent of the vertical gaze: if the upper tip of the muscle has been displaced further back than the lower one, the effect of the recession will be maximum in elevation; conversely if the lower tip of the muscle is recessed more the effect will be greater in depression.

A vertical displacement of the horizontal recti is based on the vertical effect these muscles obtain in the vertical directions of gaze: the horizontal rectus assists the elevation on looking up and the depression on looking down while its horizontal action diminishes in these directions of gaze. This side effect of the horizontal recti can be enhanced when these rectus muscles are displaced vertically: when the insertion of the muscle is displaced downwards its horizontal action is weakened favoring the depression; if the insertion is displaced upwards the horizontal action is reduced in favour of the elevation.

2. *Surgery of the vertical rectus muscles*

Surgery of a vertical rectus muscle has primarily an effect on the vertical position of the eye. This effect is greatest in the field of action of the muscle; surgery of the superior rectus will thus have its greatest effect in elevation and surgery of the inferior rectus in depression. But the secondary actions of the muscle are also influenced: the horizontal and torsional actions are reduced by a recession and increased by a resection. A recession of the superior rectus thus decreases the adduction and the intorsion in the upper field of gaze and a recession of the inferior rectus reduces the adduction and extorsion in the lower field of gaze.

These secondary actions of a vertical rectus can selectively be influenced by a lateral displacement. A temporal displacement of the muscle reduces its adducting effect but increases its torsional effect and a nasal displacement increases the adduction and decreases the torsion.

With regard to the vertical effect of this procedure one should take into account the fact that a temporal displacement tightens the muscle and a nasal displacement relaxes it.

3. *Surgery of the oblique muscles*

The action of an oblique muscle is weakened in total with a recession and strengthened with a resection: the horizontal, vertical and torsional components are all influenced by the same amount. But we can influence these components selectively by displacing the scleral insertion forwards so that the course of the muscle becomes less sagittal. This desagittalization enlarges the angle between the line of pull of the muscle and the visual axis so that the vertical and horizontal action of the muscle are weakened in favour of the torsional action.

A displacement forwards and temporalwards of an oblique muscle reinforces its torsional action not only because it enlarges the angle between the muscle and the visual axis but also because it strengthens the anterior part of the muscle which has a greater torsional action than the posterior part.

SURGICAL INDICATIONS

I. Conventional surgery

A. *General directives*

What is the advisable time for surgery? The answer is: in principle as soon as an amblyopia has been eliminated. A problem arises however when a child has a birth onset of squint. Proper diagnosis is difficult because of the poor cooperation of the child and the risk of a surgical overcorrection or undercorrection is great. On the other hand we should not lose time so that many surgeons are inclined to operate at a younger age than before, when surgery at the age of 4 or 5 was considered early.

An argument for early surgery is that it would give a better chance to obtain a functional result even though we may only obtain some degree of peripheral fusion whilst a foveal suppression of the non-dominant eye remains (29). Besides, early surgery can be indicated for psychological reasons and a long standing squint can give a contracture of the muscles, Tenon's capsule and conjunctiva.

For these reasons an operation for congenital esotropia is mandatory within the first 24 months of life and preferably during the first 12 months (7, 29) on the condition that the following criteria are met: presence of a stable and sufficiently large deviation, absence of an accommodative factor, alternating fixation behaviour after treatment of amblyopia and identification of associated vertical deviations or incomitances. Thus we may say that the ideal time for surgery is the time when the diagnosis is complete.

Concerning the choice of the appropriate surgical procedure several general rules play a part: a recession will have a greater effect than a resection of the same amount of millimeters; a recession-resection procedure will have a larger effect than a bilateral recession or a resection provided the surgery is carried out in the same session (6, 7, 8).

A recession of a single rectus muscle has to be avoided if possible. The relaxation results in a shortening of the muscle which can produce a restriction of its contractibility when the recession is a large one. In extreme cases anatomical changes can occur which limit the extensibility of the muscle. In order to avoid this complication the recessed muscle has to be tightened again by adding a resection of the homolateral rectus muscle (22) or a recession of the antagonistic medial rectus muscle (Hering's law).

As surgery induces a progressive brake against an active deviation (fig. 20 and 21) it should be carried out on the usually squinting eye. This means that a recession-resection procedure of the horizontal recti should be done. When there is a monocular squint this will give no problems. It is different however when there is an alternating squint: a bilateral medial rectus recession can have too little effect in each eye thus leading to a residual angle whereas a recession-resection procedure will have a good effect on the operated eye but not on the other one. As a consequence the patient will look straight when he fixes with the non operated eye, but he will show an undercorrection when he fixes with the operated eye. This problem can only be solved when 3 or 4 horizontal recti are operated on, which however can only be done in case of a large angle of squint.

Burian and Von Noorden (7) state that surgical procedures on the extra-ocular muscles should normalize the excursions of the eyes. Thus, in an esotropia with excessive adduction and normal abduction a maximal recession of the medial rectus muscle should be done and only a minimal resection of its antagonist. On the other hand, if deficient abduction is a prominent clinical feature, maximal resection of the lateral rectus muscle is combined with a small recession of the medial rectus muscle.

The principle of making eye movements concomitant also applies to vertical deviations: we should operate on the muscle which acts in the direction of the maximal deviation. Although vertical incomitances are best treated by means of surgery of the oblique muscles, we should bear in mind that it will not sufficiently reduce a large deviation.

The amount of surgical correction of the extra ocular muscles is notoriously unpredictable. The surgical results depend largely on the operative technique used, the manner in which the muscle is exposed and how thoroughly it is freed, whether the check ligaments are severed, placement of sutures and other factors. Each surgeon must through experience establish the approximative effectiveness of the procedure he or she routinely chooses to employ. Besides, the fact that within certain limits a residual angle can be corrected by peripheral fusion reflexes will falsify any statistical evaluation and will make the predictability of the effect of a certain procedure rather illusive.

Nevertheless there are some empirical rules that are helpful in determining the amount of surgery to perform. The effect of a given operation will be greater in young patients than in older ones, greater in variable or intermittent deviations than in constant ones, greater in deviations of short duration than in those of long duration, greater in larger deviations than in small ones, and greater when the deviation disappears under deep anaesthesia (8).

The maximum of surgery is determined by the risks of creating a duction limitation. In case of a recession the arc of contact may not be restricted to such an extent that the muscle can no longer unroll within the physiologic field of gaze. The recession is also limited by the extensibility of the check ligaments and of the postoperative adhesions. For the medial rectus the maximum recession is approximately 5 mm depending on the diameter of the globe. A recession of a vertical rectus amounts usually to 3 or 4 mm but may not exceed 5 mm and of a lateral rectus to 7 mm with a maximum of 10 mm.

In larger angles a recession with a loop may be carried out which allows the muscle to retract as far back as 10 mm without restricting the arc of contact (14). However the check ligaments are stretched proportionally increasing the risk of duction limitation.

A resection procedure is limited by the extensibility of the muscle. Beyond a certain amount the resection will exceed the limits of elasticity and the muscle can no longer be stretched sufficiently to permit a normal duction towards the opposite side. A 10 mm resection seems to be a maximum for a horizontal rectus and a 5 mm resection for a vertical rectus. However these limits are not as restrictive as for a recession and are conditioned, for instance, by the age of the patient and the appearance of the muscle.

General anaesthesia is always used for reoperations or for surgery on several muscles and of course in young patients. In general, the surgical plan should not be changed when the patient is on the operating table and general anaesthesia has caused a modification of the deviation, except when a forced duction test reveals mechanical obstacles not anticipated preoperatively.

B. *Specific directives*

1. *Primary surgery*

By primary surgery we mean surgery on a patient who has not had squint surgery before.

Treatment of horizontal deviations

Conventional surgery is limited to the non-accommodative element of the horizontal angle. This deviation can be corrected by means of a recession and/or a resection of the horizontal rectus muscles.

A bimedial recession has to be done when the following circumstances prevail: a bilateral fixation in adduction and/or a free alteration with a high AC/A ratio. Usually both medial rectus muscles are recessed the same amount. However, this is not mandatory; if adduction in one eye is significantly greater than in the fellow eye, an asymmetrical recession may be performed. When the angle is large this asymmetry can be performed by adding a loop to the recession on the non dominant eye.

If unilateral surgery is performed the medial rectus should not be recessed more than 5 mm when combined with a resection of the lateral rectus. Although we should not forget the risk of a "tight lateral rectus syndrome" (21) there are usually more problems created with resections which are too small than by those that are too large. A resection of the lateral rectus usually varies between 8 and 10 mm; less than 4 mm is of no use and a resection of more than 10 mm should only be carried out when cosmetic surgery is indicated e.g. with a blind or deep amblyopic eye. In those cases an excessive resection can be avoided by adding a loop to the recession-resection procedure; the adduction limitation which is thus created will enhance the effect of the operation and prevent a recurrence.

Considering the amount of surgery in esotropia Burian and Von Noorden (7) give the following guidelines: a minimal bimedial recession corrects 15$^{\Delta}$ to 20$^{\Delta}$ and a maximal bimedial recession up to 40$^{\Delta}$ A minimal amount of combined recession-resection in one eye can be expected to correct 20$^{\Delta}$ to 25$^{\Delta}$ and a maximal recession-resection procedure may correct 40$^{\Delta}$ to 50$^{\Delta}$. If the deviation exceeds 50$^{\Delta}$ a maximal bimedial recession is combined with a resection of the lateral rectus of the non-dominant eye; all horizontal rectus muscles are operated on, if the deviation exceeds 75$^{\Delta}$. In such large angles a bimedial rectus recession with a loop may be done, provided no limitation of adduction is created in the dominant eye.

The sensory state must also be considered. If the patient has a good functional potential for binocular vision, the surgeon should aim for complete alignment of the eyes. In those without a functional potential, less extensive surgery is required (29), since a cosmetically acceptable residual angle is desirable in order to avoid consecutive exotropia developing when the child grows older.

Recently interest has been revived in adjustable sutures which allow an increase or decrease of the effect of surgery by stretching or loosening the sutures during the postoperative period (23). However, the immediate postoperative position of the globe is not of much help in assessing the result of surgery. A perfect ocular alignment or an overcorrection or undercorrection present on the first postoperative day may disappear with time.

The dynamic part of the angle of squint can be neutralised by a posterior fixation suture. This dynamic part is the difference between the minimum and the maximum angle. The place of reattachment of the posterior fixation suture depends of course on the importance of the dynamic factor but also on the diameter of the eye and thus of the age of the patient (4). To be effective the suture must be placed far enough back without exceeding certain limits. The posterior fixation suture is placed between 12 and 15 mm behind the original insertion for a medial rectus. Of course one must consider the arc and not the chord so that the diameter of the eye should be known; according to Von Noorden (32) however the difference between both quantities may be neglected within the distance of 14 mm.

The dynamic factor frequently is associated with a static one. Thomas (31) and Ardouin (2) recommend looking for this static angle in lateroversion where it is smaller than in the primary position. This static angle is corrected by means of a classic recession-resection procedure (31); the medial rectus is recessed before the posterior fixation suture is fixed and a resection of the lateral rectus is added if necessary.

To conclude we will stress again the fact that the effect of surgery is largely dependent on the surgeon's hand: his surgical effect is determined by his training and experience so that he must adapt the choice of the surgical procedure and the amount of surgery to the results he obtains.

Treatment of diagonal deviations

By diagonal deviations we mean the vertical deviations which are most pronounced in the oblique directions of gaze. In fact they are the A and V incomitances.

The A and V incomitances can be reduced by surgery on the oblique muscles, by a vertical displacement of the horizontal recti, by a horizontal displacement of the vertical recti, or even by an oblique displacement of the horizontal recti.

Most ophthalmologists treat an elevation in adduction with a weakening of the inferior oblique muscle. After weakening an overacting inferior oblique muscle it is not unusual for an overaction in the fellow eye to become manifest (7); even a hypertropia of the non-operated eye can develop. Therefore bilateral inferior oblique weakening procedures should be carried out unless it has been clearly established that this muscle is not overacting in the fellow eye. Parks (29) recommends weakening the inferior oblique by means of a recession. This procedure corrects 15^{Δ} to 25^{Δ} of the V pattern between the primary position and up gaze, the effect increasing with the size of the preoperative deviation (7). In case there is only a slight elevation in adduction it may be neglected as it may disappear after horizontal surgery. Simply recessing the medial recti corrects approximately 10^{Δ} of V pattern.

An inferior oblique weakening procedure closes the V pattern in upward gaze and thus horizontal surgery almost always is mandatory, the amount of which should be planned according to the size of deviation in the primary position. Horizontal and oblique muscle surgery should be combined in one procedure.

If a hypoaction of the superior oblique is predominant this muscle can be strengthened. A tuck of the tendon at its insertion has the greatest effect, is safest and reduces incidence, severity and persistence of a postoperative Brown syndrome (19). It is impossible to give a number of millimeters for the correct amount of superior oblique tucking in a given case. However, it is safe to say that more errors are committed by making too small a tuck than too large. The amount to tuck varies between 12 and 22 mm depending on the vertical deviation and the laxity of the tendon.

In patients with an A pattern a weakening of the superior oblique is indicated; to counteract the predictable increase of the esotropia in downward gaze it is usual to combine horizontal surgery with this procedure. Bilateral weakening of the superior oblique should be done unless it is proven that an overaction of this muscle is strictly unilateral, since hypotropia almost invariably develops in the non-operated eye.

Weakening a superior oblique is accomplished by a tenotomy or a tenectomy, midway between the nasal border of the superior rectus muscle and the trochlea. According to Parks (29) this operation eliminates 40^{Δ} to 45^{Δ} of A pattern, the increase of the esodeviation in the primary position being approximately 15^{Δ} to 20^{Δ}. This procedure should not be used unless a large A pattern with marked overaction of the superior oblique muscles is present. Indeed a vertical deviation in the primary position is often produced postoperatively and in the patient who is able to fuse, a sustained head tilt may be adopted to compensate for the imbalance. To avoid these problems a loop recession of the tendon of the superior obliques can be carried out in less pronounced cases (19) and in slight A patterns a posterior tenectomy can be performed.

The A and V incomitances can also be reduced by adding a vertical displacement of the horizontal recti to the recession or resection of the muscle. The medial rectus should be displaced towards the closed end of the A or V and the lateral rectus towards the open end.

As for the indication for a vertical displacement, it will be carried out in A and V patterns without oblique muscle dysfunction. This procedure has been found to be effective not only in conjunction with symmetrical horizontal surgery but also with recession-resection operations on one eye (7).

Half width tendon transposition yields 15^{Δ} to 20^{Δ} change in the A or V pattern between up and down gaze. Full width transposition produces more improvement, but the frequent duction limitation in the field of action of the transposed muscle limits the usefulness of this procedure. In a V pattern we must remember that simply recessing the medial rectus muscles corrects approximately 10^{Δ} of the V; an infraplacement of the insertions corrects an additional 15^{Δ} and a recession of an associated overacting inferior oblique muscle corrects another 15^{Δ} of the V pattern (29).

Horizontal transposition of the vertical rectus muscles has been suggested as an alternative surgical approach (28). The quantity of transposition varies from half to full width of the tendon. In an A esotropia, the superior rectus is transposed temporally, thereby increasing its abductive effect in up gaze. When a V esotropia is present, the inferior rectus muscles are transposed temporally to increase the abduction in down gaze. However, since patients with an A or V pattern usually require horizontal surgery, most surgeons at present prefer to transpose the horizontal rectus muscles rather than risk anterior segment ischemia by operating on several rectus muscles in the same session.

Some authors have advocated a slanted recession and resection of the horizontal rectus muscles (25). In a V esotropia the lower margin of the medial rectus muscle is recessed further backwards or the lower margin of the lateral rectus muscle is resected more than the upper margin. In an A esotropia on the contrary, more recession is required of the upper margin of the medial rectus muscle and more resection of the upper margin of the lateral rectus muscle.

Treatment of torsional deviations

An excyclotropia can be treated with a weakening of the inferior oblique muscle but one has to consider the vertical side effect of this surgery. We can however selectively emphasize the torsional effect of the superior oblique muscle by displacing the anterior third of the tendon forwards and temporalwards (fig. 19). To this procedure a recession of the anterior part of the inferior oblique muscle can be added. The displacement reduces 3° of cyclodeviation per mm and a recession corrects 2° per mm.

An incyclotropia can be reduced by weakening the superior oblique but if we want to avoid the vertical side effect of this intervention the anterior part of the inferior oblique can be displaced forwards. A tenotomy of the anterior part of the superior oblique can be associated.

Treatment of vertical deviations

Incomitant vertical deviations are best corrected by surgery on one or two of the synergic muscles which have their vertical action in the direction of maximum deviation. If only one of the synergic muscles is operated on we should bear in mind that surgery of the vertical recti has a greater effect than surgery of the oblique muscles. We should also remember that a combination of two muscles has a greater effect if performed in one session than when they are operated on in different sessions.

An incomitant vertical deviation can however be influenced by correcting the horizontal deviation: a hypertropia decreases when an elevation in adduction is associated and a hypotropia diminishes when there is an associated depression in adduction (fig. 23).

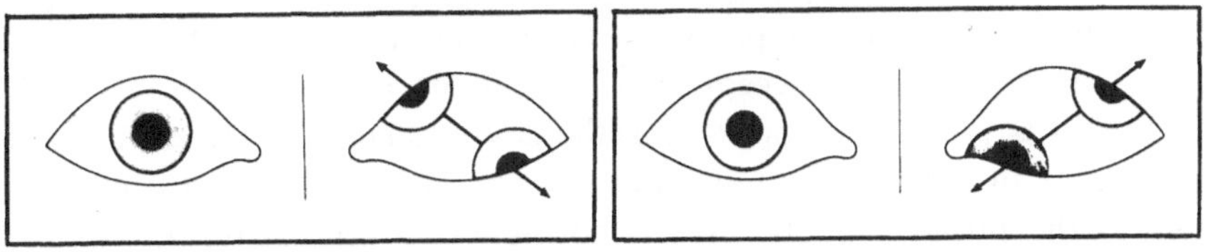

Fig. 23. — When a vertical incomitance is present the eye follows the arrow when the horizontal deviation changes.

When a comitant vertical deviation is present together with a horizontal one, it is unnecessary to attempt to correct both deviations at the same time. The most pronounced deviation could be corrected first and later, if necessary, the smallest deviation. Small comitant vertical deviations can also be reduced by a vertical transposition of the antagonistic horizontal rectus muscles (1); it would be best to displace their insertions together with a recession-resection procedure. To lower an eye both insertions are lowered; to raise an eye they are raised. A transposition by one muscle width can correct a deviation of 8^{Δ} to 13^{Δ}. Large concomitant vertical deviations require surgery of the vertical recti. It must be pointed out that surgery on the vertical rectus muscles is infinitely more effective and more predictable than surgery on the horizontal rectus muscles. As for the maximum amount of surgery, we should not exceed 4 or 5 mm recession or resection, depending on the size of the eye.

According to Brown (6) concomitant vertical deviations can best be corrected by an equivalent procedure on both elevator or depressor muscles of the non fixing eye.

A factor which matters from a cosmetic point of view is the fixing eye in case of a vertical deviation: a hypertropia is more obvious than a hypotropia because of the white crescent which appears under the cornea. Therefore, if a hypertropic eye cannot be made dominant, the vertical deviation must be corrected surgically without considering the risk of an overcorrection. On the contrary if the hypertropic eye is the dominant one the surgeon should be cautious in correcting the vertical deviation.

2. *Secondary surgery*

By secondary surgery we mean surgery on patients who have had squint surgery before.

Patients should be told beforehand that a reoperation may be necessary to prevent them losing faith in their surgeon. They should especially be warned about a possible overcorrection, as this is psychologically more difficult to accept than an undercorrection.

We do not reoperate too soon as the deviation can decrease and even disappear in the months following surgery. We usually wait 6 months unless the position of the eyes is cosmetically very disturbing or the deviation increases; in that case we wait at least 2 or 3 months until the eye has become quiet so that excessive bleeding can be avoided.

a. *Undercorrections*

An undercorrection will only require furher surgery if the residual angle is cosmetically disturbing. Especially a child who is teased at school will need further surgery. In general an angle up to $+7°$ will not be seen, but the interpupillary distance and the angle kappa play a part. Of course the deviation has to be measured without dissociating the eyes, for example using the corneal reflex test, so as to be close to reality.

Residual deviations are treated by performing a similar operation on the fellow eye if the primary surgery consisted of a recession-resection procedure or by resection of both lateral rectus muscles if the primary operation consisted of a bimedial recession. We can also use a secondary loop (fig. 12) on the previously recessed muscles (16) but we should bear in mind that this may give a duction limitation; so the loop has to be placed on the squinting eye whereas a loop will only be added on the dominant eye in large angles.

After monocular surgery the amount of surgery of the fellow eye can be determined on the basis of the correction achieved in the first eye (7). After a bilateral recession of the medial rectus muscles the resection of both lateral rectus muscles amounts from 5 to 8 mm (29).

Often a vertical deviation is the cause of an operation's failure; it should thus be looked for very carefully and treated together with the horizontal deviation. A recurrence of a vertical deviation after oblique muscle surgery is often due to a remaining posterior part. This means that the posterior fibres of the oblique muscle are still attached to the posterior pole of the eye, either because they were not cut or because they became reattached. This posterior attachment has to be excised very carefully and often a further weakening is indicated according to the degree of the deviation: concerning the inferior oblique this means that a disinsertion will follow after a recession; in case the superior oblique was weakened by a recession with a loop, a new loop can be placed on the pseudotendon which has been formed on the first loop. A disinsertion is only carried out in extreme cases, though we should not be afraid that the tendon may retract too far back as adhesions will prevent this. Concerning the vertical recti, a resection can be repeated and a recession can be enlarged with a secondary loop. We should however take into account that the effect of surgery is enhanced by the adhesions which are more extensive in case of a reoperation.

b. *Overcorrections*

A horizontal overcorrection seems to occur more often when early surgery is performed. It is our experience that in young children the result is complete success or failure: the eyes are either perfectly straight or they show a marked under or overcorrection. An overcorrection will also appear more often after a bimedial recession than after a recession-resection (8); this is probably due to a duction limitation on the dominant eye.

An unexpected advantage of an overcorrection is that, from a functional point of view, it actually may be more beneficial than an undercorrection. The functional results are at least as good and perhaps better than those in the overall group (8). It seems that this favorable effect can be enhanced if the consecutive exotropia is allowed to persist for some time; this has led some ophthalmologists to strive intentionally for an overcorrection.

Overcorrections should be treated according to Cooper's law (8), that is as if they were new cases, and surgical decisions should be based on the result of the examinations and not on prior surgery. Consequently the rules for primary surgery are to be applied here.

We prefer not to undo a recession of a medial rectus, a recession of the lateral rectus being much safer as a recurrence to the original deviation wil be prevented by the previously recessed medial rectus (16). The tightened check ligaments and the adhesions of the medial rectus act as a progressive brake which will decrease the risk of a recurrence of the esodeviation. On the other hand the recession of the lateral recti will tighten the check ligaments of these muscles and produce adhesions which induce a progressive brake and thus prevent a recurrence of the exodeviation (fig. 24). For these reasons the primary surgery should include a recession of the medial rectus of the non dominant eye; indeed in case of a bilateral lateral rectus resection without a recession there will be no progressive brake against the adduction which could prevent a recurrence to the original deviation.

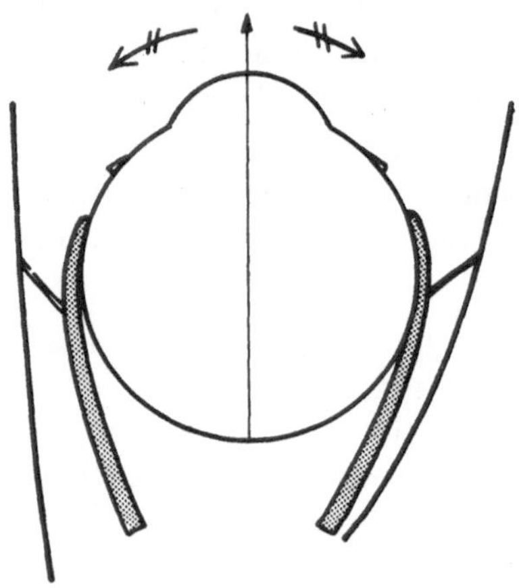

Fig. 24. — When a recession of one rectus muscle is followed by a recession of its antagonist the check ligaments of both muscles are tightened and act as a parapet; they help to keep the eyes straight.

Proportionally more surgery is necessary to restore a consecutive exotropia than was performed in the first instance. This means that essentially both lateral recti need to be recessed even if only one medial rectus was operated on before.

There are however exceptional cases in which the first operation has to be undone. This is so when a large adduction limitation is present, especially in the dominant eye as this will cause a horizontal incomitance (Hering's law). The recessed medial rectus has to be placed back at the original insertion and a weakening of both lateral recti should be added. If the adduction limitation is due however to an excessive resection of the lateral rectus the resected muscle has to be recessed.

Vertical deviations need to be carefully looked for and should be reduced together with the horizontal deviation. Vertical overcorrections are treated as though they were due to a paresis of the operated muscle by weakening the direct antagonist and/or the contralateral synergist. In case however the vertical overcorrection is the consequence of a duction limitation, the original surgery will have to be undone. If a contracture of the antagonist has developed, for instance if the deviation was left untreated for several years, this muscle of course has to be recessed in addition.

II. Simultaneous horizontal and cyclovertical surgery

A. *General directives*

As we try to straighten the eyes by removing the obstacles to the motor fusion reflexes, surgery will be determined by these obstacles. They can be situated on a central or a peripheral level. On a central level suppression is the most important obstacle. Therefore it is very important to overcome amblyopia preoperatively with a well carried out occlusion therapy and postoperatively with a part time occlusion of one or several hours a day until the age of 10 years. Even in alternating squint we occlude postoperatively but then the occlusion alternates for half an hour a day. The reason is that preoperatively alternation can be maintained by the angle of squint which is no longer the case after a surgical correction of this angle. If microtropia subsists, suppression of the fovea may lead to amblyopia and even without an angle of deviation bifoveal fixation may be lacking so that a straight eyed amblopia may develop.

At motor level the obstacles to fusion consist of deviations in the horizontal, diagonal and vertical plane (12). They maintain suppression and thus weaken the fusion reflexes. However, the influence of a deviation is not always in relation to its size because it may partially be compensated.

The horizontal deviations are reduced by a weakening of the horizontal recti, the medial recti in case of convergent strabismus and the lateral recti in case of divergent strabismus.

As surgery to measure is impossible we aim systematically for an overcorrection relying on the motor fusion reflexes to compensate for this overcorrection. It is indeed our clinical experience that the fusion reflexes can overcome an overcorrection much easier than an undercorrection. The recessed rectus muscle being relaxed will shorten by an adapted contraction; the muscle can even adjust anatomically to its new length especially when the patient is young, the child growing as it were into orthophoria.

We strongly advise against shortening of a rectus muscle, the procedure being traumatic and thus favoring adhesions. Besides, an overcorrection produced by a resection will be less easily compensated, the more so if the resection exceeds the limits of the muscle's extensibility. Finally a resection can lead to an unsightly enophthalmos especially if combined with a weakening of an oblique muscle.

The diagonal deviations are a matter of the oblique muscles. In our opinion these deviations can be caused by a sagittalization of the oblique muscles (15). With sagittalization we mean that one oblique muscle has a more sagittal course than its antagonist. Therefore we treat the diagonal deviations by means of a desagittalizing surgery which makes the line of pull of the muscle less sagittal.

The vertical deviations are reduced by weakening the vertical recti taking into account the horizontal side-effect of the operation. The vertical deviation we talk about here is the real vertical deviation (RVD) in the primary position. We measure the RVD on the synoptophore, the eyes being placed in a symmetrical position (13, 16).

As our surgery aims at the removal of the obstacles to fusion it is important to avoid creating new obstacles. This implies that all obstacles should be removed in one operating session because otherwise the fusion reflexes cannot adjust the effect of our surgery; a possible under or overcorrection is then consolidated and represents a new obstacle.

It is also very important to avoid creating adhesions as they often form insuperable obstacles. The tendency to make adhesions varies of course from patient to patient and is dependent on the patient's age: the older the patient the stronger and more disturbing the adhesions will be. A very important factor however is the traumatism induced by surgery. Therefore the surgeon's dexterity plays an important role: if he is unexperienced the tissues will be manipulated excessively and the operation will last longer. Postoperatively the mobilisation of the eyes will be delayed enhancing the chance for adhesions to be formed within the physiological field of gaze.

B. *Specific directives*

1. *Primary surgery*

Treatment of horizontal deviations

The horizontal deviations are treated with a bilateral medial rectus recession. As we aim for a horizontal overcorrection the muscle is placed back as far as possible without impeding its function; a recession has limits indeed outside which the muscle cannot function properly. The limits for the horizontal recti are determined by the check ligaments and adhesions rather than by the arc of contact. Thus our recessions of the medial recti always amount to 5 mm even when the angle is small or intermittent. If the angle exceeds +20° we add a loop to one or both recessed muscles. The following scheme shows our indications:

<+20°	: 5 mm recession of both medial rectus muscles
+20°/+24°	: 5 mm recession of both medial rectus muscles + a small loop on the non dominant eye
+25°/+34°	: 5 mm recession of both medial rectus muscles + a large loop on the non dominant eye
+35°/+39°	: 5 mm recession of both medial rectus muscles + a small loop on the dominant eye + a large loop on the non dominant eye
⩾+40°	: 5 mm recession of both medial rectus muscles + a bilateral large loop.

The angle which is taken into account is the angle as measured at the Maddox cross. The child is placed at 1 metre of the cross without wearing glasses. The examiner is seated under the light, his back against the cross and he moves his finger along the graduated scale. The child must follow the finger until the corneal reflex is correctly placed on the non fixing eye. The position of the finger on the graduated scale indicates the angle of squint.

When the eyes are orthotropic in the primary position and we have to operate on the oblique muscles we perform a central tenotomy of both medial recti. A desagittalization reduces indeed the abducting effect of the oblique muscles causing an esodeviation and suppression which prevent the eyes from being straightened again.

In the rare cases where an eso and an exodeviation alternate, we recess the medial as well as the lateral rectus. If the esodeviation predominates we perform a bimedial recession with a lateral rectus recession on the squinting eye. If the exodeviation predominates a recession of both lateral recti is combined with a medial rectus recession of the squinting eye.

In amblyopic eyes the deviation has a strong tendency to recur so that a loop is indicated more readily. In spite of the fact that amblyopes also easily show an overcorrection, we do use a loop as we create a strong progressive brake against adduction; this will prevent a return to the original deviation after treatment for an overcorrection.

As the effect of surgery is highly dependent on the hand of the surgeon he has to adapt his indications to his results. If he frequently obtains an overcorrection he should reduce the amount of his recessions being guided by the duction limitations he creates. These are looked for in lateroversion the adducting eye being made to fix: if the abducting eye suddenly moves quicker than the adducted eye the recession of the medial rectus has introduced too strong a brake which favors the occurrence of an overcorrection through the horizontal incomitance it induces.

Treatment of diagonal deviations

A diagonal deviation is reduced by a desagittalization of the oblique muscles. An elevation in adduction is treated with a desagittalization of the inferior oblique. As a sagittalization is present on both eyes this operation is always carried out bilaterally even if the elevation in adduction only shows up in one eye; it can be present in a latent form and appear after occlusion or after unilateral oblique muscle surgery. Even the V patterns without vertical incomitances are treated with a bilateral desagittalization, a diagonal overcorrection being easily compensated.

The amount of surgery is influenced by the size of the deviation: if it is small a posterior myectomy will be sufficient, if it is more marked an anteropositioning of the muscle is indicated and with large deviations a disinsertion will be necessary (fig. 17). The indications depend in first instance on the overaction of the inferior oblique but the function of the superior oblique must also be taken into account: an obvious underaction necessitates a more pronounced surgery on the inferior oblique; on the contrary, if there is only a slight hypofunction we should be more cautious. The horizontal deviation in the primary position should also be considered: in a large esotropia an elevation in adduction is usually marked and it decreases when the horizontal deviation diminishes. This means that the same diagonal deviations will need more surgery when the horizontal deviation is small than when it is large.

A depression in adduction is treated with a desagittalization of the superior oblique muscle. The procedure is also performed bilaterally even when the deviation is only present in one eye or when the A pattern is purely horizontal without a depression in adduction.

Concerning the amount of surgery it varies from a posterior tenectomy over an anteropositioning with a loop to a disinsertion according to the size of the deviation (fig. 18). Here too the dosage is influenced by the function of the antagonist: the more marked the hypofunction of the inferior oblique the more surgery will be needed on the superior oblique. The horizontal deviation in the primary position also has to be considered: the desagittalization of the superior oblique should be more pronounced in a large esotropia than in a small one, the depression in adduction being masked in esotropia.

If an elevation in adduction in the upper field of gaze is combined with a depression in adduction in the lower field of gaze all four oblique muscles are desagittalized. As these incomitances are often small a symmetric desagittalization will be indicated. If however the incomitance is more marked in one field of gaze than in the other asymmetric surgery can be performed: if the elevation in adduction predominates more surgery is performed on the inferior obliques and reversely if the depression in adduction predominates more will be done on the superior obliques. We also perform a desagittalization of the four oblique muscles if there are no diagonal incomitances, thus when the esotropia is concomitant. We think indeed that almost everyone has a sagittalization of one oblique with regard to its antagonist and that concomitance of the eye movements depends on a good fusional compensation of the incomitances. But as we do not know whether there is a latent elevation or a latent depression in adduction we desagittalize all four oblique muscles. Of course this does not change the mutual relation of the obliques so that a torsional imbalance is not removed. However the torsional reflexes can now compensate either an incyclo or an excyclo deviation without disturbing horizontal and vertical side effects.

Treatment of vertical deviations

A real vertical deviation (RVD) is often the cause of failure of our surgery and therefore something should be done about it especially if it is pronounced.

In case of a RVD associated with a V pattern we weaken the inferior rectus of the hypotropic eye in addition to a desagittalization of both inferior obliques; according to the degree of the RVD we perform a central tenotomy or a recession. If however the vertical deviation increases in adduction, surgery of the superior oblique of the hypotropic eye may be considered; we then carry out a posterior tenectomy or a recession with a loop of this muscle, whilst surgery on the inferior rectus is reduced or omitted as simultaneous surgery on both depressors greatly enhances the effect.

In case of a RVD associated with an A pattern we perform a central tenotomy or a recession of the superior rectus of the hypertropic eye in addition to the desagittalization of both superior obliques. Here too, surgery of the vertical rectus can be replaced partly or completely by a posterior myectomy or a recession of the inferior oblique if the hypertropia is larger in adduction as compared with abduction taking into account the increased effect of a simultaneous surgery on both elevators.

In case of a RVD associated with a symmetrical X pattern, the desagittalization of all four oblique muscles is combined with a weakening of the superior rectus of the squinting eye if it is higher and of the inferior rectus if it is lower.

One should also realize that a weakening of a vertical rectus greatly enhances the effect of the desagittalization of the contralateral antagonist, so that a vertical overcorrection easily occurs. This is especially so if the vertical rectus of the dominant eye is operated on. Perhaps it is therefore better to neglect a small vertical deviation especially if it is expected to decrease after the correction of the esodeviation (fig. 23). If the RVD is more marked an asymmetric desagittalization of the oblique muscles may be sufficient when the deviation is greatest in the field of action of those oblique muscles.

We can also take the influence of Hering's law into account: the desagittalization of the inferior oblique of the dominant eye will cause a contraction of the contralateral synergist which will reduce hypotropia and increase hypertropia of the squinting eye; in the same way the desagittalization of the superior oblique of the dominant eye will reduce hypertropia and increase hypotropia of the squinting eye.

Finally we should warn against the risk of an unexpected and marked hypertropia which can arise after weakening an inferior rectus on the non dominant eye, especially if this eye is amblyopic. In those cases we should remember that a hypotropia of the squinting eye is cosmetically less disturbing than a hypertropia.

2. *Secondary surgery*

Again we make a distinction between deviations at a horizontal, diagonal or vertical level. Of course an undercorrection at one level can occur together with an overcorrection at another level; they are considered separately but corrected in the same operation.

a. *Undercorrections*

Treatment of horizontal undercorrections

A horizontal undercorrection is treated with a secondary loop (fig. 12). If this muscle has had a loop recession before, we place a new loop on the pseudotendon which has been formed between the retracted tendon and the sclera.

We place a secondary loop on the medial rectus depending on the angle of deviation as measured on the Maddox cross at 1 metre and without wearing glasses:

$< +10°$: a large loop on the non dominant eye
$+10°/+20°$: a small loop on the dominant eye
+ a large loop on the non dominant eye
$> +20°$: a large loop on both eyes.

A reoperation on a muscle easily leads to adhesions and duction limitations: hence we are cautious on placing a loop on the dominant eye.

Treatment of diagonal undercorrections

A diagonal undercorrection is treated with a further desagittalization of the concerned oblique muscle. A recurrence of an elevation in adduction requires a reoperation on the inferior oblique and when there is a recurrence of a depression in adduction, a reoperation of the superior oblique is required. When there is no associated RVD we perform bilateral surgery even if a recurrence of the deviation is only visible in one eye. When a small RVD is present surgery on one oblique may suffice leaving a weakening of a vertical rectus to a more pronounced RVD.

As for the amount of surgery we proceed to a higher level on the graduated scale.

In case of the inferior oblique we pass:
- from a posterior myectomy to an anteropositioning;
- from an anteropositioning to a disinsertion;
- from a disinsertion to a redisinsertion.

For the superior oblique we pass:
- from a posterior tenectomy to an anteropositioning with a loop;
- from an anteropositioning with a loop to a disinsertion;
- from a disinsertion to a redisinsertion.

If a diagonal undercorrection is due to uncut or reattached posterior fibres it may be sufficient in small deviations to cut these strands. If a pseudotendon has been formed after an anteropositioning with a loop on the superior oblique we may hang this pseudotendon in a new loop. A redisinsertion we can only carry out if the muscle became reattached to the sclera; if this is not so, a central tenotomy of the contralateral antagonist may be carried out if the deviation is large enough to justify surgery on a vertical rectus muscle.

Treatment of vertical undercorrections

A small RVD can be neglected or treated by means of an oblique muscle surgery if a diagonal deviation is associated. If the RVD is important an operation on a vertical rectus is added. We perform a reoperation on the vertical rectus concerned: the superior rectus of the hypertropic eye in an A pattern and the inferior rectus of the hypotropic eye in a V pattern. Here we also proceed to the next graduated step and we pass:

– from a central tenotomy to a recession;
– from a recession to a secondary loop.

In borderline cases a central tenotomy can be repeated because the tendon usually has crept back towards the original insertion.

b. *Overcorrections*

Treatment of horizontal overcorrections

Except in small angles a horizontal overcorrection is treated with a bilateral 5 mm recession of the lateral rectus; a loop is added to the recession when the deviation is large.

The indication for a loop depends on the angle of squint as measured after maximal decompensation:

$< -5°$	: 5 mm recession of the lateral rectus of the non dominant eye + a central tenotomy of the lateral rectus of the dominant eye
$-5°/-14°$	: 5 mm recession of both lateral rectus muscles
$-15°/-19°$	: 5 mm recession of both lateral rectus muscles + a large loop on the non dominant eye
$\geqslant -20°$	: 5 mm recession of both lateral rectus muscles + a bilateral large loop.

If an adduction limitation with a horizontal incomitance in the lateral gaze is present more extensive surgery is needed: in small angles the central tenotomy of the dominant eye is replaced by a 5 mm recession and in angles which exceed $-5°$ a loop is added to the recession of the hyperactive lateral rectus. If the limitation of adduction is pronounced a loop may be added even if an esodeviation is found in the primary position.

Treatment of diagonal overcorrections

A diagonal overcorrection is due to a postoperative paresis of an oblique muscle. This is treated with a weakening of the homolateral antagonist or of the contralateral synergist; both are operated on if the deviation is large. The homolateral antagonist is not desagittalized this time but weakened: for the inferior oblique this means a recession or a disinsertion; for the superior oblique this means a recession with a loop or a disinsertion.

The amount of weakening depends on the size of the diagonal overcorrection, but we should not be too cautious because the muscle we have to counterbalance is a paretic one.

Treatment of vertical overcorrections

A vertical overcorrection can be due to an overcorrection of an oblique muscle or of a vertical rectus.

Concerning the treatment we may neglect a small RVD especially if it is expected to disappear after the correction of the horizontal angle (fig. 23). When the RVD is moderate, surgery will more likely be done on one oblique muscle without adding a vertical rectus muscle, especially if the deviation is incomitant. When the RVD is more marked surgery will preferably be limited to a vertical rectus muscle adding an oblique muscle only in large angles as this combination enhances the effect.

In case the RVD is due to a postoperative paresis of an oblique muscle the contralateral synergist of this muscle is weakened and in case the RVD is due to an overcorrection of a vertical rectus the homolateral antagonist is dealt with. In general an overcorrection changes an A pattern into a V and vice versa. In that case there is no problem concerning the choice of the vertical rectus; it will be the inferior rectus of the hypotropic eye in a V pattern and the superior rectus of the hypertropic eye in case of an A pattern.

As for the amount of surgery we perform a central tenotomy or a recession, depending on the importance of the RVD.

SURGICAL COMPLICATIONS

1. *Conjunctiva and capsular tissue*

A shrivelled conjunctiva is not only cosmetically unacceptable but it can also limit the duction to the opposite side. Often this shrivelling can be seen at the lateral canthus; it can be due to a traumatic surgery or to a large resection of the lateral rectus. The conjunctiva can also be shortened by a longstanding large deviation; it is smooth and appears normal but on carrying out a forced duction test we feel a resistance; we can often see a tightenend conjunctival strand running from the limbus to the canthus. The treatment consists of a careful freeing of this shrivelled conjunctiva. In a first step the conjunctiva is detached from the underlying tissue checking from the outside that we do not perforate the conjunctiva (fig. 25). Care should be taken to put the scissors just underneath the conjunctiva thus leaving no scar tissue adhering to it; it is indeed difficult to free the conjunctiva of superfluous connective tissue in a second attempt. Once the conjunctiva is free, the scar tissue can easily be cut away from the sclera. After closing the wound the eye is pulled towards the opposite side with two forceps in order to check if the conjunctiva no longer offers resistance. If this is the case a fenestration should be carried out: level with the limbus the conjunctiva is incised over half the circumference so that it can retract (fig. 26). If desirable a transverse cut can be made at the end of the incision to allow further retraction. The crescent of sclera which thus appears is easily epithelialised. If necessary the conjunctiva can be fixed to the sclera. The freeing of a shrivelled conjunctiva may not be done together with muscle surgery which places the eye in the involved zone: the conjunctiva would wrinkle again in the postoperative period and thus adhere again in an unsightly way.

An attraction of the plica towards the limbus is a complication which can be very unaesthetic; it may even give the aspect of a squint. This attraction can occur after a resection of the medial rectus or when this muscle is placed back at its original insertion. Postoperatively the eye is in an adducted position so that the conjunctival incision and the muscle stump lie close together and can adhere; when the eye straightens afterwards the plica is pulled with it (fig. 10). To prevent attraction of the plica one could use the limbal incision. Personally we prefer an

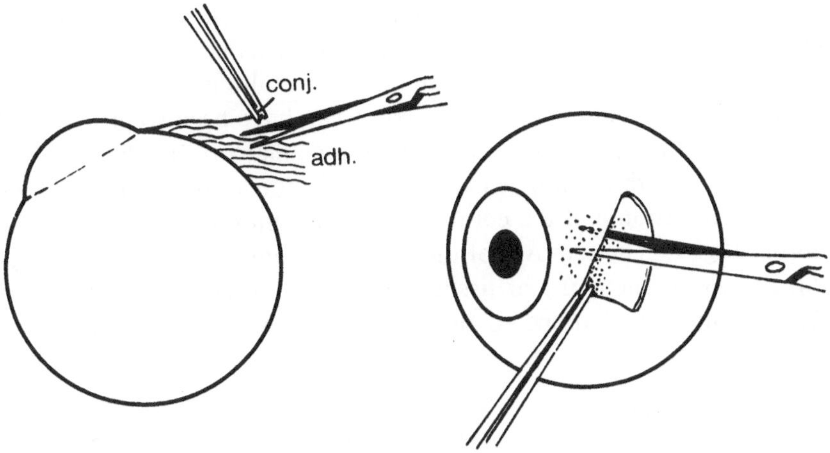

Fig. 25. — Detachment of the conjunctiva from the underlying scar tissue while from the outside the conjunctiva is checked for perforation.

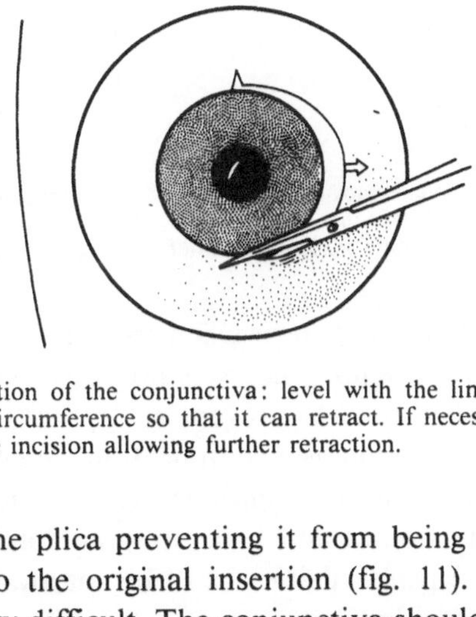

Fig. 26. — Fenestration of the conjunctiva: level with the limbus the conjunctiva is incised over half the circumference so that it can retract. If necessary a transverse cut is made at the end of the incision allowing further retraction.

incision next to the plica preventing it from being attracted by fixing the conjunctiva to the original insertion (fig. 11). To restore an attracted plica is very difficult. The conjunctiva should be freed from the underlying tissues and a semicircular fenestration performed level with the limbus; the plica is kept in its normal place by attaching the nasal lip of the fenestration wound to the original insertion of the medial rectus muscle.

Besides a shrivelled conjunctiva hypertrophic capsular tissue can lead to a ugly scar. This happens with a recession when Tenon's capsule is incised at the height of the muscle's tendon so that it curls up and retracts towards the limbus (fig. 27a). In case of a resection the capsular tissue is pulled forward with the muscle and folds near the limbus (fig. 27b). The tissue absorbs blood and swells resulting in a vascularised thickening near the limbus. The swelling can have been so pronounced that the conjunctiva remains prolapsed over the cornea. The best way to prevent this thickening is cutting away Tenon's capsule between the muscle's insertion and the cornea so that it cannot retract towards the limbus (fig. 1). The removal of the thickness consists of carefully excising all subconjunctival scar tissue making sure to cut away any superfluous conjunctival tissue so that it will no longer prolapse over the cornea.

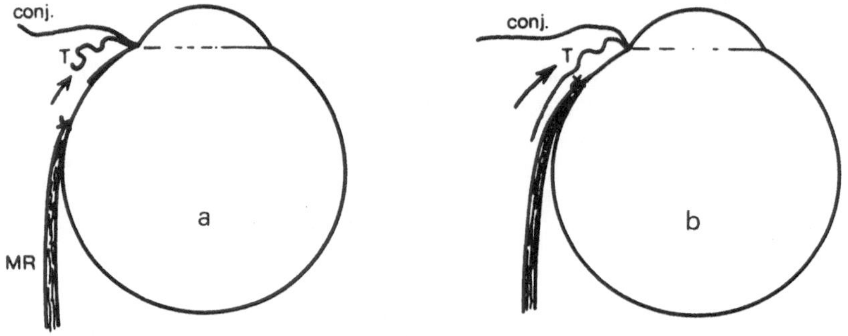

Fig. 27a-b. — When Tenon's capsule (T) is not excised it can fold up near the limbus resulting in a vascularised thickening. This happens after a recession when the capsule is incised at the level of the muscle's insertion or after a resection when the capsule is pulled forwards.

Subconjunctival cysts can appear when epithelial cells or foreign bodies are bedded in the wound. The cysts are filled with clear fluid and have to be removed in total to prevent recurrence.

A pedunculated granuloma is a complication which may occur after a long-lasting and traumatic intervention: the swollen capsule of Tenon prolapses out of the wound and becomes granulomatous. To prevent this, the prolapsed capsular tissue has to be cut away; pushing it back into the wound is often ineffective as postoperative swelling may cause it to protrude again. Once the granuloma is formed it should be excised with the peduncle and the conjunctival wound should be carefully closed.

An allergic reaction to a thread is a good natured complication. The reaction can be acute or appear as a delayed foreign body reaction occurring six to eight weeks later. Swelling and redness may show up as a chronic granuloma. It can disappear with time but this often occurs very slowly and incompletely. The treatment consists of local steroids and cold compresses. In some cases the remaining granulomatous tissue has to be cut away for aesthetical reasons.

An abscess on the sutures is a very rare complication and is probably due to infected suture material. It appears as a local swelling occurring within the first week after surgery. Treatment consists of draining the abcess followed by an appropriate topical antibiotic treatment after culture.

Orbital cellulitis is a rare but life threatening complication. It develops within a few days after the operation; therefore surgeons who discharge their patients quickly from hospital should be aware of this complication. Culture and sensitivity determination have to be done and the proper systemic and topical antibiotic treatment carried out.

2. *Muscles*

Complications related to the muscles can lead to a duction limitation. As causes we can mention: too much tightening of the check ligaments, adherences between the muscle and surrounding structures, a loss of the muscle, too much shortening and fibrosis of the muscle itself.

The forced duction has to be done. We should not only check whether the forced duction is restricted, but we should also evaluate the resistance the eye offers when pushing it in the orbit (fig. 28a and b). This test gives valuable information in localizing the site of these complications.

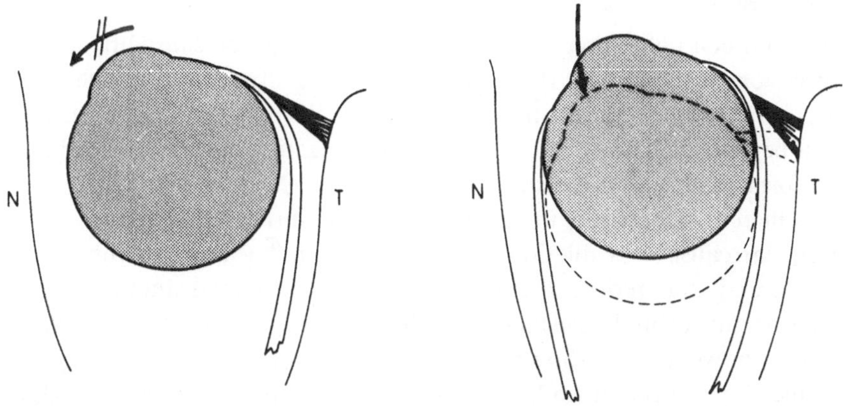

Fig. 28a. — The forced duction can be limited (crossed arrow) but the resistance against pushing the eye into the orbit can be normal (uncrossed arrow).

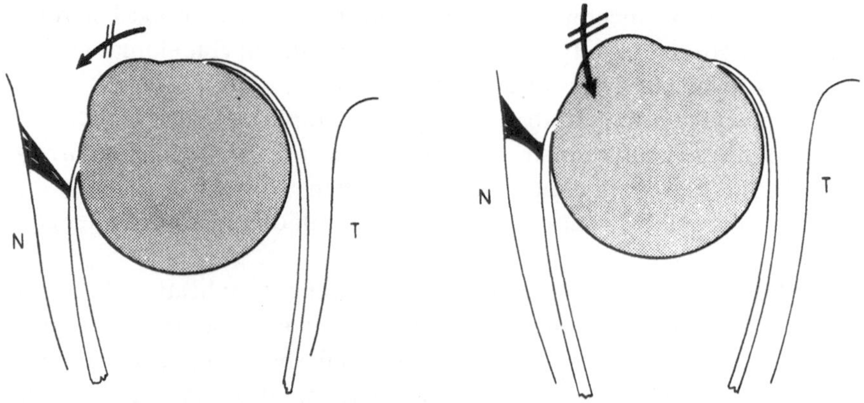

Fig. 28b. — The forced duction as well as the resistance against pushing the eye into the orbit can be limited (crossed arrow).

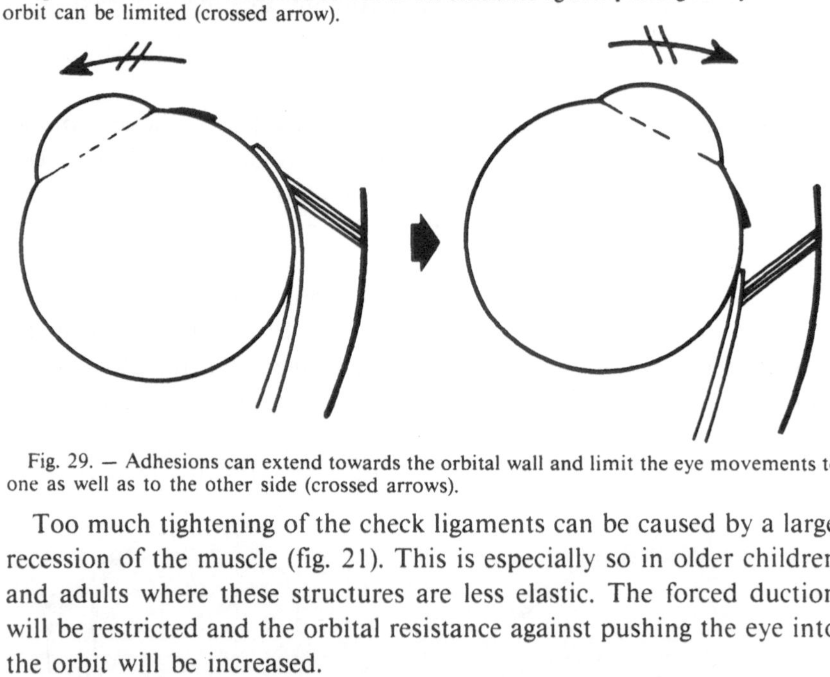

Fig. 29. — Adhesions can extend towards the orbital wall and limit the eye movements to one as well as to the other side (crossed arrows).

Too much tightening of the check ligaments can be caused by a large recession of the muscle (fig. 21). This is especially so in older children and adults where these structures are less elastic. The forced duction will be restricted and the orbital resistance against pushing the eye into the orbit will be increased.

Adherences between the muscle and the surrounding tissues are a frequent cause of a duction limitation. The adhesions can run to the sclera and thus reduce the arc of contact. The forced duction test as well as the orbital resistance will be normal. The posterior fixation suture however has shown that the arc of contact can be extremely reduced with little or no limitation of movement as a result. Adhesions can also extend towards the orbital wall and limit the eye movements to the same as well as to the opposite side (fig. 29). The forced duction test will be abnormal as well as the orbital resistance. If adhesions stretch towards the orbital floor as can happen after surgery of the inferior oblique, the elevation will be limited; a retraction of the globe on attempted elevation can even be associated (fig. 30). Adhesions are often due to traumatic surgery whereas the individual tendency of the patient to form them also plays a part. As the removal of these adhesions can be difficult and disappointing it is of the greatest importance to perform a smooth and atraumatic surgery.

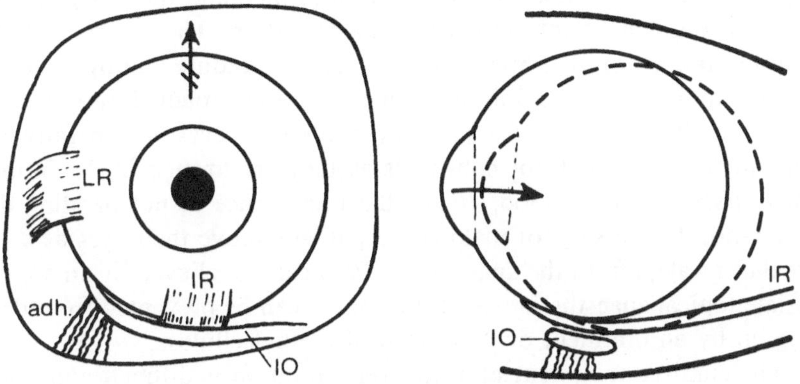

Fig. 30. — If adhesions stretch towards the orbital floor the elevation can be limited (crossed arrow). In extreme cases even a retraction of the globe can be added to the limitation (uncrossed arrow).

The loss of a muscle is a serious but fortunately rare complication. Both the forced duction test and the orbital resistance will be normal. Especially after a resection, a muscle can slip as the tightened muscle fibres can easily tear out of the suture. With a recession, a muscle can slip already before it has been reattached to the sclera. The tendon then retracts into the perimysium so that the muscle is only suspended in the suture via this perimysium (fig. 2).

If a resection exceeds the stretching limits of a muscle the duction towards the opposite side can be reduced (fig. 20); the forced duction test is limited but the orbital resistance is normal. Especially a resection of the lateral rectus when being very large can lead to this complication (21), the more so in older patients when the tissues are less elastic. Too much shortening of the superior oblique can also lead to a duction limitation which is particularly pronounced in the upper nasal field of gaze thus leading to an acquired Brown's syndrome.

Fibrosis of a muscle is an irreparable complication. The forced duction towards the side of the lesion and the orbital resistance are normal.

The forced duction towards the opposite side may be limited if the muscle cannot be stretched any more. This complication is due to traumatic surgery. We have seen it several times after a marginal myotomy; the fact that one cuts into the muscle and that an interstitial bleeding occurs is perhaps responsible for this fibrosing of the muscle.

The treatment of duction limitations is primarily preventive. We should take care in choosing an atraumatic surgical technique. The duration of the operation plays an important role (27): the longer the operation lasts the more oedema will be formed and the more the eye movements will be inhibited after the operation. The operation time can be speeded up by respecting the correct procedure and by reducing all manipulations to a minimum. The age of the patients is also important: the older they are the less they move their eyes postoperatively; this increases the risk for adhesions as they are formed in the immediate postoperative period. Hence the importance of not padding the eyes and, if necessary, of making the patients move their eyes as soon as they awaken from the anaesthesia. Pain can be relieved by an appropriate topical anaesthesia whilst the cornea can be prevented from drying up by an ointment or by a drop of methylcellulose.

The curative treatment of a duction limitation is difficult and often disillusioning. A small duction limitation can be treated by creating a similar duction limitation on the synergic muscle by, for example, recessing it with a loop. For large duction limitations the concerned muscle will need to be reoperated. If a recession is the cause of a duction limitation we undo it. We must take care not to mistake connective tissue adhering to the original insertion for the tendon; a resection of this connective tissue would anchor the eye to the orbital wall thus increasing the duction limitation (fig. 31).

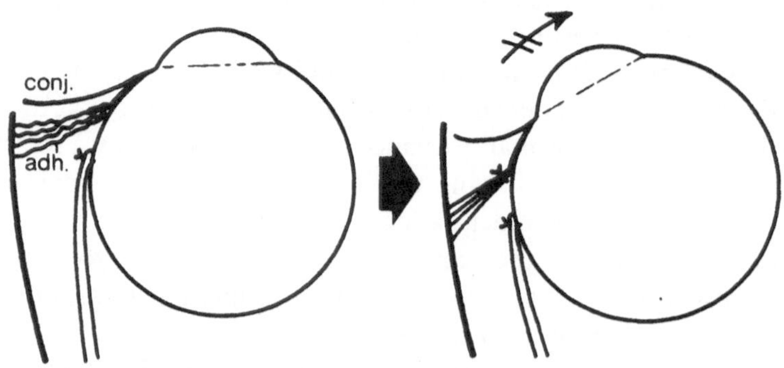

Fig. 31. — A bridge of connective tissue can connect the original insertion with the orbital wall (left). When mistaken for the tendon and resected, it will anchor the eye (right).

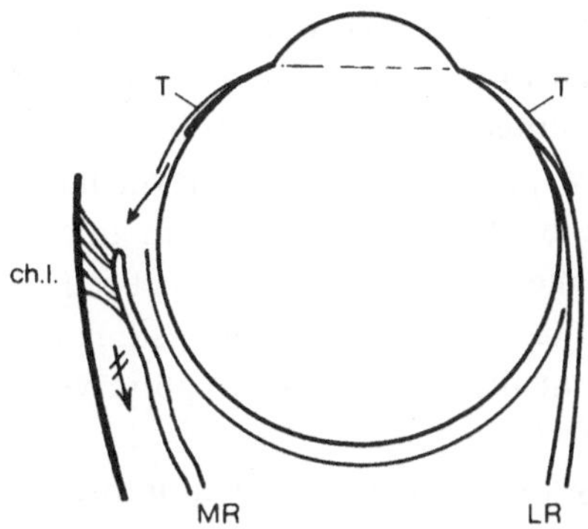

Fig. 32. — A slipped muscle remains attached by its check ligaments just outside Tenon's capsule.

If a slipped muscle is the cause we put it back into place. We should remember that a slipped muscle has to be looked for outside Tenon's capsule where it remains attached by its check ligaments (fig. 32). If the muscle has become too short and unelastic we attach it at the point to where it can be stretched with ease, the eye being pulled completely to the opposite side; sometimes the muscle is so short that it can only be reattached by means of a loop.

When the medial rectus has to be placed back at its original insertion, it is necessary to weaken the lateral recti. Three factors play a part in the amount of weakening:

- the position of the eye after the medial rectus is reattached: if the eye is still in an abducted position a great amount of surgery is necessary on both lateral recti; if on the other hand the eye is in an adducted position we should be careful;
- the contractibility and the extensibility of the medial rectus: if the contractibility is poor and the muscle is atrophic and slack we should put the accent on the weakening of the contralateral synergist to prevent a recurrence of the limitation. If the extensibility of the medial rectus is restricted we should be careful when weakening the ipsilateral antagonist because the latter may no longer be able to overcome the restricted extensibility so that a duction limitation in the opposite direction occurs;
- the adhesions: if there are a lot of adhesions around the medial rectus and especially if they cannot be totally removed, a recurrence of the limitation can be predicted: a marked weakening of the contralateral synergist is then indicated.

If too large a resection is the cause of a duction limitation the muscle should of course be recessed. To free the muscle from the surrounding tissues it is essential to find the plane of cleavage between the perimysium and the adhesions. We should look for this plane at the height of the tendon, as a perforation at this level has no consequence: we then have only made a hole in the tendon in an area where there will be no bleeding. Once the plane of cleavage has been found it is easy to free the muscle further backwards as the adhesions and the accompanying blood vessels stop at the limit with the perimysium and do not penetrate the muscle itself.

It is unnecessary to say that a good mobilisation of the eyes in the immediate postoperative period is of the greatest importance. Especially with adults this may cause problems: they often keep their eyes immobile, afraid of pain. A drop of tetracaine can then be helpful.

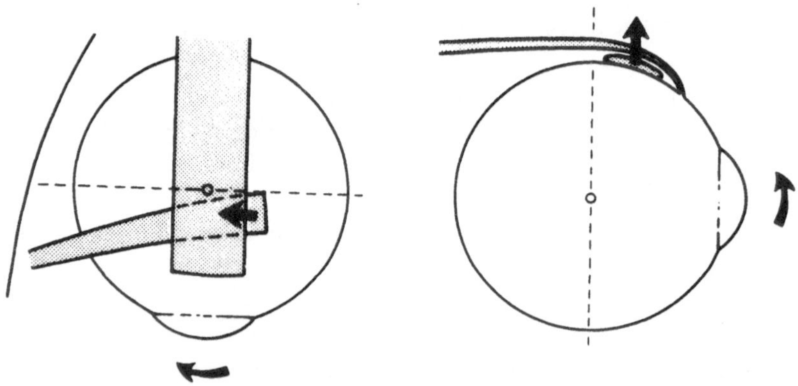

Fig. 33. — When the superior oblique readheres to the sclera in front of the equator it pulls at the anterior pole instead of the posterior pole of the eye. As a consequence the horizontal and vertical actions of the muscle are reversed.

Finally we should mention a very special form of complication which can occur after a desagittalization of the superior oblique muscle, namely the reversal of its secondary actions (fig. 33). When the muscle adheres to the sclera in front of the equator of the globe it is the anterior pole instead of the posterior pole of the eye which is pulled at. As a consequence the horizontal and vertical actions are reversed: the superior oblique becomes an adductor and an elevator and will counteract the inferior rectus with a limitation of depression as a result; the clinical picture which thus arises is one of a V pattern of the eye movements combined with a retraction of the abducted eye and a depression of the adducted eye when looking down and to the side. To avoid this complication we should take care to prevent a reattachment of the tendon in front of the equator of the globe; therefore we should always carefully push the tendon backwards before closing the wound. If the reversal has occurred it is very cumbersome to undo it; the tendon should be freed from the sclera and reattached behind the equator of the eye.

3. *Bulbus*

A perforation of the sclera is probably more common than generally realised. Retina surgeons of course will advise to surround the site of perforation by diathermy or cryocoagulation; this requires an excessive manipulation however while the operation lasts longer enhancing the risk of adhesions and of failure of the squint surgery. McLean (26) and McNeer (27) claim that in the normal eye with a sound vitreous a perforation is well tolerated probably because hemorrhage seals the site until fibrous adhesions form. We therefore agree with Helveston (19) when he states that simple perforations may be left untreated. In case of doubt one may consider of course a cryocoagulation right at the site of the perforation. Larger defects should be closed and a ring of cryocoagulations should be placed around the perforation. The retina should be examined at the time of surgery and at close intervals during the postoperative period.

Endophthalmitis is fortunately an extremely rare occurrence which is probably related to scleral perforation. An aseptic technique is of course of great importance and a long exposure of the wound has to be avoided (27). Preventively we give local antibiotics for one week, starting the day before surgery. In case of a scleral perforation it is perhaps wise to add systemic antibiotics; we should also check if the red fundus reflex remains normal.

Optic atrophy can occur due to excessive and prolonged traction on the retrobulbar blood vessels and nerves. Thomas (31) has described this complication after a posterior fixation suture in which case of course there is strong traction on the globe. That is why we have to observe the pupil and when mydriasis shows up traction should be released.

Anterior segment ischaemia is a serious complication caused by a section of the ciliary vessels of three or four rectus muscles of one eye at a time. The tolerance to a reduction of blood supply to the anterior segment is higher in children than in adults. Especially patients with arteriosclerosis consitute a high-risk group. Treatment consists of intensive systemic and topical administration of corticosteroids and vasodilatators.

Dellen are small areas of corneal thinning caused by localized drying of the cornea. They are usually the consequence of an interruption of the corneal tear film by a prolapse of the conjunctiva over the cornea. They can be prevented by resection of excessive conjunctiva and capsule of Tenon to prevent tissue swelling near the limbus.

4. *Eyelids*

Surgery of the vertical muscles can have influence on the eyelids by means of their connections with the tarsus. The superior rectus is connected with the upper eyelid through its connections with the levator palpebrae and the inferior rectus with the lower eyelid by means of the tarsal connections of Lockwood's ligament. An excessive recession of a vertical rectus muscle can thus give a retraction of the eyelid and an excessive resection will pull the eyelid forwards (fig. 34).

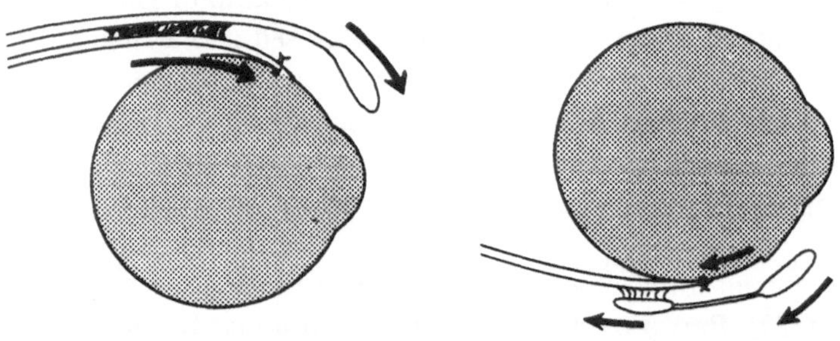

Fig. 34. — A resection of a vertical muscle causes the eyelid to be pulled forwards (left) and a recession retracts the eyelid (right) because of the connections between the muscle and the tarsus.

These complications can be prevented by cutting the connections with the eyelids. This is difficult with the superior rectus as we may damage the levator palpebrae. Therefore a recession should not be too large, especially where the dominant eye is concerned, as a weakening of the superior rectus will induce an extra stimulus to the levator palpebrae because of the synkinesis between both muscles. In case of extensive surgery of the inferior rectus, the connections with the inferior oblique should be cut. This has to be done atraumatically, taking care not to damage the nerve of the inferior oblique which enters the muscle at the crossing with the lateral border of the inferior rectus. One should however take into account that vicious adhesions can replace

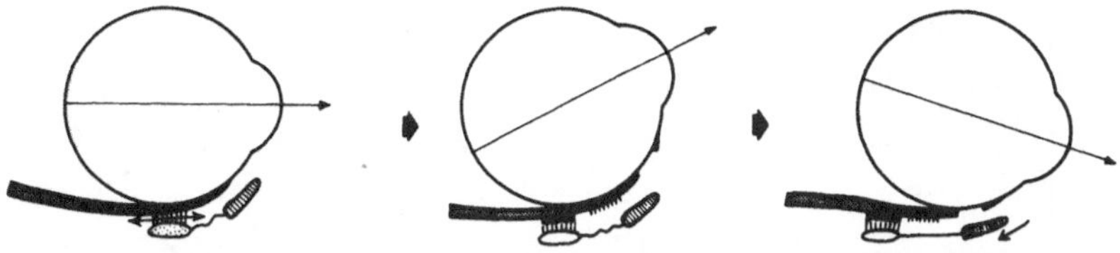

Fig. 35. — When the connections between the inferior oblique and the inferior rectus are cut (arrow), they can readhere further back to the inferior rectus resulting in an increased retraction of the lower eyelid.

the sectioned connections with the eyelid (fig. 35). The eye is directed upwards during the anaesthesia and the following sleep so that the severed ligaments can adhere further back to the inferior rectus making the remedy worse than the disease; indeed upon awakening, when the eye moves downwards the lower eyelid will retract more than if the ligaments were not cut. If after traumatic surgery the risk of adhesions is enhanced we should wake the patient as soon as possible and make him move his eyes in depression.

In order to restore the position of the eyelids it is often necessary to undo the causal surgery.

5. *Palpebral fissures*

Surgery of the eye muscles can alter the palpebral fissure. The position of the eye in the orbit is determined by the opposite traction of the recti and the oblique muscles, the rectus muscles pulling the eye backwards and the oblique muscles pulling it forwards.

The position of the eye in the orbit determines the width of the palpebral fissure. A strengthening of a rectus muscle and a weakening of an oblique cause a relative enophthalmos with a narrowing of the palpebral fissure as a result (fig. 36). Contrarily, a weakening of a rectus muscle and a strengthening of an oblique muscle will bring the eye forward thus widening the palpebral fissure (fig. 37). This effect of eye muscle surgery on the palpebral fissure should not be neglected: if we operate on two muscles which have the same effect on the palpebral fissure, for example a weakening of an oblique muscle together with a resection of the lateral rectus, a severe enophthalmos can be the consequence.

To avoid such a narrowing of the palpebral fissure we always combine a weakening of an oblique muscle with a weakening of a horizontal rectus muscle: the medial rectus if an esodeviation is present and a lateral rectus if an exodeviation is present. When there is no horizontal

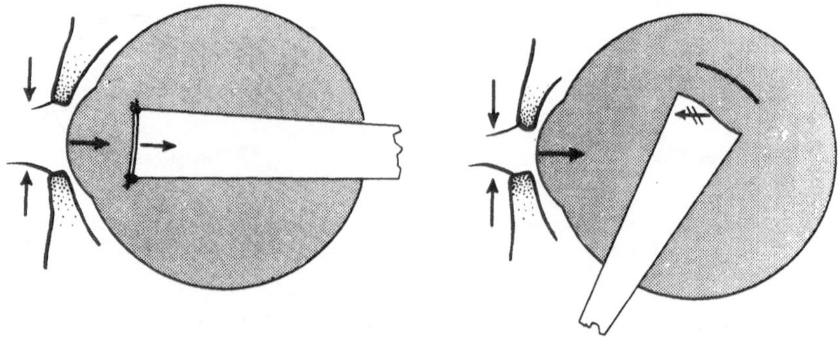

Fig. 36. — A strengthening of a rectus muscle increases the force which pulls the eye into the orbit (uncrossed arrow) and a weakening of an oblique muscle releases the force which pushes the eye forwards (crossed arrow), in both cases resulting in a narrowing of the palpebral fissure.

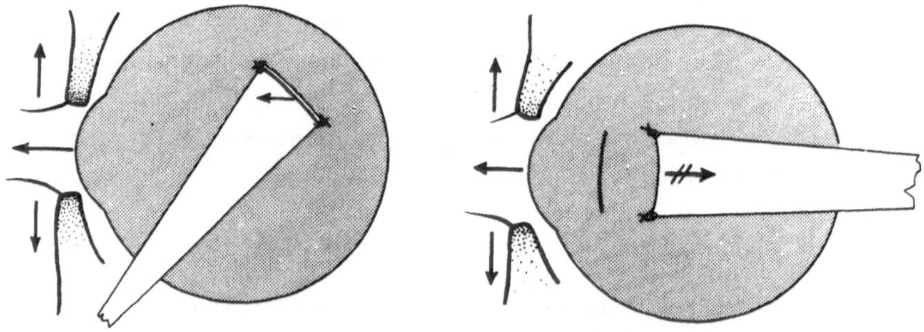

Fig. 37. — A strengthening of an oblique muscle increases the force which pushes the eye forwards (uncrossed arrow) and a recession of a rectus muscle decreases the force pulling the eye into the orbit (crossed arrow), resulting in a widening of the palpebral fissure.

deviation we perform a central tenotomy of both antagonistic horizontal recti.

Therapeutically we can normalize the palpebral fissure by adapting our muscle surgery if possible. We can perform a "widening" procedure on the enophthalmic eye and a "narrowing" procedure on the other eye. When no horizontal deviations are present we can consider a recession or a resection of both antagonistic horizontal recti.

6. *Postoperative diplopia*

We should make a distinction between transitory and permanent diplopia. The transitory and easily ignored diplopia is due to an image falling outside the suppression area but being localized on the retina-half which was suppressed in early childhood. This suppression will return gradually and the double image will fade. A large incomitance will of course impede this suppression as the image constantly wanders over the retina thus attracting attention.

A permanent and thus very disturbing diplopia is due to an overcorrection with the double image being formed on the non suppressed retina-half which the patient is unable to suppress because of his age. This overcorrection may occur in the primary position or only in lateroversion in case of a duction limitation. With a duction limitation indeed diplopia will occur every time the patient looks aside where the double image falls on the non suppressed retina-half; the patient's attention is thus attracted repeatedly to the double image which he will continue to see when the eye moves back to the primary position, even though an undercorrection shows up there.

To treat a transitory diplopia the ophthalmologist has to reassure not only the patient but more over himself; if the eye surgeon hesitates the patient will become worried and instead of neglecting the diplopia, become impatient.

Permanent diplopia will disappear together with the overcorrection. We have to look for this overcorrection very carefully; often it is only present upon looking in the far distance or in extreme lateroversion.

The treatment consists in removing the overcorrection and all incomitances present. We should of course wait long enough to enable the overcorrection to disappear spontaneously.

7. *Anaesthesia*

Complications from anaesthesia are fortunately extremely rare. In addition to cardiac arrest and asphyxia, hereditary or idiopathic malignant hyperthermia were cited as life threatening complications (5). Malignant hyperthermia is especially seen in children, adolescents and young adults; infants do not appear to be affected, no case having been reported under the age of 18 months. Other genetically-determined diseases are of direct importance in relation to anaesthesia such as porphyria and suxamethonium sensitivity. Worth mentioning is also the congenital pseudocholine-estherase deficiency which can result in a prolonged apnea, a situation which is annoying, but, if well managed, will present no real danger to the patient. Added to this should also be the danger of drugs with an irreversible anticholine-estherase action such as Diflupyl and Phospholiniodide: succinyl-choline is no longer broken down and a prolonged apnea will result. These drugs should thus be stopped long before the anaesthesia.

Another but sometimes very annoying complication which can appear during the operation is the bleeding caused by the anaesthesia. We can classify the causes of such a bleeding at three levels: too high an arterial pressure, too high a venous pressure and a CO_2 retention.

Too high an arterial tension is found when the anaesthesia is not deep enough and when pain stimuli can cause increased sympathetic tone. These problems will often appear at the beginning of the anaesthesia: the eyes appear congestive and the abundant tear production indicates that the anaesthesia is not deep enough. All vessels will bleed considerably during the operation, the large vessels as well as the capillaries.

Too high a venous pressure is found when the intra-thoracic pressure is high or when the jugular veins are compressed. Care should be taken to use an intubation system which offers little resistance and to apply it correctly. A frequent and often neglected cause of raised intra-thoracic pressure is the fact that the tube touches the carina: the distance between the larynx and the carina is very short in children so that the tube can easily touch the carina blocking the lumen. In case of increased venous pressure the blood vessels are swollen and bleed the moment they are touched. The free passage of the intubation system should then be checked and in case it is suspected that the tube touches the carina it should be pulled out a little. The pressure on the jugular veins can be removed by adjusting the position of the head whilst the patient can be brought into antitrendelenburg position.

A CO_2 retention may be caused by an increased expiratory resistance but especially by too deep an anaesthesia which will delay the evacuation of CO_2 because of respiratory depression. We should think of this possibility when suddenly diffuse blood appears from tissues which have been cut before without bleeding.

When we cannot find the cause, careful hyperventilation may be used: the surplus of CO_2 is eliminated and a superficial anaesthesia becomes deeper. The disadvantages of a larger dose of anaesthesia is compensated for by the shorter duration of the operation which is made possible by the absence of bleeding.

BIBLIOGRAPHY

(1) ALVARO, M. — Simultaneous surgical correction of vertical and horizontal deviations. *Ophthalmologica*, 1950, *120*, 191-197.

(2) ARDOUIN, M., URVOY, M. and SALMON, M. — Technique simple de l'opération du fil de Cüppers. *Bull. Soc. Ophtal. France*, 1977, *5-6*, 577-578.

(3) BERARD, P., MOUILLAC-GAMBARELLI, N. and SPIELMAN, A. — Opération du fil de Cüppers. *Arch. Ophtal. (Paris)*, 1977, *37*, 6-7, 417-438.
(4) BERARD, P., SPIELMAN, A. and REYDY, R. — Opération du fil de Cüppers. *Bull. Soc. Ophtal. France*, 1976, *12*, 1111-1116.
(5) BRITT, B. — Recent advances in Malignant Hyperthermia. *Anesth. Analg. Current Researches*, 1972, *51*, 5, 841-849.
(6) BROWN, H. — Prévention et traitement des complications de la chirurgie oculaire. Fasenella R. editor, Masson, Paris, 1960, 195-205.
(7) BURIAN, H. and VON NOORDEN, G. — Binocular vision and ocular motility. C.V. Mosby Co., St. Louis, Toronto, London, 1974, 298-350 and 448-483.
(8) COOPER, E. — The surgical management of secondary exotropia. *Trans. Amer. Acad. Ophthal. Otolaring.*, 1961, *65*, 595-608.
(9) CUPPERS, C. — The so-called "Fadenoperation". Second Congress of the International Strabismological Association, Fells P. editor. Marseille, Diffusion Générale de Librairie, 1976, 395-400.
(10) DE DECKER, W. and CONRAD, H. — Fadenoperation nach Cüppers bei Komplizierten Augenmuskelstörungen und nicht akkommodativen Konvergenz excess. *Klin. Mbl. Augenheilk.*, 1975, *167*, 217-226.
(11) DELLER, M. — Les techniques de l'opération du fil. *J. Fr. Orthopt.*, 1978, *10*, 89-96.
(12) FINK, W. — The role of developmental anomalies in vertical muscle defects. *Amer. J. Ophthal.*, 1955, *40*, 529-552.
(13) GOBIN, M. — Semeiologie des deviatons cyclo-verticales. *J. Fr. Orthopt.*, 1981, *13*, 123-130.
(14) GOBIN, M. — Recession of the medial rectus muscle with a loop. *Ophthalmologica*, 1968, *156*, 25-27.
(15) GOBIN, M. — Nouvelles conceptions sur la pathogénie et le traitement du strabisme, 1e partie. *J. Fr. Ophtalmol.*, 1980, *3*, 10, 541-556.
(16) GOBIN, M. — Nouvelles conceptions sur la pathogénie et le traitement du strabisme, 2e partie. *J. Fr. Ophtalmol.*, 1981, *4*, 1, 7-18.
(17) HAASE, W., MALCHARTZECK, C. and RICKERS, J. — Ergebnisse der Fadenoperation nach Cüppers. *Klin. Mbl. Augenheilk.*, 1978, *172*, 313-324.
(18) HARADA, M. and ITO, Y. — Surgical correction of cyclotropia. *Jap. J. Ophthal.*, 1964, *8*, 88-96.
(19) HELVESTON, E. — Strabismus surgery. C.V. Mosby Co., St. Louis, 1977, 183-197.
(20) ING, M., COSTENBADER, F., PARKS, M. and ALBERT, D. — Early surgery for congenital esotropia. *Amer. J. Ophthal.*, 1966, *61*, 1419-1427.
(21) JAMPOLSKY, A. — A simplified approach to strabismus diagnosis. Symposium on strabismus. Trans. New Orleans Acad. Ophthal., C.V. Mosby Co., St. Louis, 1971, 34-92.
(22) JAMPOLSKY, A. — Surgical leashes and reverse leashes in strabismus surgical management. Symposium on strabismus. Trans. New Orleans Acad. Ophthal., C.V. Mosby Co., St. Louis, 1978, 244-267.
(23) JAMPOLSKY, A. — Current techniques of adjustable strabismus surgery. *Amer. J. Ophthal.*, 1979, *88*, 406-418.
(24) KNAPP, P. — Vertically incomitant horizonal strabismus: the so-called A and V syndromes. *Trans. Amer. Ophthal. Soc.*, 1959, *57*, 666-699.
(25) LAVAT, J. and BONS, G. — Reculs obliques dans la chirurgie des syndromes A et V. *Bull. Soc. Ophtal. France*, 1972, *72*, 3, 317-320.
(26) McLEAN, J., GALIN, M. and BARAS, I. — Retinal perforation during strabismus surgery. *Amer. J. Ophthal.*, 1960, *50*, 1167-1169.
(27) McNEER, K. — Complications of strabismus surgery. Symposium on strabismus. Trans. New Orleans Acad. Ophthal., C.V. Mosby Co., 1978, 292-300.
(28) MILLER, J. — Vertical recti transplantation in the A and V syndromes. *Arch. Ophthal.*, 1960, *64*, 175-179.
(29) PARKS, M. — Ocular motility and strabismus. Harper and Row, Hagerstown, 1975, 107-109 and 135-141.
(30) SPIELMAN, A. — L'opération du fil de Cüppers. Principe, Technique, Indication, Expérience personnelle. Studiegroep voor Strabisme, Lab. Cusi, Brussel, 1976.

(31) THOMAS, C., SPIELMAN, A. and BERNARDINI, D. — L'expérience de trois années de «l'opération du fil» de Cüppers dans les interventions contre l'ésotropie avec phénomènes innervationnels de blocage. *Bull. Soc. Fr. Ophtal.*, 1977, 173-180.
(32) VON NOORDEN, G. — Posterior fixation suture in strabismus surgery. Symposium on strabismus. Trans. New Orleans Acad. Ophthal., C.V. Mosby Co., 1978, 307-320.
(33) QUERE, M., CLERGEAU, G., PECHEREAU, A., FONTENAILLE, N. and BRASSEUR, G. — Le sanglage musculaire rétro-équatorial (note préliminaire). *Arch. Opht. (Paris)*, 1977, *37*, 8-9, 531-538.
(34) QUERE, M., CLERGEAU, G. and PECHEREAU, A. — Le sanglage musculaire rétroéquatorial. *Bull. Soc. Ophtal. France*, 1977, *5-6*, 573-576.

INDEX

B

C

D

R

S

W